Casebook of Exemplary
Evidence-Informed Programs that
Foster Community Participation
After Acquired Brain Injury

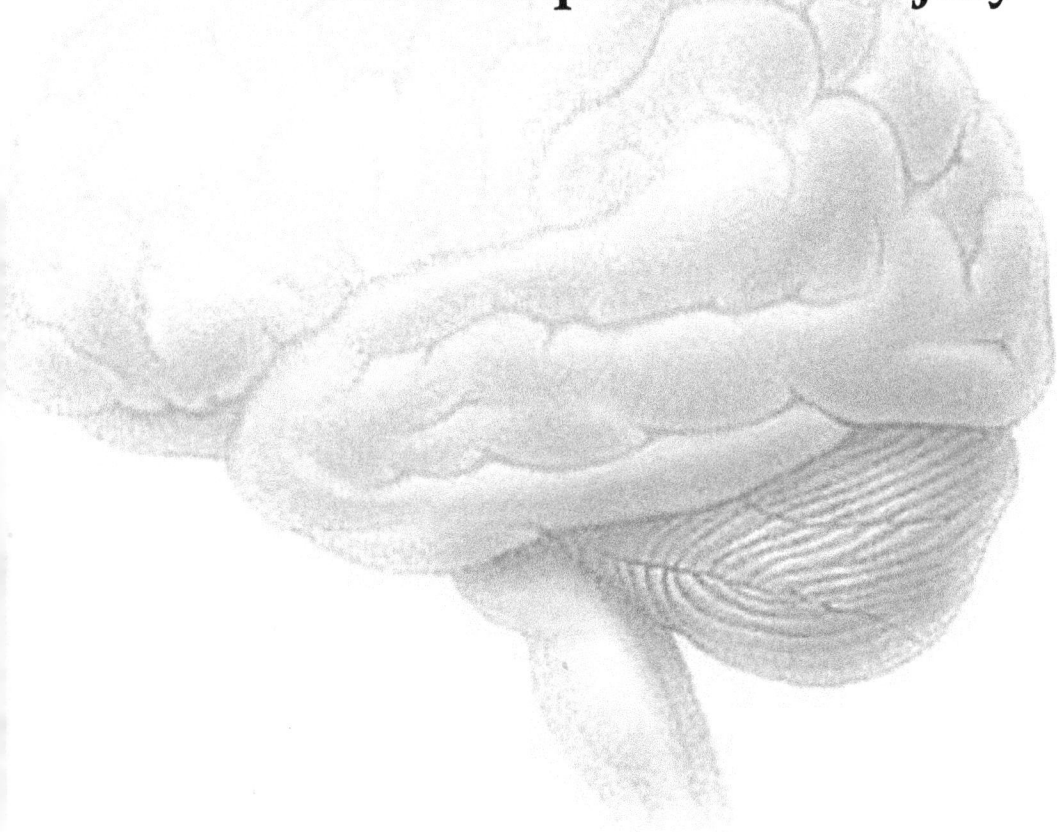

Casebook of Exemplary Evidence-Informed Programs that Foster Community Participation After Acquired Brain Injury

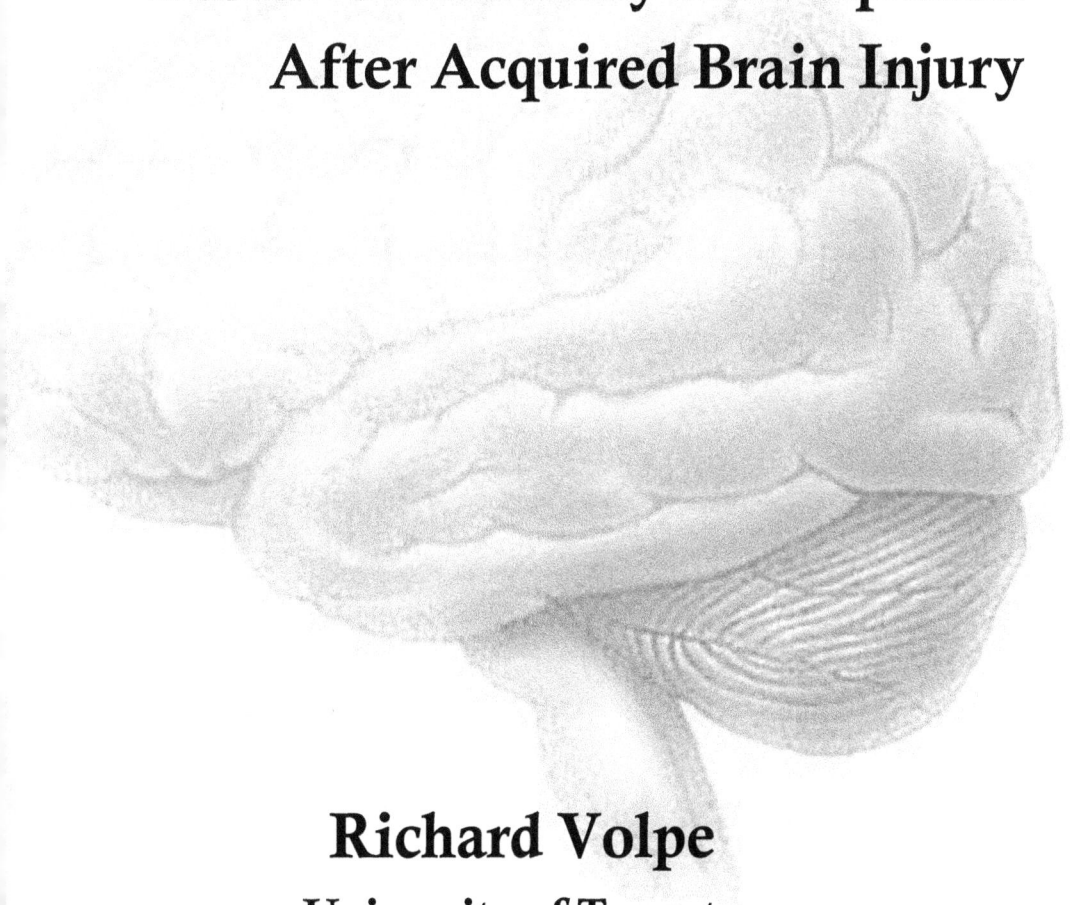

Richard Volpe
University of Toronto

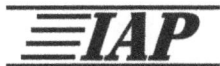

≡**IAP**
INFORMATION AGE PUBLISHING, INC.
Charlotte, NC • www.infoagepub.com

Library of Congress Cataloging-in-Publication Data

Casebook of exemplary evidence-informed programs that foster community
participation after acquired brain injury / [edited by] Richard Volpe,
University of Toronto.
      pages cm
   Includes index.
   ISBN 978-1-62396-289-0 (pbk.) – ISBN 978-1-62396-290-6 (hardcover) –
ISBN 978-1-62396-291-3 (ebook) 1. Brain damage–Patients–Rehabilitation.
2. Community mental health services–Citizen participation. 3. Community
health services–Citizen participation. I. Volpe, Richard, editor of
compilation.
   RC387.5.C373 2013
   617.4'81044–dc23
                                                          2013009021

Printed in the United States of America

Contents

Acknowledgements

We would like to thank the Ontario Neurotrauma Foundation for providing the funding for this research. Our appreciation is extended to members of the international community of practice, especially to those who acted as representatives of the research's external advisory group—a community who provided valuable information and resources and who helped to identify many of the programs that were brought forward for review.

Special thanks go out to the many key informants who shared their knowledge, time, insight, and vision about programming that aims to improve the lives of people who are survivors of brain injury.

We gratefully acknowledge the support of Christine Davidson in the Dr. R.G.N. Laidlaw Centre for research at the Dr. Eric Jackman Institute of Child Study, University of Toronto.

Research Team

Negar Ahmadi

Sherry Ally

Heather Finch

Georgios Fthenos

Danielle Hryniewicz

Natasha Jamal

Gaayathiri Jegatheeswaran

Helen Looker

Rakib Mohammed

Tanya Morton

Kelsey Ragan

Priyanka Raj

Jami-Leigh Sawyer

Amanda Stewart

Ontario Neurotrauma Foundation
Fondation ontarienne de neurotraumatologie

Life Span Adaptation Projects
Dr. Eric Jackman Institute of Chlid Study
University of Toronto

CHAPTER 1

By Richard Volpe

INTRODUCTION

Acquired brain injury (ABI) describes damage to the brain that occurs after birth, caused by traumatic injury such as an accident or fall, or by non-traumatic cause such as substance abuse, stroke, or disease. Today's medical techniques are improving the survival rate for people of all ages diagnosed with ABI, and current trends in rehabilitation are supporting these individuals returning to live, attend school, and work in their communities. Yet strategies on the best way of fostering community participation vary among rehabilitation experts. Because many of these individuals do not and will not return to the status quo of their former lives, it is important to examine what constitutes exemplary and promising practices in this area. This casebook is the world's first compilation of evidence-informed programs that foster community participation in people of all ages with brain injury. The service settings that we sought, investigated, and cased were comprehensive programs rather than individual practices that were essentially community based or focused. Further, these programs needed to consider the individual from a holistic perspective by taking into account psychological and social components that affect the health of the individual such as quality of life and sense of well-being, along with the physical and cognitive components. Our overarching goal has been to help others learn about exemplary programs by making information about them accessible to service providers, policy makers, and researchers for possible replication and/or adaptation. The search was worldwide and involved a systematic process to select those programs that are evidence-informed and exemplary in fostering community participation using pre-identified criteria. We considered community-based programs to be programs where individuals and families actively participate in their own therapy (rehabilitation) and take responsibility for their own health or that of a family/community member.

Evidence and Exemplary Programs

The preceding paragraph contains the terms evidence and exemplary that should be defined at the onset of this introduction. The British National Health Services (**British Medical Association, 1995**) defined evidence as:

> .....The best current research information available based on a systematic analysis of the effectiveness of a treatment, service or any other intervention and its use, in order to produce the best outcome, result or effect.

Although this definition is useful, it is also idealistic in view of the complexity of assessing community participation as an outcome in human services. Consequently, our notion of evidence incorporates the definition provided by the **Canadian Health Research Foundation** (2000):

> Evidence is information that comes closest to the facts of a matter. The form it takes depends on context .....The evidence base for a decision is the multiple forms of evidence combined to balance rigor with expedience—while privileging the former over the latter.

Adopting this view has given evidence a place among our selection criteria that is realistic and balanced. The case studies that have resulted from our review process are program descriptions that should enable decision makers to make well-informed decisions.

We have also taken what we consider to be a more realistic and practical approach to the labeling of programs by describing them as exemplary/promising as opposed to best/innovative. The idea of a compilation of cases is based on the observation from previous casebooks in the prevention of head and spinal cord injury that carefully documented case histories can provide excellent guidelines for policy-making and for planning new initiatives. Documenting exemplary programs is a valuable source of knowledge because the cases provide alternative solutions that can improve decisions by providing policy-makers and practitioners with deeper insight into the many different aspects of community participation. If the cases are held up as examples, as sources of inspiration, planning can be based on what really works in real life practice.

In gathering this information, we extensively went into the details of each practice. We focused on the ways that the practice has been adapted and applied as well as on the way the knowledge is transferred and disseminated. Many people are working on projects in which community participation plays an essential and practical role. It is very important that information about these kinds of projects is made available worldwide so that other people can learn from the experiences. Calling programs "exemplary" suggests that they could be replicated, that useful ideas can be generated from them, and that they can contribute positively to both policy and practice. In contrast, designating a program as a best practice implies that the programs surveyed were in a hierarchical competition. Moreover, the designation exemplary was also important because although our review process has been systematic and as comprehensive as possible, it cannot be seen as exhaustive. Because this review relied on nominations and published reports it is likely that some very good programs have been missed. Because they could have been have included but were not, describing the ones that did get cased as the "best" seems inappropriate.

Conceptualizing Community Participation

The concept of community participation implies that people after brain injury will be involved in aspects of their lives with the least amount of restriction as possible. This kind of involvement includes enabling survivors to make decisions about the care and services they receive that allow them to become a part of community life that is meaningful, satisfying and socially productive. The casing of programs has been an attempt to help clarify and concretize community participation in actual program descriptions. To this end the following section reviews the major conceptual schemes that have been explicitly employed by the designers of the exemplary programs reviewed.

Although community-based programs in the US increased ten-fold between 1981 and 1991, much conflict existed between medical models and non-medical models; the polarity did not serve the ABI population well because people with complex needs ideally required a blend of specialist inputs from professionals with medical allied health backgrounds in addition to non-professional community members, support and education for care givers, and attention to the social lives of people with ABI. Models that were either medically grounded or socially grounded, therefore, were insufficient alone to optimize community integration.

Whatever It Takes (WIT)

Willer and Corrigan (1994) proposed a model that extended the traditional rehabilitation model to bridge the divide between institutional care and providing professional care within communities complemented by social supports non-medical in nature. The "Whatever It Takes" model described by Willer and Corrigan provided a program ideal based on ten principles:

1. No two individuals with acquired brain injury are alike

2. Skills are more likely to generalize when taught in the environment they are to be used

3. Environments are easier to change than people

4. Community integration should be holistic

5. Life is a place-and-train venture

6. Natural supports last longer than professionals

7. Interventions must not do more harm than good

8. The service system presents many of the barriers to community integration

9. Respect for the individual is paramount

10. Needs of individuals last a lifetime; so should their resources (**Willer & Corrigan,** p. 650-657, 1994).

Willer and Corrigan acknowledged that some needs for those with ABI required the adjustment of pre-existing services to be inclusive of ABI needs, rather than duplicating another service or level of it dedicated to ABI clients. Substance abuse is one such example where community services may already exist, but need modification to accommodate the needs of people with ABI. **Willer and Corrigan** (1994) assert that community-based program models should serve as an extension of the traditional rehabilitation model for individuals with acquired brain injury (ABI), and have as a goal community integration. The "Whatever It Takes"(WIT) model incorporates principles which support and encourage independence, emphasize the importance of real life skill development, and advocate for life-long access to resources. A foremost feature of WIT is maximum self-determination for each individual with ABI, acknowledging the unique characteristics of each individual before, and after, brain injury. The model's ten principles each highlight a critical feature of a program designed to overcome barriers in community participation. "Whatever It Takes" insists on individuality in the assessment, goal setting, planning, and execution. **Willer and Corrigan** (1994) argue that skills are most successfully developed and taught in the context in which they are used, and that every effort should be made to identify environmental manipulations that assist the individuals in reintegration. Furthermore, a holistic approach to community integration should be undertaken, including the ascertainment of the individual's desired level of integration. They highlight the importance of natural support as being more sustainable and beneficial as compared with professional support, and therefore an effort to identify circles of support is necessary. Interventions should be approached critically and with caution, while making certain to identify and overcome system-based barriers to care such as ignorance, fragmentation of services, and limited funding. Finally, the WIT model emphasizes respect for each individual and supports access to resources for as long as is necessary. Overall, the "Whatever It Takes" model proposes that community-based programs can facilitate the integration and continued support of individuals with acquired brain injury through holistic approaches that respect the individual and emphasize integrated behaviours in normalized settings.

Social Capital

The model advanced by Willer and Corrigan falls into the social capital conception of human services (**Putnam**, 2000). **Condeluci** (2002) elaborated this concept in application to persons with disability through his notion of cultural shifting, the process of becoming part of a community that involves connecting and extending circles of support and reciprocity. Social capital has its foundation in the idea that human relationships and connections are positively linked to health and opportunity (**Putnam**, 2000). The amount of social capital that a given individual possesses has concrete benefits in terms of quality of life, and community-based rehabilitation programs for individuals with acquired brain injury should aim to foster an environment in which social capital is built. The value of these new relationships is measured in the opportunities and benefits following from the feelings of reciprocity and trustworthiness that arise from being part of a social network (**Flaherty**, 2008). It is the creation of this environment of reciprocity that results in individuals feeling connected, which is of particular importance to individuals living with acquired brain injury as they often experience feelings of exclusion and isolation. The event of brain injury often leads to a loss of social capital, with a concurrent decrease in feelings of hope and opportunity. Social capital as applied to community-based programs serving an ABI population should have as a goal the creation and strengthening of social networks, an initiative that offers benefits in the form of new relationships, which often feedback positively to offer further opportunities for creating a social network. **Condeluci** (2002) describes this process as cultural shifting, a joining with others that involves connecting and extending circles of support and reciprocity. The inclusion of this principle into programs for individuals with ABI offers a non-traditional, individual-based approach to improving health and quality of life.

Clubhouse Model

A Clubhouse represents a specific model for delivering community support to adults living with the effects of an Acquired Brain Injury (ABI) (**Cornerstone Clubhouse**, n. d.; **Jacobs**, 1997). International Standards for Clubhouse programs define the Clubhouse model (**Cornerstone Clubhouse**, n.d., p. 3). End-users who participate in the Clubhouse community are called members rather than patients or clients, because the program is primarily a club with members having all associated right of access and decision-making ability (**Macias, Schroder, Jackson, & Wang, 1999**). Community participation in a Clubhouse arises out of the need to serve the members' common cause, similar to what would happen in any other structured organization with an agenda. The Clubhouse model recognizes the value of meaningful work, with members being relied upon and expected to do that work by other members and staff. The Work-Ordered Day mandates the nature of activities undertaken, work units, and the daily working hours. Hence, members develop their skills and relationships with each other in a natural ecology rather than a protected setting. They run their Clubhouse by participating in essential activities that keep it operating (**Macais, Jackson, Schroder, & Wang, 1999**). Someone is needed to clean up, prepare food, answer the telephone, pay bills, and perform other activities in order to keep the house operational. Members select work units they feel would be a good fit given their particular interests and abilities. Individuals' unique talents and contributions to the Clubhouse effort (e.g., artistic, cooking, computer skills) are valued. Individual long-term goals are broken down into smaller, more manageable pieces to give clear benchmarks for progress. Within a Clubhouse, community participation is manifested as members taking responsibility for building their own capacity and that of their community; feeling accepted and regarded as useful contributors by a group of peers; and identifying, accessing and interacting with local resources as necessary to accomplish their goals. The Clubhouse model possesses a number of key features that promote community participation.

World Health Organization's International Classification of Functioning, Disability, and Health (ICF)

The **International Classification of Functioning, Disability and Health**, known more commonly as ICF, is a classification of health and health-related domains. These domains are classified from body, individual, and societal perspectives by means of two lists: a list of body functions and structure, and a list of domains of activity and participation. Since an individual's functioning and disability occurs in a context, the ICF also includes a list of environmental factors. The ICF is the WHO's framework for measuring health and disability at both individual and population levels. The ICF puts the notions of "health" and "disability" in a new light by acknowledging that every human being can experience a decrement in health and thereby experience some degree of disability. The ICF thus "mainstreams" the experience of disability and recognizes it as a universal human experience. By shifting the focus from cause to impact it places all health conditions on an equal footing allowing them to be compared using a common metric—the ruler of health and disability. Furthermore, ICF takes into account the social aspects of disability and does not see disability only as a "medical" or "biological" dysfunction.

Community Approach to Participation (CAP)

The Community Approach to Participation (CAP) has flexible, client-centric values at its core and is built on participatory interventions (**Sloan, Winkler, & Callaway, 2004**). Therapy includes a client's family and friends and also relevant community contacts to promote integration according to client goals and interventions to optimize abilities. Therapy can span many years, adapting to client needs over the life span, so the therapeutic relationship plays a significant role in the degree of success achieved in interventions planned and designed to make participation possible in life roles important to a client. Skill development and environmental modifications are also deployed to minimize limitations to participation. Participation can lead in any direction that a client considers most important for achieving quality of life and may relate to being a family member, a hobbyist, able to work for pay, or becoming active within a community, for instance. Validation of the client's personal perspective on life is paramount and is supported through encouragement and constructive feedback as, and when, the client is ready to receive it. The fundamental tenet of CAP is that brain-injured individuals can achieve independence and satisfaction in life despite the influence of complex, sometimes permanent impairment affecting physical and psychological health.

Operationalizing Community Participation

The various conceptualizations reviewed above have spawned a number of measures that have been employed in the evaluation of programs that seek to foster community participation. It is now widely accepted that community participation is an outcome worth measuring. Efforts to tie conceptualizations to empirical indicators often refine and concretize concepts. However, despite nearly two decades of scale development, a single widely used and accepted measure of participation has not been agreed upon. The following outlines the leading measures of community participation both in and beyond the exemplary programs cased in this review.

Community Integration Questionnaire

The *Community Integration Questionnaire (CIQ)* was developed by Willer in order to provide a measure of community integration after traumatic brain injury that could be incorporated into the National Institute on Disability and Rehabilitation Research's (NIDRR) TBI Model Systems program (**Dijkers, 2000**; **Salter et al., 2008**). It was designed to respond to the limitations of traditional outcome measurement (**Willer et al., 1993**). Through consultation with a steering group on the assessment of community integration, a foremost consideration in the development of the CIQ was to reflect aspects of participation that were most important to the individuals who experienced traumatic brain injury (TBI). Further to this goal, the CIQ was designed to allow consumers to describe their situation rather than rely on the evaluation by a third party. Due to the cognitive deficits experienced by individuals who have suffered a TBI, the scale was developed to be brief in order to avoid problems associated with attention span, fatigue, and memory (**Willer et al., 1993**). For the purposes of this tool community integration is divided into three aspects: integration into a home-like setting, social integration, and the regular performance of productive activities including employment. The current CIQ consists of 15 multiple-choice questions covering these three areas; they are designed to reflect behavioural indicators rather than self-perceived emotional status (**Willer et al., 1994**; **Dijkers, 1997**).

Craig Handicap Assessment and Reporting Technique

The *Craig Handicap Assessment and Reporting Technique (CHART)* was developed by **Whiteneck et al. (1992)** to quantify the extent of handicap in individuals. It is based on the World Health Organization's (**WHO**) concept of *handicap* existing when an individual is unable to fulfill expected social roles. The WHO has subsequently revised their terminology to use the word '*participation*' to describe the concept of '*handicap*' and thus CHART is still considered as a participation scale (with handicap being the absence of social participation) (**Mellick, 2000**). The 27 item instrument is designed to be administered by interview, focus on observable criteria (i.e. not feelings) and worded to maximize clarity (**Whiteneck et al., 1992**). The original **WHO ICIDH** model contained six dimensions: physical independence, mobility, occupation, social integration, economic self-sufficiency, and orientation. CHART was developed for individuals with spinal cord injury but has since been shown to be reliable and valid in other groups, including individuals with traumatic brain injury (**Hall et al., 2001**; **Mellick et al., 1999**; **Walker et al., 2003**; **Zhang et al., 2002**). **Walker and colleagues (2003)** showed that CHART-R discriminated among the categories of impairment (SCI, TBI, MS, amputation and stroke) in a direction that would parallel increasing disability and therefore showed it to be valid across impairment types. It is possible to calculate scores on each of the subscales as well as a global score using CHART. The WHO model includes a sixth dimension of handicap called "Orientation" which was not addressed in the original CHART. The revised CHART-R contains this sixth domain entitled 'Cognitive Independence' (**Mellick et al., 1999**).

Community Integration Measure

McColl and colleagues (2001) developed the *Community Integration Measure (CIM)* following extensive research and interviews with individuals with TBI focusing on their perceptions and attitudes toward community participation (**McColl et al., 1998**). As such, CIM is traumatic brain injury (TBI) specific and is grounded in the perspectives of individuals with TBI. Despite this background, the CIM has been criticized for its lack of evidence supporting scale reliability and validity (**Salter et al., 2008**). The CIM is made up of 10 items which are declarative statements based on the definition of community integration provided by brain injured individuals (**McColl et al., 2001**). The CIM is considered a subjective assessment of participation relating to the dimensions of home, socializing, and productive activity. Each statement is rated on a 5-point scale with the maximum amount of points (50) indicating the highest integration score. The strength of the CIM is that it does not reflect societal norms with respect to expectations of brain injured individuals (i.e. assumptions as to the relative importance of activities are not made (**McColl et al., 2001; Linden et al., 2005**). Another strength of the scale is the use of consumer language to increase comprehension and response.

Reintegration to Normal Living Index

The *Reintegration to Normal Living Index (RNLI)* is similar to CIM in that it aims to capture the subjective experience of the individual with brain injury with respect to achieving reintegration after their injury. It is a short 11-item tool composed of declarative statements with higher scores indication higher levels of perceived integration. **Wood-Dauphinee et al. (1988)** define reintegration to normal living as "the reorganization of physical, psychological and social characteristic of an individual into a harmonious whole so that one can resume well-adjusted living" (p. 39). Unfortunately, despite being one the first tools intended to measure integration the RNLI has not been well studied and thus its reliability and validity have not been demonstrated across different populations of TBI individuals (**Salter et al., 2008**).

Sydney Psychosocial Reintegration Scale

The *Sydney Psychosocial Reintegration Scale (SPRS)* was designed to assess individuals with traumatic brain injury while taking into account previous life roles and values (**Tate et al., 1999**). This scale was developed after CIQ and CHART and was designed to reflect the conceptual base provided by the World Health Organization's model of Impairments, Disabilities and Handicaps. Specifically, it was designed to measure psychosocial functioning of individuals in comparison to their pre-brain injury levels (**Tate et al., 1999**). The SPRS measures three domains: occupational activities, interpersonal relationships and independent living skills. Each domain is addressed by four questions, resulting in 12 statements overall. Behavioural descriptors are attached to the responses, which are made on a 7-point scale reflecting change from the pre-injury state, from 0 (extreme degree of change) to 6 (no change). The total score for the SPRS ranges from 0 to 72, with scores for each of the three domains ranging from 0 to 24. Higher scores indicate better degrees of psychosocial functioning (**Tate et al., 1999**).

Participation Objective, Participation Subjective Scale

The *Participation Objective, Participation Subjective (POPS)* measure was developed in 2004 at Mount Sinai School of Medicine as part of a National Institute on Disability and Rehabilitation Research (NIDRR) funded project. POPS works with the World Health Organization's updated ICF model with an emphasis on participation and the need for measures of rehabilitation efforts that more adequately and accurately reflect the perspective of the individual whose life it is (**Brown et al., 2004**). The updated version of the WHO's model shifts the language from "community integration" to "participation" with the latter emphasizing involvement in a life situation as opposed to simply the execution of a task or action by an individual (**WHO, 2001**). The POPS is designed to reflect the perspective of the individual with the disability (subjective) as well as the societal norm (objective). In this sense it combines approaches used by earlier scales addressing only one dimension or the other. The POPS consists of a list of 26 items which are sorted into five categories of participation: Domestic Life; Major Life Activities; Transportation; Interpersonal Interactions and Relationships; and Community, Recreational and Civic Life. For each item, an objective and subjective question is asked.

Mayo Portland Adaptability Inventory

The *Mayo Portland Adaptability Inventory* (MPAI) was designed for assessment during the post-acute/post-hospital) period following acquired brain injury and for the outcome evaluation of rehabilitation programs (**Lezak, 1993**). MPAI-4 items cover physical, cognitive, emotional, behavioural, and social problems that people may encounter after ABI. MPAI-4 also provides an assessment of major obstacles to community integration associated with the social and physical environment. The fourth revision, the MPAI-4 provides three subscales (Ability Index, Adjustment Index, Participation Index) that are well developed and documented for both clinical and research applications. The 8-item Participation Index provides a short measure of social participation. The MPAI has been designed for completion by professional staff, people with ABI and their significant others. Recent research establishes the reliability of these rater groups. The MPAI-4 offers the possibility for combining results of the inventory completed by two or three rater groups that may provide a more reliable tool. Other traditional measures such as the functional independence measurement and functional activity measurement system (FIM/ FAM) and the Disability Rating Scale (DRS) are sensitive to improvements in physical and cognitive status during acute rehabilitation, but have limited ability to track long-term changes in vocational and psychosocial functioning (**Sanders et al., 1999**). In particular, the Disability Rating Scale does not provide satisfactory measure of the psychosocial domain as a single item only addresses it. The Glasgow Outcome Scale (GOS) and Neurobehavioral Rating Scale are also not appropriate, as they do not assess psychosocial factors. Items that measure community participation on any given scale must be evaluated in the context of the specific population and program being evaluated. For example, it has been suggested the most widely used scale, the CIQ, may not be appropriate for use with young males as they will likely receive very low scores on items related to household activities, which is not necessarily reflective of a lack of participation, but more so a lack of relevance to their personal situation. Given the spectrum of traumatic brain injuries, and the complexity of measuring a concept such as participation, discretion should be used in interpreting and reporting participation measures.

REVIEW RATIONALE

Traditional approaches to integration often focus on promoting independent living for survivors of ABI, including supporting their employment options or helping them to adapt to school. This approach is described as "strengthening the host." Such interventions aimed at the individual to help him or her resume previous social roles and responsibilities—return to the status quo—are generally found to be narrow in perspective and unsatisfactory to stakeholders who foster community participation because they imply a return to an unsustainable state. The study of life span human development offers some insights to be employed in this report that may be useful to understanding what constitutes a successful effort at community participation. This is reasonable because many traditional rehabilitation interventions do not take place in the real world.

The literature on community participation among people with acquired brain injury has grown rapidly in recent years. **McColl (2006)**, in a review of fifteen years of post acute programming for community participation, concludes that the services typically offered to survivors of brain injuries include traditional rehabilitation, cognitive and social skills development to help the individual return to school, employment, family life, and independent living as a contributing member of society. While this standpoint has been useful in rehabilitation work, it assumes that the challenges of ABI have to be faced by individuals independent of their extended social context. Recent studies of disability as a social construction through the life span—where quality of life is assessed, sense of well-being is measured, and participation is considered a necessity—reveal the importance of conceiving community participation not as a state, but as a complex process; in other words, the context in which a person whose life has been changed by ABI must adapt. Adaptations are distributed and imply the need for both person and environment changes. Many ABI intervention programs focus on the attainment of specific program objectives outcomes as both their means and end and not the more inclusive long-term goal of community participation.

Aims and Objectives

The major aim of the following casing of programs is to help clarify and concretize community participation in actual program descriptions. **Rifkin (1986)** provided our working definition:

> "...Community participation is the process by which individuals and families assume responsibility for their own health and welfare and those of the community, and develop capacity to contribute to their and the community's development. They come to know their own situation better and are motivated to solve their common problems. This enables them to become agents of their own development instead of passive beneficiaries of development aid..."

Because achieving community participation is a complex process, it requires a comprehensive case study framework for describing programs with it as their main objective. Consequently, all of the programs and strategies profiled below were organized into the BRIO and Life Space case framework discussed below that help capture the major areas of community participation.

This casing framework facilitates the complex systems associated existing programmatic efforts to foster community participation to be cased in way that combines emphasis on the individual, the social, and the service systems. This approach helps to capture community participation as a process of change that that does not divorce ABI survivors from their contexts, and where participation efforts facilitate positive change in the social and political context.

Specific research objectives were to:

a)   survey the range of community participation and programs;

b)   identify examples of effective, evidence-informed practice;

c)   describe, analyze, and evaluate these in terms of their effectiveness for diverse age groups;

d)   develop and strengthen networks by mobilizing public support and encouraging the participation of stakeholders;

e) provide a compilation of exemplary, evidence-informed community participation efforts;

f) create a means of distributing the compilation and resource documents;

g) analyze evidence for program sustainability;

h) derive general principles for the community participation.

Study Design

To gauge and identify exemplary programs in community participation, we engaged in a multi-phase process. Our expectation was born out that this review involved more gray literature and word of mouth contacts than previous Internet-based reviews of traditionally published reports. Information for the review was gathered by interviewing program representatives face-to-face, by telephone, and through the Internet. Further collection of information was obtained from a variety of methods developed in previous reviews that are described in the following three phases. Phase 1 outlines the tangible steps that were taken to establish case selection and identify possible exemplary programs. Phase 2 describes the data gathering methods that were employed throughout the course of the research that follow the BRIO Model; it also includes an outline of the case analysis framework based on the complex systems conceptual scheme of human development research known as the Life Space Framework. Lastly, Phase 3 establishes the final set of criteria used to identify chosen programs as "Exemplary".

Methodology

Phase 1: Steps to Identify Exemplary Programs

Investigation

Various search tools were utilized to provide a broad picture of community participation on a global level and which include a meta-search of the World Wide Web, academic literature reviews, nominations from consortium members and partners, and legislative and regulatory information. Specifically, meta-searches on the web enabled us to access relevant worldwide information. National centres for rehabilitation and community participation research acted as information resources regarding community participation programs on national levels. Based on their respective expert knowledge of the field, ONF Advisory Group members and partners provided contact information of key informants directly involved in strategies that may be considered exemplary.

Referrals were garnered through literature reviews and key informants. Based on past experience in the evaluation of best practices for other projects (e.g., **Volpe, Lewko, & Batra, 2002**), we have learned that knowledge of unpublished yet worthwhile programs is often gained by networking with program personnel.

Systematic reviews were obtained from the relevant published and unpublished reports in an effort to uncover community participation programs/models on an international scale. The Advisory Group was asked to help nominate unpublished national and international programs for possible investigation. The Advisory Group helped connect the review team to other stakeholders that included consumers, community leaders, non-governmental organizations, government agencies, field practitioners, consultants, and researchers. Community participation programs identified and that fell within the identification standards (including efforts at all levels, such as legislative, environmental, community, and individual) were considered for nomination.

Nomination

The aim of the nomination phase was to form a broad picture of programs that seemed promising and deserving of further study. Key informant contacts were identified and/or established through program documents such as annual reports and evaluations requested, so that further referral information could be obtained.

Only programs that satisfied collaboratively agreed upon criteria from the Advisory group were investigated and ultimately evaluated for the review. The following *Nomination Criteria* was suggested to the Advisory Group for use during this stage of the project:

1. Credibility of source: a rating of the authority of the source in the field.

2. Community reputation: a rating of the program's standing among members of the field.

3. Frequency of referral: the number of times a specific program is nominated by different referral agents.

4. Country and region: the geographical location of the program.

5. Position and demonstrated experience: length and degree of experience of the program since its inception.

6. Consumer participation: whether consumers have roles in the program.

Program Selection

Documented information received from programs that met the nomination criteria was further examined to determine if they met the selection criteria, the purpose of which is to help us further develop a profile of what constitutes an exemplary program. This set of criteria was created by the combined research knowledge and expertise of the research team and contacts established within the community participation field. They include:

➢ replicability and adaptability to Ontario

➢ sufficient documented information

➢ innovative strategies

➢ open and cooperative participation in the case writing process.

Phase 2: Data Gathering Methods

Programs that met the requirements of Phase 1 became candidates for more in-depth investigation. In Phase 2, we began by using a semi-structured questionnaire (primarily a telephone interview) that follows the BRIO Model (Background, Resources, Implementation, Outcome) in order to provide a consistent way of describing each case so that a comprehensive yet succinct understanding of the program's structure and operation can be made explicit. The second half of Phase 2 is to understand how the program fits into the Life Space Case Analysis framework, using the Complex Systems Conceptual Scheme.

The BRIO Model and Life Space Case Study Analysis Framework

Components of the BRIO Model

Background : According to the BRIO Model (**Volpe et al., 2002**), exploring the background of a program is to uncover its history, and the environment and events that have shaped the program development and implementation (e.g., legal mandates in a community, special funding opportunities, community reactions to the program.) Background inquiries aim to understand why the community participation program takes a particular form, and how, for example, relevant policies, legislation and community needs have influenced the objectives of the program. Sample questions that probed the background of the nominated programs include:

a) What were the community participation issues at the program site prior to program implementation?

b) Who initiated the program?

c) What were the original goals and objectives of the program?

d) What events surrounded the development of program?

e) What were the community reactions to the program at the time of program development?

f) What were the reactions of program personnel at the time of development?

g) How do associated professionals and sponsors perceive the program?

h) Who (if any) are the chosen community partners?

i) What is evidence for program sustainability?

j) What is the evidence that shows the general principles of community participation?

Resources : The term Resources calls for an investigation of the program design and resource allocation, particularly, how the program intends to achieve the articulated objectives. Financial resources and the strategies adopted to promote community participation are critical inputs to the program that should be clarified. Knowledge of alternative implementation and community participation is useful to gauge the fit of the chosen strategies. The following are examples of questions that examined resources:

a) What community participation strategies are employed in the program?

b) What financial resources are committed to the program?

c) What kinds of resources are developed for and allocated to the program?

Implementation : When discussing program implementation, we refer to the operationalization of a program, comparing the intended program design and how the program is actually practiced. A look at process examines how and why a community participation program does or does not adhere to the original plans for program governance, administration, management, implementation, and practice. Questions probing implementation issues included:

a) What checks on program process have been made?

b) What evidence exists as to the relation between what was intended in the program's design and what exists today?

c) How and when are adjustments to the program made?

d) How is feedback structured and given to management and front line service providers?

Outcome : To understand a program's *Outcome* is to determine the impact of the program. This component asks how stakeholders operationalize the objectives of the program and provides evidence of the program's attainment. Long- and short-term outcome measures of the program, including intended and unintended positive (e.g., improved community participation) and negative outcomes, are of interest. Examples of questions that explored the outcome of a program include:

a) What does the program do in terms of enhancing community participation?

b) How do practitioners, participants and observers judge the attainments of the program?

c) What are the short-term and long-term outcomes of the program?

d) How does the program measure success or effectiveness?

Life Space Case Study Analysis Framework

While the BRIO model structures the story of a program, the Life Space Study Framework (**Volpe, 2005**) provides the features for its analysis in terms of four interrelated components: interpersonal relations, intrapersonal (internal) states, the physical environment, and the sociocultural environment. This division into these features is arbitrary and serves primarily analytic purposes. In reality the life space is a complex fusion of elements. The facilitation of community participation requires that multidimensional programs enable individuals as opposed to one-dimensional interventions that focus merely on adjustment or adequate functioning.

The four components capture complex system changes in human development: 1) the sources of interpersonal support accessible to an individual; 2) the personal resources that an individual can command—intelligence, appearance, strength, health, and temperament—investments of effort that the individual makes on his or her own behalf; 3) what the physical environment offers in terms of stimulation, support, and security; and 4) the sociocultural opportunities available or the obstacles encountered as influenced by social class, ethnic membership, age, gender, personal contacts, social calamity, economic adjustment, and technological change. Although the content of systems is highly variable, the common structural features within each case shows how change is brought about in the course of human development over the entire life span. In this framework, change is seen as a relationship between resource and challenges in the life space. Community participation efforts were depicted as a resource mobilized in response to the challenge of ABI. Each complex system is different and varied in its approach, but developed according to the needs of individuals or communities targeted in programmatic efforts.

All of the programs and strategies profiled using the BRIO Model were then organized into the Life Space Case Study Analysis Framework and classified according to the major areas of community participation. The Life Space Framework allowed us to understand what community participation means to stakeholders. This approach captures how a program addresses the resources and challenges associated with community participation. (See Appendices for BRIO and Life Space Table Summaries for each case.)

Phase 3: Final Criteria for Determining An Exemplary Program

In this phase, actual "Exemplary Programs" criteria were identified, revised, and defined in consultation with the Advisory Committee, other stakeholders, previous reviews, and the team's professional experience. The following set of exemplary program criteria was used to make an argument to the research group for a program to be cased as either an exemplary or promising program. The final decision to case a program was based on the research group reaching a consensus.

   a) Avowed Support of Community Participation
       How does the program prove its commitment to community participation?

   b) Multidisciplinary Framework and Multilevel Approaches
       Does the program use a multidisciplinary framework or approach?

   c) Environmental and Behavioural Strategies
       Does the program employ a combination of environmental and behavioural strategies?

   d) Developmental Approaches, Flexibility and Adaptability
       Does the program incorporate a developmental perspective?

   e) Implementation and Outcome Evaluation
       Is the program's methodology grounded in credible and appropriate sources? Can the program be defined in terms of its implementation?

f) Broad-Based Community Support and Capacity Building
Does the program have active community support?

g) Cost-Effectiveness Analysis
Does the program employ a cost analysis? Can it adopt one with a long-term perspective?

h) Sustainability
How has attention to the long-term viability of the program been addressed? How adequate are efforts to continue, maintain benefits and build capacity?

i) Contribution to Community Participation
How does the program's evaluation research contribute to the refinement and elaboration of the conceptualization of community participation?

Initially, the Advisory Group supplied names of significant individuals who are working in the field of ABI. These individuals were contacted by the Principal Investigator (PI) and provided an extensive list of potential key informants. The project was also announced in the Summer 2009 Newsletter of the **Brain Injury Association of America** (BIAA), after which a number of groups specializing in community-based treatments were in touch with the PI. This led to a contact database with more than 130 organizations. Contrary to what was originally thought, the volume of potential programs was substantial. A member of the research team contacted each organization, and preliminary BRIO charts were prepared for programs that fit the profile of what constitutes an exemplary program in community participation. Programs are described in terms of publicly available information with full administrative consent of involved organizations whose key informants (usually the executive director) voluntarily co-create their exemplary program case study and retain final approval on any public documentation. Participation of organization key informants is voluntary and collaborative; all discussion of their programs is in terms of information they are willing to share publicly.

The following case studies constitute a unique casebook of evidence-informed exemplary programs that foster community participation for people across the life span who have acquired brain injury. To reiterate from an earlier paragraph, these are not simply individual practices, but comprehensive programs that consider the individual from a holistic perspective. Two of the programs were deemed to be "promising practices" because, although highly innovative, they have not been sufficiently evaluated. They were, however, exemplary in their capacity to deal with the psychological and social components that affect the health of the individual affected by ABI—such as quality of life and sense of well being– along with the physical and cognitive components. These programs also consider that individuals actively participate in their own intervention and take responsibility for their own health or that of the family or community member.

The achieved aim of this two year study was to compile a casebook of evidence-informed programs that facilitate community participation in people across the life span with ABI, with a goal to help others learn about these programs by making information about them accessible to service providers, policy makers, and researchers for replication and/or adaptation. The wide range of programs from around the world that were surveyed encouraged the participation of a variety of stakeholders and program key informants to articulate both their aspirations and implementations of efforts to foster community participation. Our hope is that the cases of effective, evidence- informed practice that were identified, analyzed and evaluated that are reviewed in the following chapters will inspire and act as exemplars for program change.

Overview of Cases

As discussed in prior sections, individuals who have experienced acquired brain injury often exhibit a wide range of challenges in their physical functioning cognition, affect, and behaviour. Recognition of these issues that may remain long after hospitalization and primary rehabilitation makes it imperative to provide comprehensive attention to the post trauma sequelae. The programs cased in the subsequent chapters all attend to this period in terms of social participation and community integration. **Collacut-McGrath (2007)** has advanced the view that facilitating social and economic adaptation in this period is a moral imperative of modern rehabilitation medicine. Although the programs reviewed all address this post injury period in terms of community participation, they do not present or measure it in a consistent way. This was expected because, as earlier, community participation is a complex and somewhat elusive concept. Olico-Okui contends that the reason for this is because "the community participation concept is power laden, it is a process of change and context specific, and it is a slow process...[it is] an abused concept because of the cosmetic, simplistic and superficial impression it is given by its advocates" **(Olico-Okui, 2005)**. Consequently, our efforts to capture exemplary program features have been guided by a heuristic: An overriding organizing notion that fostering community participation involves conceiving of it as bringing about change in complex systems that includes the role of power human relations **(Volpe, 2005)**. As used here, power refers to an individual's or family's control over situations. Because examining power is central to understanding human service programs, the ordering of the case studies in Chapters 2 to 15, and summarized below, has not been random. That is, we found it useful to employ the **Arnstein Ladder of Citizen Participation (1969)** to order and better understand the role of power in the practices associated with efforts to foster community participation.

Arnstein equates participation with an individual's level of power in a sociopolitical system. Adapted here, the original Arnstein eight rungs of the ladder of citizen participation, arranged from lower to higher, are management, therapy, informing, consultation, placation, partnership, delegated power, and client control. The lower rungs (management and therapy) describe levels of "non-participation" that often substitute for genuine participation. They are not designed to enable people to participate. Rather, they are situations that control or hold people in place for treatment or therapy. Further up the ladder the rungs (information, consultation, and placation) refer to situations that enable passive education and opportunities to speak but not necessarily be heard. The next level (partnership, delegated power, client control) allows for full participation, negotiation and actual control over situations.

CASE STUDIES

Previews Ordered by Level of Participation

The case studies begin in Chapter 2 with **communityworks, inc.**, a program that provides services to individuals of all ages with TBI (full range of injury severity), cerebrovascular accidents, multi-diagnosis situations, CNS disorders, and spinal cord injuries. The program was established to address the need for a new approach to rehabilitative services, one that gives control back to the individual and does "whatever it takes" for consumers to live in the community. Consumers are in control of their own rehabilitation services. They interview and choose their own staff, decide where they want to live and work and decide on their own rehabilitation goals. Communityworks collaborates with consumers, their families, physicians and hospitals, and government and mental health agencies, to ensure that the consumer is connected to all possible community resources. The program's multidisciplinary framework and system continues to work for the consumer even when professional services are no longer needed. Consumers have long-term access to services and are able to re-enter the program if and when new needs and goals emerge.

Two examples of the **Clubhouse** service model are featured in Chapter 3. **Cornerstone Clubhouse** provides normalized, inconspicuous support that members use to improve their quality of life. With a focus on individual abilities and unique contributions, the Clubhouse model is flexible in terms of the size of community it can serve. The **Side-by-Side** program exists to support the members, and, in turn, the members use it voluntarily for the purpose(s) they need. Thus, the Clubhouse is not to create artificial jobs; it is to encourage people to work in the community. Clubhouse activities are dynamic in nature. Roles, tasks, and relationships grow out of the need to operate the Clubhouse. Members have the opportunity to participate in every facet of the Clubhouse; administration, research, outreach, HR issues, advocacy, education and orientation are typical areas in which members become involved. For example, support is offered for members who are experiencing psychological distress at any point in time. The members assume responsibility for the Clubhouse and its direction. The Clubhouse is physically located in an area where access to local transportation can be assured. The convenient location is helpful in terms of members' independent access to the Clubhouse and Transitional Employment (TE) opportunities. Transitional Employment, Supported Employment and Independent Employment programs facilitate return to paid work. Employment is *not* offered through in-house businesses or sheltered settings. Individual long-term goals are broken down into smaller, more manageable goals to give clear benchmarks for progress. Annually, the Clubhouse conducts two member satisfaction surveys, one family satisfaction survey, one-community partners' survey and an employment placement survey. Evaluation results are both qualitative and quantitative. The Side-by-Side service follows an established exemplary program: the Clubhouse exists to support the members and, in turn, the members use it voluntarily for the purpose(s) they need. Thus, the Clubhouse is not to create artificial jobs; it is to encourage people to work in the community. Clubhouse members participate in an individualized approach that assists them with their lives outside of the clubhouse. Eliciting the support of local businesses, employers and community partners, the Clubhouse's community participation strategy is enhanced by increased awareness among the public of the lifelong effects of brain injury. Side-by-Side Brain Injury Clubhouse serves individuals of 14 different ethnicities.

Chapter 4 examines the **Skills To Enable People and Communities** (STEPS) program that aims to develop social support networks for people (adults ages 18-65 years) with brain injuries and their families in efforts to enhance quality of life and community participation. The STEPS program consists of two sequential phases: the **STEPS Skills Program** and **STEPS Network Groups**. The **STEPS Skills Program** is a six-week group program led by leaders and facilitators. One leader is a "peer leader" with lived experience of ABI, while the other, a "professional" leader, is an allied health professional with an interest in community rehabilitation. The Program adopts a self-management approach sequentially exploring three themes: how I look after myself, how I live in my community, and how I work with services. The sessions contain participation and discussion in groups, a workbook and reflection on a range of topics (e.g., learning self-management techniques to manage stress and transition toward independent living) relevant to these areas. The workbook is written in such a way that caregivers and friends can also participate. The **STEPS Skills Program** culminates in a community outing organized by participants. A plan is then established as to whether the group would like to continue meeting, and in what capacity. Ultimately, the group becomes their own

Network Group. **STEPS Network Groups** was designed for individuals who have completed the six-week Skills program. The groups provide an ongoing source of support for group participants. Groups assume ownership of their own group and make key decisions such as the format of group meetings, topics, and frequency of meetings and whether newcomers can join the group. Most groups welcome newcomers. Within each phase, difficulties in the community regarding stigma and restrictive attitudes are identified and examined. Community awareness projects, including attitudes and accessibility, are undertaken. All resources required to participate in the **STEPS Program Leader Training**, to deliver the **STEPS Skills Program** and to coordinate a **Network Group** are provided. Program materials include brochures, leader manuals, posters, activity planners, DVDs, group workbooks, referral forms, attendance records, and so on.

Simply Self-Sustaining System is reviewed in Chapter 5. This promising program employs a non-medical rehabilitation model, which represents an innovative departure from the rehabilitation of deficits to the development of capacity. Program services aim at providing persons with an ABI (both traumatic and non-traumatic) the opportunity to relearn skills, re-access social groups and modify behaviour sufficiently to be able to be included in work—namely, a small business. Following clinical assessment, local community members, serving as mentors, create the business structure. These "sympathetic but not professional" mentors coordinate services. Mentors may sew, design, cook, woodwork, and so on, and have to teach, guide and alter behaviour, while performing their skill. The program serves to educate ABI and TBI survivors, the community and the mentors themselves. Workshops centre on the performance of simple and repetitive tasks (i.e., how to make items for sale) and the development of functional and self-sustaining skills (e.g., learning punctuality, task completion, safety, respectful behaviour and social conflict resolution). Having participated in the workshops, clients enter a buddying system in which they are effectively integrated into applicable social settings. Community members may also volunteer and offer support. For example, farmers may bring food to the facility. A Simply Self-Sustaining System focuses primarily on survivors of ABI who live in rural areas. The facility is housed in a rural town in renovated stables for workshops.

Chapter 6 examines **Community Head Injury Resource Services** (CHIRS), a multi-service agency that provides a broad range of supports to an adult clientele (ages 18-60) with diverse and complex needs. From its origins as a transitional group home, **CHIRS** has evolved into a multi-service agency that provides a broad range of supports to an adult clientele (ages 18-60) with diverse and complex needs. **CHIRS** also provides leadership in the development of brain injury services across the province and participates in regional and provincial planning for government-funded ABI services. **CHIRS** provides services for persons who have sustained an ABI based on the principle that services, supports and life opportunities must be provided to correspond as much as possible to the individual's community environment, in a manner which enhances the individual's well-being, dignity, self-respect, and physical and emotional security. Prior to participation in a program or service, a "Service Plan" (a comprehensive assessment of the client's goals and needs) is created. Services and programs provided by **CHIRS** include: Ashby Community Support Services (ACSS), Adult Day Services (ADS), and Family-Centered Services, Aging at Home, Residential Services. Adult Day Services (ADS) provides mentorship and offsite programming opportunities. Clients are able to volunteer their time to see what strengths and interests they have. Having volunteered, they are invited to become mentors, and may assist with the lunch preparation, club coverage and operations of the Club. Offsite programming is designed to launch clients into the community; participation within adapted programs promotes community participation through the building of community connections and autonomy. Many of the programs are run in partnership with local organizations and private businesses that provide their expertise, equipment and facilities. The Continuum of Vocational Placements (from an error-free workshop setting to competitive supported employment) was developed by CHIRS program managers is an example of this approach. This program has resulted in numerous community collaborations, including charitable groups and commercial enterprises. In conjunction with the Supported Employment Program, a CHIRS' Job Developer works with clients to determine their areas of interest and to design individualized work assessments enabling the client, his/her family and CHIRS staff to assess their vocational skills. The Job Developer also undertakes an extensive job search, partnering with interested community employers. Once a client obtains a placement, a Job Coach provides a variety of work site supports to assist the client in learning his/her job and maintaining employment. Work site supports can include travel training, job-site and task analyses, ongoing assessment, employer education, social skills training and the development of individualized strategies.

Community Approach to Participation (CAP), described in Chapter 7, is a private practice of occupational therapists, neuropsychologists, physiotherapists, family therapists, dieticians, speech pathologists, medical doctors and case managers that seek to rehabilitate ABI survivors in a holistic and comprehensive manner. Home-centred therapies eliminate geographic disadvantage to rural clients and allow for services to fully incorporate the client's family, friends, neighbours and other community members. Positive, individualized support that is flexible, goal-oriented and balanced is delivered in client homes. Client norms and values are central to customizing a mutually agreed upon plan of therapy. Interventions seek to address both physical and psychological states of health to optimize participation within communities. Coping mechanisms, use of cues and environmental modifications to barriers facilitates community participation. Communications with clients are structured to be encouraging, open and collaborative, as the client's strengths are the primary focus in "building self-identity". Participation, then, builds from the client's sense of belonging and experiences of achievement. Long-term intermittent support is available to the clients.

Chapter 8 reviews the **ABI Partnership Project** that coordinates a continuum of community-based services for adults with ABI so that their clients "may live successfully in their communities with improved quality of life." The program's services and programs enable clients, families and caregivers to receive education, rehabilitation, life enrichment, respite, and residential and vocational services, in the community in which they live. Two specific services offered are Outreach and Aboriginal ABI Community Support. Members of the Outreach Team meet regularly with clients to help establish and maintain personal relationships, to learn clients' goals and to connect clients to services and programs that will support them in achieving their individual goals. Services are individualized to meet the expressed needs and goals of each client. The Aboriginal ABI Group facilitates the formation of new connections and relationships between adults with ABI and community elders, ceremonial groups from various reserves, cultural centres, urban services, and Aboriginal agencies and community programs. Its mission is to decrease feelings of isolation among its clients while simultaneously strengthening their community ties and spirituality through participation in traditional practices. Program activities are community-based and culturally focused. Promotional materials are translated into Cree and Dene for Northern Aboriginal clients.

Acquired Brain Injury Ireland (ABII), described in Chapter 9, is a national program that provides a range of flexible and tailor-made services to adults (ages 18-65) with ABI. The **Side by Side Day Resource Service**, one of the services offered, places a strong emphasis on individual development and person-centred planning (the client is fully involved in all decisions that affect his/her life). Holistically driven efforts foster and facilitate individual development, which is conceptualized as self-esteem, independence, community involvement, responsibility, empowerment and personal growth. The **Side by Side Day Resource Service** is 'inserted in the community', with many facilities located nearby. A **Rehabilitation Team** consisting of clinical staff, Local Services Managers, ABI Case Managers and Rehabilitation Assistants is responsible for assessing the individual needs of a client and for developing a person centred program of rehabilitation and support. A **personal development plan** (PDP) is created in partnership with each client and clearly identifies the areas in which the client is independent, where support is needed along with any potential risks. It is then implemented and prioritized with realistic and achievable goals identified.

Chapter 10 looks at **School Transition and re-Entry Program** (STEP). This promising program seeks to improve identification of school-aged children (ages 5-18) with a TBI or ABI when they are in the hospital. Based on the "Back to School" model, **STEP** uses a multi-faceted approach to facilitate communication and cooperation between all points of contact in the child's community: hospital, school and parents (family). A comprehensive hospital–school transition intervention, which includes hospital, school and family components, provides a systematic and coordinated approach to the development, validation, and dissemination of effective measures and transition intervention practices, facilitating clients' participation in their schools and communities. STEP project recruiters are placed within the hospital to engage families with children who have suffered a TBI or ABI. "Transition facilitators"—mainly Physical Therapists, Special Education Teachers and Social Workers who work for the Board of Education—liaise with the hospital and produce individual educational plans for each client. One of the program's interventions is a website for parents, developed to address a range of concerns common to parents with an injured child. The information provided by STEP promotes empowerment of parents and teachers to understand, encourage, and advocate for the child over the life course—within grade school and beyond. The program is sufficiently flexible to accommodate different areas of the United States.

Chapter 11 reviews the **Pediatric Acquired Brain Injury Community Outreach Program** (PABICOP), which represents an innovative approach to providing support and training to children and families with an ABI through an Acquired Brain Injury Rehabilitation and Reintegration Outreach Team. The Travelling Acquired Brain Injury Rehabilitation and Reintegration Team bridges the gap between rehabilitation services that are currently at **Children's Hospital of Western Ontario** (CHWO) and those in smaller rural communities in Southwestern Ontario. The program's philosophy and model of operation is holistic, parent and family/client-centred, community-based, and inclusive of the community at large in the ongoing care and management of the child or youth with an ABI. Three primary objectives govern program operations: to improve integration and acceptance of children with an ABI into their home communities, to improve the quality of life of children and their families with an ABI, to minimize problems and maximize the quality of life of each individual child with an ABI as they enter adolescence and adulthood. **PABICOP** also encompasses the concepts of continuity, accessibility, knowledge, collaboration, empowerment and advocacy within its services, which are individualized, inclusive of home and school environments, long-term and centred on the needs identified by the client. **PABICOP**'s practice is culturally sensitive and the client and his/her family help to guide its team of experts in understanding what is meaningful to them, in order to effectively plan, support and educate.

TIRR Memorial Hermann's Challenge Program (TIRR), examined in Chapter 12, is a specialized outpatient program for persons with a TBI or ABI. The program's guiding philosophy is to treat clients holistically and to help them to return to work. The objective of the program is to identify something the client can do to meet an individual goal at the end of the treatment. Clients are continually involved in decision-making and assessment of their rehabilitation program. Community reintegration becomes a key focus as compensatory strategies are learned, following a focus on restoration therapy. Physical, Occupational, Speech, Cognitive, Psychotherapy, and Community Integration Therapies are integrated with one another and offered two-to-four days a week, in a group format. Group therapy is thought to facilitate the development and furthering of a client's self-awareness and social skills, as peers provide feedback and a sense of community to learn more strategies. The family is regarded as a key component to the client's rehabilitation. Family members are invited and encouraged to collaborate with the staff (members of the rehabilitation team). Staff, in turn spend a considerable amount of time educating and working with the family so that the client can become more independent at home. A track-based method (e.g., employment track, volunteer ready, education track and Independent living readiness) based on what clients can accomplish during the course of their rehabilitation is utilized. Clients are connected with supportive community-based partner organizations in order to practice their skills and to work towards their community reintegration goals.

Chapter 13 looks at a program offered through the **Krempels Center** that facilitates growth and improvement in various aspects of the client's life, including functional goals and social skills. Clients form primary relationships with other clients, program staff, volunteers, student interns, and members of the community throughout their involvement with the program. Field trips and community events are encouraged to broaden the client's physical environment and ties to the community. Further, community outings help to increase the client's knowledge of various societal and cultural norms. Family members are encouraged to become involved in the programming. A holistic approach is adopted to improve the overall quality of life for clients.

Chapter 14 examines the **Biscayne Institute of Health and Living** (BIHL) program that follows the **Biscayne HealthCare Community Model**. This undertaking emphasizes health care delivery for frontline community-based care. More specifically, the BIHL model is primarily focused on the care of the whole person through individualized treatment by a community team of professionals. Physical, cognitive, social and behavioural aspects are addressed within a model that "lies in between individual practitioners and hospitals on a continuum of healthcare delivery." A full continuum of services ranging from primary care and health and wellness promotion to the community is offered in the form of a 3-stage program. In Stage 1 (Assessment and Treatment Plan), each client's evaluation is performed and an interdisciplinary care plan developed. Weekly team rounds within the BIHL facility (a centre situated in "peaceful surrounding" with rooms that resemble rooms in a home) assess the client's progress and set new goals. Ongoing forms of healing include a tailored cognitive retraining program; biofeedback, physical, occupational and speech therapies; Chinese medicine; modules to assist with taking medication; performing activities of daily living and maintaining safety; and individual, family and group therapy. Stage 2 (Consolidation of the Learned Skills) features field trips and interactions within the community. Finally, Stage 3 (Life after Rehab) facilitates the client's return to his/her home environment. The client is continually monitored at home, while he/she participates in protected and supported work and volunteering environments. BIHL is a community-based model: consumers and their families are able to participate in their own programming, and work with a team of professionals to choose services. Clients are followed long-term in the community and are able to return to BIHL (even as volunteers), if they so choose

Chapter 15 reviews the **Brain Integration Program** (BIP), developed by the **Rehabilitation Centre Groot Klimmendaal** in the Netherlands with the aim of achieving optimal community integration for ABI survivors with complex behavioural or psychiatric problems. BIP is a structured residential program. The main objective of the program is to re-integrate "difficult to treat" individuals with chronic ABI back into their communities. The program allows participants to achieve a balance in their daily activities between domestic life, work, leisure and social interaction, through participation in 3 modules: an independent living module which emphasizes training in specific abilities; a social-emotional module which facilitates the setting of new, adjusted and achievable life goals; and, the work module whose focus is on the development of vocational aims. The client's family participates in the activities associated with the social-emotional module. Likewise, community employers facilitate the training and employment subsumed within the work module. At each stage, clients at the residential facility support one another through continued social interaction. Clients return home each and every weekend to practice their acquired skills.

Finally, Chapter 16 provides an overview of the cases, insights, and conclusions derived from this investigation of exemplary programs. The programs detailed in the following chapters are among the world's best efforts to foster community participation after acquired brain injury.

REFERENCES

Arnstein, S. R., (1969). **A ladder of citizen participation**. *Journal of the American Planning Association*, 35(4), 216-224.

British Medical Association. **Report of the working group on medical education.** London: BMA, 1995

Brown, M., Dijkers, M., Gordon, W., Ashman, T., Charatz., Cheng, Z. (2004). **Participation Objective, Participation Subjective: A Measure of Participation Combining Outsider and Insider Perspectives**. *Journal of Head Trauma Rehabilitation*. 19(6), 459-481.

Canadian Health Research Foundation, (2000). *Annual Report*. Ottawa, CIHR.

Collacut-McGrath, J. (2007). **Ethical practice in brain injury rehabilitation**. Oxford; New York : Oxford University Press, 2007.

Condeluci, A. (2002) *Cultural Shifting: Community Leadership and Change*. St. Augustine : TRN.

Cornerstone Clubhouse (n.d.). *Cornerstone Clubhouse member handbook*. London, On: Cornerstone Clubhouse.

Dijkers, M. (2000). *The Community Integration Questionnaire*. The Center for Outcome Measurement in Brain Injury. **http://www.tbims.org/combi/ciq**

Dijkers, M. (1997). **Measuring the long-term outcomes of traumatic brain injury: A review of the Community Integration Questionnaire.** *Journal of Head Trauma Rehabilitation*, 12, 74-91.

Flaherty, P. (2008). **Social capital and its relevance in brain injury rehabilitation services.** *Journal of Vocational Rehabilitation*, 29 (3), 141-146

Hall, K.M., et al. (2001). **Assessing traumatic brain injury outcome measures for long-term follow-up of community-based individuals.** *Archives of Physical Medicine and Rehabilitation*, 82: 367-374.

Jacobs, H. E. (1997). **The Clubhouse: Addressing work-related behavioral challenges through a supportive social community.** *Journal of Head Trauma Rehabilitation*, 12(5), 14-27.

Lezak, M. D.(1993). **Newer contributions to the neuropsychological assessment of executive functions.** *Journal of Head Trauma Rehabilitation*, 8:24-31.

Linden, M.A ., Crothers, I. R., O'Neill, S. B., McCann, J. P. (2005). Reduced community integration in persons following traumatic brain injury, as measured on the Community Integration Measure: An exploratory analysis. *Disability and Rehabilitation*, 27, 1353-1356.

Macias, C., Jackson, R., Schroeder, C., & Wang, Q. (1999) **What is a Clubhouse? Report on the ICCD 1996 Survey of USA Clubhouses.** *Community Mental Health Journal*, 35(2), 181-190.

McColl, M. A., Davies, D., Carlson, P., Johnston, J., & Minnes, P. (2001). **The Community Integration Measure: Development and preliminary validation.** *Archives of Physical Medicine and Rehabilitation*, 82(4), 429-434.

McColl, M. A. & Jongbloed, L. (Eds.) (2006). *Disability and social policy in Canada* (2nd ed). Toronto: Captus Press.

McColl, M. A., Carlson, P., Johnston, J., Minnes, P., Shue, K., Davies, D., Karlovits, T. (1998). The definition of community integration: Perspectives of people with brain injuries. **Brain Injury**, 12, 15-30.

Mellick, D. (2000). *The Craig Handicap Assessment and Reporting Technique.* The Center for Outcome Measurement in Brain Injury. **http://www.tbims.org/combi/chart**

Mellick, D., Walker, N., Brooks, C. A., Whiteneck, G. (1999). Incorporating the cognitive independence domain into CHART. *Journal of Rehabilitation Outcomes Measures*, 3,12-21.

Olico-Okui, M. (2005). **"Community Participation: An Abused Concept?"** Makerere University Institute of Public Health, Uganda: 1- 4.

Putnam, R. D. (2000) **Bowling Alone: The Collapse and Revival of American Community.** New York: Simon & Schuster.

Rifkin, S. B. (1986) **Lessons from community participation in health programmes.** *Health Policy and Planning*, 1(3) 240-249.

Salter, K., Foley, N., Jutai, J., Bayley, M., & Teasell, R. (2008). Assessment of community integration following traumatic brain injury. **Brain Injury** : 22(11), 820-835.

Sloan, S., Winkler, D., Callaway, L. (2004). **Community integration following severe traumatic brain injury: outcomes and best practice.** *Brain Impairment*, 5(1), 12-29.

Tate, R., Hodgkinson, A., Veerabangsa, A., & Maggiotto, S. (1999). **Measuring psychosocial recovery after traumatic brain injury: Psychometric properties of a new scale.** *The Journal of Head Trauma Rehabilitation,* 14(6), 543-557.

Volpe, R. (2005). The conceptualization of injury prevention as change in complex systems. Toronto: SMARTRISK Foundation.

Volpe, R., Lewko, J. H., & Batra, A. (2002). *A compendium of effective, evidence-based best practices in prevention of neurotrauma.* Toronto, Canada: University of Toronto Press.

Walker, N., Mellick, D., Brooks, C. A., & Whiteneck, G. G. (2003). **Measuring participation across impairment groups using the Craig handicap assessment reporting technique.** *American Journal of Physical Medicine & Rehabilitation / Association of Academic Physiatrists*, 82(12), 936-941.

Whiteneck, G. G., Charlifue, S. W., Gerhart, K. A., Overholser, J. D., & Richardson, G. N. (1992). Quantifying handicap: A new measure of long-term rehabilitation outcomes. *Archives of Physical Medicine and Rehabilitation,* 73(6), 519-526.

Willer, B., & Corrigan, J. (1994). Whatever It Takes: a model for community-based services. **Brain Injury**, 8(7), 647-659.

Willer, B., Ottenbacher, K. J., & Coad, M. L. (1994). **The Community Integration Questionnaire: a comparative examination.** *Am J Phys Med Rehabil*, 73(2), 103-111.

Willer, B., Rosenthal, M., Kreutzer, J., Gordon, W., & Rempel, R. (1993). **Assessment of community integration following rehabilitation for TBI.** *Journal of Head Trauma Rehabilitation*, 8, 11-23.

Wood-Dauphinee, S. L., Opzoomer, M. A., Williams, J. I., Marchand, B., & Spitzer, W. O. (1988). Assessment of global function: The reintegration to normal living index. *Archives of Physical Medicine and Rehabilitation*, 69(8), 583-590.

World Health Organization. (2001). **International Classification of Functioning, Disability and Health: ICF.** Geneva: World Health Organization.

Zhang, L., et al. (2002). **Comparison of the Community Integration Questionnaire, the Craig Handicap Assessment and reporting technique, and the disability rating scale in** traumatic **brain injury.** *The Journal of Head Trauma Rehabilitation*, 17(6), 497-509.

CHAPTER 2

communityworks, inc.

by Amanda Stewart

communityworks inc.

Population Served : Life Span	
Contributing Author Contact Information	
Janet M. Williams, PhD	Hope E. Atchison
President	Administrative Assistant to the President
7819 Conser Place	7819 Conser Place
Overland Park, KS 66204	Overland Park, KS 66204
Phone: (913) 789-9900 ext. 101	Phone: (913) 789-9900 ext. 130
Email: **janetw@communityworksinc.com**	Email: **hopea@communityworksinc.com**

BACKGROUND

History and Development

Dr. Janet M. Williams, president and owner of **communityworks inc.**, is a long-time advocate for community participation within Kansas. Williams first began to develop strategies in 1982 to promote independent living in the community for people living with brain injuries. At this time, Williams was working as a social worker at a rehabilitation centre. Through this role, she witnessed firsthand the challenges and frustrations experienced by individuals living with traumatic brain injuries. In particular, Williams noted that the traditional medical model approach to providing services was inadequate in supporting self-sufficiency and community membership. Instead, the service system was focused on "fixing" individuals through the use of deficit-based assessment and planning (**Williams, 2008**). Essentially, the system was grounded in the notion that individuals living with brain injuries require intervention before they can "earn" the right to re-enter the community (**Williams, 2008**). Consequently, Williams observed that the overwhelming numbers of requests from consumers to make the transition back home and into the community were often ignored. This perception was reaffirmed through her time as the Director of Family Services at the **Brain Injury Association of America** (BIAA). From 1985 to 1989, Williams helped the BIAA provide information and support to individuals living with brain injuries and their families. This was accomplished by responding to requests from the newly established 1-800 information number at the BIAA. Williams reported that within one year of establishing the information hotline, the BIAA received approximately 20,000 calls. She noted that the majority of callers were directed at seeking assistance in returning home. She resolved to address this issue by establishing a program that would adopt a revolutionary approach to rehabilitation services—one that gives control back to the individual.

Driven by this vision, Williams devoted her time toward researching rehabilitation programs for people with brain injuries. In 1990, she visited rehabilitation programs in Norway, Denmark, The Netherlands, and Germany. Her experiences highlighted the disparities that existed at this time between the services provided in these countries verses the services provided in the United States. Specifically, Williams noted these countries allocated the resources of the community to better meet the needs of people living with brain injuries. She further examined the concept of independent living for people with brain injuries through her dissertation research at the **University of Kansas**. Her research revealed that the most influential factor in achieving independent living for people with brain injuries was the allocation of financial resources to the community sector.

Ultimately, Williams' research emphasized the importance of developing social capital for people living with brain injuries.

Williams founded **communityworks, inc.** in 1991 following the implementation of the **Medicaid Home and Community Based (HCBS) waiver**. The waiver stated that people must live in their home and receive services in the community. The HCBS waiver is grounded in the independent living philosophy (**State of Kansas Department of Social and Rehabilitation Services, 2004**). A key tenet of this philosophy is that individuals with disabilities should have the same civil rights, options, and control over choices as individuals without disabilities. Consumers are encouraged to take active roles and participate in decision making rather than assuming the passive role of the patient. Essentially, the locus of control is placed on the consumer. The implementation of the HCBS waiver reflected the shift from the medical model to the independent living model by changing the focus from professionally driven services that aimed to "fix" the cognitive and physical impairments of the individual toward more flexible consumer driven services devoted to the individuals rights and social capital of the individual (**Williams, 2008**). Ultimately, the implementation of the HCBS waiver represented an opportunity to initiate an agency dedicated to supporting full community inclusion and customer autonomy.

Program Objective

The mission statement of communityworks, inc. is to "support people to live, work, and play in the community" (**Williams, 2008**, p. 158). This primary objective is supported by the "North Star" approach, which represents the organization's vision of where they wish to go as individuals and as an agency. In essence, the North Star symbolizes a vision of people with brain injuries "living in their homes, doing something they want to do, with as few paid supports as possible" (Williams, 2008, p. 158). The very name of the agency captures this fundamental goal. The small letters of the name emphasize the role of the consumer rather than the agency, and therefore symbolize the shift from professionally driven to consumer driven services. The notion of inclusion is also represented by combining "community" and "works" as one word, which signifies the goal of blending into the community. Finally, the name itself highlights the fact that community works for everyone, and is a reminder of our similarities.

Philosophical Principles

Williams conceived that a more flexible, consumer driven approach must be adopted in order for individuals with TBI to be fully part of the community. Her research, along with her experience in assisting individuals with brain injuries, led her to develop a series of philosophical principles that now guide the ultimate program design of communityworks, inc. First, she reasoned that programs must be designed to promote decision making on the part of the consumer and family in order to effectively draw on the person's strengths and personal goals (**Racino & Williams, 1994; Williams, 2008**). Second, services must be designed to foster both community connections and autonomy (Racino & Williams, 1994; Williams, 2008). Third, the environment was identified as a critical factor in skill training. In other words, interventions must take place in the very environments in which the skills will be put into practice (Racino & Williams, 1994; Williams, 2008). Fourth, services must be self-directed (Racino & Williams, 1994; Williams, 2008). This principle highlights the shift from the expert medical model to the consumer driven model, as it affirms that consumers must be in charge of the hiring and firing of service providers. Services must also be designed to assist consumers in discovering meaning in their lives by assisting them in finding their places in the community (Racino & Williams, 1994; Williams, 2008). Attention is given to the importance of facilitating the development of personal connections, which ultimately represent "natural" supports in the community (Racino & Williams, 1994; Williams, 2008). In order for people to achieve these connections, Williams asserts that people must be truly "of" the community and live in generic housing options of their own choosing. Tied to this principle is the notion that the housing of consumers must be kept separate from the agency in order to promote autonomy and to achieve a sense of permanency in the community (Racino & Williams, 1994; Williams, 2008). These philosophical principles are summarized as follows:

1. People using services and families know themselves best.

2. Services must promote self-sufficiency and community membership.

3. People using services manage their own personal assistants.

4. Services should be functional and take place in relevant environments.

5. All people have a place to contribute in the community. It is our job to assist in finding that place.

6. Support resources include "natural supports," community supports and personal assistance services.

7. People must live in generic affordable housing within communities and neighborhoods.

8. The provision of support services is separate from housing. We do not own or operate property where people live.

Description of Consumers

communityworks, inc. provides services to anyone who needs in-home supports, resource coordination, therapies, and employment services. The consumer population includes individuals with the following conditions: TBI, cerebrovascular accidents, ABI, complex multi-diagnosis situations, CNS disorders, spinal cord injury, and injuries on the job. The level of services provided range from intensive support (i.e., requiring 24-hour care) to minimal support. In terms of the TBI population, communityworks serves individuals with a full range of injury severity (i.e., mild to severe). Currently, communityworks serves approximately 480 consumers in 20 counties of Kansas. The consumer population ranges in age from 8 to 70 years old. Of these 480 consumers, 227 are currently receiving intense rehabilitation, 58 require 24-hour support, and 123 have achieved independent living and are receiving assistance directed at fostering community connections.

RESOURCES

Reimbursement for services at communityworks, inc. is determined on a fee-for-service basis. Services can be funded through a variety of methods, including existing contracts with insurance agencies, worker's compensation, private settlements, private pay, and the **Kansas Home and Community Based Waiver Services** (Traumatic Brian Injury, Physical Disability, and Frail Elderly). Communityworks, inc. has received funding from the following sources: **Blue Cross & Blue Shield of Kansas City**, **Johnson County Vocational Rehabilitation Service**, **Kansas Medicaid**, **Kansas Traumatic Brain Injury Waiver**, **Missouri Traumatic Brain Injury Program**, TRIWEST, **United Healthcare**, **Mutual of Omaha**, **Veterans Administration**, and **Workers Compensation** by Case. Importantly, the consumer is provided with assistance in seeking alternative sources of funding (such as funds from the federal state and community resources) when funding from privates sources runs out. The program is designed to meet the long-term needs of consumers. Therefore, consumers have the option of re-entering the program as new goals and needs emerge in the future.

Medicaid Home and Community Based Waiver

As previously mentioned, in 1991 Kansas implemented the **Medicaid Home and Community Based (HCBS)/ Traumatic Brain Injury (TBI) waiver**, which was the first in the nation to support people with brain injuries to live in the community. Medicaid is a public assistance medical care program designed to help states meet the health care costs of populations in need. The HCBS/ TBI waiver provided states with the flexibility to offer eligible individuals with alternatives to institutional care (i.e., hospitals, nursing facilities, etc.). The following eligibility criteria must be met for individuals to receive services under the HCBS/TBI program: (1) individual must be between the ages of 16 to 65 years; (2) individual meets criteria for placement in a brain injury rehabilitation hospital; (3) individual has an external, traumatically acquired non-degenerative structural brain injury (**State of Kansas Department of Social and Rehabilitation Services, 2004**). An important component of the HCBS/TBI program is the requirement that consumers be allowed to self-direct their own in-home care services. Consumers that choose to self-direct their own care services are responsible for recruiting, training, and managing their attendants.

In order to receive approval for HCBS waiver programs, the **Department of Social and Rehabilitation Services** (SRS) must guarantee the federal **Centers for Medicare and Medicaid Services** (CMS) that "on an average per capita basis, the cost of providing home and community-based services will not exceed the cost of care for the identical population in an institution" (**State of Kansas Department of Social and Rehabilitation Services, 2004**, p. 3). With regard to the TBI population, cost-effectiveness is determined by comparing community-based programs with the **TBI Rehabilitation Facility** (TBIRF) (State of Kansas Department of Social and Rehabilitation Services, 2004). In the event that the average costs of the HCBS/TBI waiver programs exceed the cost to serve individuals in a TBIRF, Kansas will no longer meet approval to provide services under the HCBS/TBI waiver (State of Kansas Department of Social and Rehabilitation Services, 2004). In addition to demonstrating cost-effectiveness, documentation of the safeguards in place to protect the health and welfare of beneficiaries must be provided. Provider agencies are required to develop individual Plans of Care, which are entered into the **Medicaid Management Information System** (MMIS) in order for reimbursement to be provided to the professionals providing services within the agencies (State of Kansas Department of Social and Rehabilitation Services, 2004). The individual Plan of Care must include the following information: medical and other services provided; frequency, scope, and duration of services; identification of providers responsible for each service; and the cost of each service (State of Kansas Department of Social and Rehabilitation Services, 2004).

IMPLEMENTATION

Services

communityworks inc. maintains that every individual is unique, and that vast differences exist between people in terms of how they adjust to rehabilitation. Hence, the services provided at communityworks are individualized. Communityworks assigns each consumer a case manager. The case manager carries out an individual assessment prior to the consumer's return home, which entails collaborating with the consumer, family, and physician in order to identify rehabilitation goals. A key part of this process involves simply asking the consumer what he or she wants to achieve, and then coordinating the community resources that will be necessary in order for the consumer to reach these self-identified goals. The consumer returns home as soon as possible and receives services that are tailored to him or her. Communityworks offers families and consumers the following services: independent living skills, case management, personal assistance, information and referral to community resources, peer support, physical therapy, occupational therapy, cognitive therapy, speech therapy, drug and alcohol counseling, overnight support, nursing, medications management, 24-hour supervision, medical consultation, and employment support. The intensity of services gradually decreases over time as the person develops proficiency in daily living skills. Williams points out that while the initial cost of providing intense therapy is significant, having the ability to decrease services over time when they are no longer necessary decreases costs in the long-term.

Application of Philosophical Principles

The implementation of services at communityworks, inc. is guided by a series of eight philosophical principles (see background section). The following section describes the ways in which each of these principles is put into practice in the day-to-day operations of the program:

1. People using services and families know themselves best.

communityworks inc. strives to shift away from the medical "fixing" culture, which implicitly teaches individuals to depend on professionals for even the most basic decisions. In contrast, communityworks maintains that the customer must be the key actor in all decision making, as it is ultimately the consumer that possesses knowledge pertaining to his or her personal goals and strengths (**Williams, 2008**). In addition, the input from family and friends is taken into consideration. This principle is put into practice by ensuring that the consumer is always at the center of every decision and interaction. For example, the consumer is the leader of team meetings and is always present when issues pertaining to him or her are discussed.

2. Services must promote self-sufficiency and community membership.

communityworks, inc. defines self-sufficiency as learning both how to do things for oneself and how to reach out to others (**Williams, 2008**). The primary role of staff is to aid consumers in establishing community connections. In this way, staff members are viewed as coaches that support customers in carrying out the necessary actions to develop friendships and support networks in the community (Williams, 2008). In practice, this may entail going to local places in the community to make friends, joining clubs/ sports team along with the consumer, etc.

3. People using services manage their own personal assistants.

In accordance with the consumer driven model, communityworks, inc. upholds the belief that the "consumer knows best" (**Williams, 2008**). The organization fulfills this principle by supporting consumers to manage their own staff. For example, consumers receive support in writing help ads, creating interview questions, conducting job interviews, creating training videos demonstrating the attendant needs they are seeking, and providing performance feedback. **communityworks, inc**. acts as a payroll agent to the staff hired by the consumers.

4. Services should be functional and take place in relevant environments.

A primary concern when teaching life skills is generalizability. In other words, skills must generalize to the home environment and community. Paid staff ensure that the skills that are relearned are transferrable by assisting consumers to practice these skills in the environments in which they will be put into practice. For example, consumers may practice cooking in their own kitchen, walking on their own streets, etc.

5. All people have a place to contribute in the community. It is our job to assist in finding that place.

The services at **communityworks, inc**. are designed to allow consumers to discover meaningful roles in various realms of community life. The "coach" encourages the consumer to explore new activities and provides support during these new experiences.

Ultimately, the goal is for the consumer to discover what works for him or her and to attain a stable support network (**Williams, 2008**).

6. Support resources include "natural supports," community supports and personal assistance services.

"Natural supports" are defined as people who are willing to help but are not paid to do so (such as family, friends, neighbours, etc.), while paid supports receive compensation from the consumer or from a form of third party payment (e.g. Medicaid). **Williams (2008)** points out that the division between natural and paid supports may become blurred, due to the fact that family members can be paid to provide personal assistance services in Kansas. In order to effectively deal with this challenge, communityworks, inc. encourages frequent discussions about the pros and cons of paid family assistants.

7. People must live in generic affordable housing within communities and neighborhoods.

It is critical for people to live within the community in order to build social support networks. Thus, communityworks, inc. promotes a range of housing options, (such as single family homes, condominiums, cooperative housing, individual apartments, etc.) and strives to eliminate barriers that may prevent the establishment of community connections (**Williams, 2008**). For example, special services that may prevent consumers from blending into the community are not carried out (such as group outings, staff vans, etc.)

8. The provision of support services is separate from housing. We do not own or operate property where people live.

communityworks, inc. separates housing from the services they provide in order to allow consumers to maintain autonomy from the organization. In this way, consumers are able to achieve a sense of permanency and are able to negotiate choices pertaining to the services they receive (**Williams, 2008**).

Community CLUES Framework

In addition to the philosophical principles guiding the delivery of services, the team members at communityworks follow the "**Community CLUES**" framework. This framework allows the team members at communityworks to effectively tailor services to people in their homes and communities. The framework is as follows:

➤ **Create** positive environments with control and choice. Team members implement environmental manipulations in order to assist individuals with independent living. For example, environmental adaptations may include a ramp if the person uses a wheelchair, reminders if the person experiences memory difficulties, etc. Choice and control are provided to the individual by ensuring that he or she puts decision-making skills into practice on a daily basis. For example, the consumer decides where he or she will live, who will provide personal care attendant services, and the goals he or she will work on.

➤ **Listen** to the consumer and develop goals based on what you hear, not on what assessments reveal. Goals are driven by what the consumer wishes to accomplish. Team members facilitate the support the person requires to achieve these goals by analyzing the tasks and breaking them down into manageable steps. As a result, the person is given the opportunity to receive real-life feedback and learn what goals are realistic, the challenges and strengths he or she brings to the task, and what steps will be necessary for future success. Importantly, this real-life experience allows consumers to begin to build confidence in their independent living skills.

➤ **Understand** what is happening from the person's perspective. True understanding is achieved by reflecting upon the quality and "best fit" of services. Team members are encouraged to reflect upon the following issues: whether the services are designed to capitalize on the person's strengths and compensate for his or her weaknesses, whether the services are ones that the team members themselves would want to receive if the roles were reversed, and if the services truly promote success.

➤ **Expect** that everyday life will bring pitfalls, surprises, and success. This element of the framework serves as a reminder that a number of outcomes may unfold in the natural setting of the community. Team members are trained to provide immediate support to help consumers effectively deal with any pitfalls and surprises they may encounter in the home and community.

➤ **Support** the person to make the best of family supports during the marathon of brain injury. Consumers and families are provided with the necessary tools and education to support each other in the long-term. For example, consumers and families are taught how to access resources and reach out to others in similar situations. The importance of social capital and social networks is also emphasized in order to highlight the underlying goal of community inclusion.

Staff Roles and Responsibilities

Multidisciplinary Team

Communityworks offers a multidisciplinary framework. The staff includes: case managers/social workers, certified transitional specialists, cognitive therapists, physical and occupational therapists, speech therapists, behaviour therapists, personal care attendants, drug and alcohol counselors, and employment counselors. Case managers are responsible for coordinating the myriad of resources. Essentially, case managers connect consumers with the support they will require to meet their individual goals. For example, case managers may assist with Social Security, equipment needs, and the identification of staff. Certified transitional specialists assist consumers to live in the community. Cognitive therapists design innovative strategies to assist consumers to live in the community. This role involves engaging consumers in problem solving, with the ultimate goal of helping them establish connections in the community. Physical therapists, occupational therapists, speech therapists, and behaviour therapists assist consumers in relearning functional skills in the home and community. Personal care attendants assist consumers with daily living activities that promote independence. Drug and alcohol counselors provide counseling and support to consumers and families experiencing addictions. Finally, employment counselors assist consumers with job-seeking and job-keeping skills. Employment counselors assist consumers with finding job opportunities, job interview preparation, and customizing work adaptations. The multidisciplinary framework at communityworks, inc. allows consumers to receive individualized services that are tailored to their unique needs.

Staff Standards

A set of staff standards was developed by the staff at communityworks, inc. in order to ensure consistency in services. These standards were also designed with the aim of reminding staff of their roles in consumers' lives. The standards are as follows:

1.   **Be the coach, consultant and support, not the boss or expert**. Staff members are reminded that their roles are to be observers, not instructors (**Williams, 2008**). This standard highlights the contrast between the traditional medical model and the community-based model upheld by communityworks, as it shifts the focus from "fixing" people to assisting them in achieving their personal goals.

2.   **You are paid to help the person get a life, not paid to be their life**. This standard highlights the distinction between paid supports and natural supports. Team members are reminded that their roles are to help the consumers establish friendships and build their social networks (**Williams, 2008**).

3.   Do whatever it takes to help someone be connected in the community. Team members follow a number of guidelines to ensure that consumers blend

into the community. First, communityworks maintains that the consumer and staff must not appear as consumer and staff (**Williams, 2008**). For example, team members do not wear names or engage in discussions pertaining to their paid roles in public. Instead, team members participate in community activities with the consumer (rather than "supervising"). As well, team members expect consumers to speak for themselves, and therefore only step in when necessary.

4.   Work yourself out of a job so you can have the benefit of working with more people. Team members employ a number of creative strategies to support independence, with the underlying goal of "fading themselves out" once this has been achieved (**Williams, 2008**). A key focus is on ensuring that consumers possess the necessary tools to perform independent living skills in the absence of the staff. For example, reminders for medication may be put up to eliminate the need for the staff to do the reminding.

Minds Matter LLC Joins the Program

Minds Matter is a training and consulting company designed to support the needs of professionals who work with people with disabilities in the community. Linda Wilkerson is the CEO of the company. **Minds Matter** was established in 2005 as the sister company of communityworks, inc. in order to respond to requests from individuals and agencies requiring services and training. **Minds Matter** provides short-term services in the consumer's home and community with the goal of decreasing challenging behaviours and increasing community participation. Services and training are delivered on the following issues: independent living needs, positive behaviour support, cognitive therapy, and physical therapy.

Challenges

Williams (2008) asserts that "the greatest challenges to running an agency focused on Social Capital is managing growth and maintaining focus" (p. 162). She began as the sole employee of communityworks, inc. at the inception of the program in 1991. Under her direction, communityworks, inc. has grown tremendously and now provides services to 480 consumers in 20 Kansas counties. In addition, the agency currently has more than 300 employees and continues to hire. The agency has ensured that its initial objective and philosophical principles are maintained by standardizing training and continuing to focus its concentration on the North Star.

OUTCOME

Evaluation Methods

Review of Individual Plan of Care

Communityworks measures the attainments of the participation strategies on an individual basis. Specifically, communityworks considers the following factors in measuring the outcome for each consumer: duration in program, reason for ending services, the number of goals that were achieved, the current employment status of the consumer, and the level of intensity of services currently required by the consumer. These factors are considered in the annual review of each individual plan of care, and adjustments are made accordingly.

Cost Analysis

Cost analysis is carried out on an annual basis. As previously discussed, in order to continue to meet approval to provide services under the HCBS/TBI waiver, programs must demonstrate that the cost of providing home and community-based services does not exceed the cost of providing services in institutions. The **Kansas Department of Social and Rehabilitation Services** reports a savings of $40,000 per person, per month for individuals using communityworks, inc. services paid for by Medicaid as compared with individuals in institutional settings. Thus, communityworks has been shown to be highly cost-effective. The following table presents the results of the cost analyses conducted between 2005 and 2010 on the cost differences between consumers in rehabilitation facilities versus consumers utilizing HCBS state waiver programs.

Table 1: Results from 2005–2010 Cost Analyses

Year	Average # of People on HCBS/TBI Waiver (monthly)	Avg. cost per person per month for people on waiver	Avg. # of people in TBI rehab facilities (monthly)	Avg. cost per person per month for people in TBI rehab facilities
2005	151	$3,351.00		$23,282.00
2006	167	3,096.00		$22,576.00
2007	183	$3,703.00		$26,142.00
2008	196	$3,690.00	27	$26,253.00
2009	243	$3,505.00	30	$23,543.00
2010	323	$3,196.00	39	$21,550.00

Consumer Satisfaction Surveys

communityworks, inc. assesses consumer satisfaction three times a year through the use of a brief survey. The survey consists of two questions, and is designed to provide the staff at communityworks with a sense of consumers' overall satisfaction with services, as well as the levels of satisfaction concerning assistance from case managers. Consumers are asked to respond on a 5 point scale ranging from "poor" (i.e. 1) to "great" (i.e. 5). At the bottom of the survey, there is a space for consumers to write comments, and list their three favorite things about working with communityworks. The survey questions and average responses gathered from 2004 to 2008 are reported below:

Question 1: You originally met with a person to help you become eligible for services. Were you satisfied with the assistance you received about our services?

> AVERAGE ANSWER: 4.5

Question 2: You currently have a case manager providing coordination and assistance. Is the case manager meeting with you regularly and assisting your needs?

> AVERAGE ANSWER: 4.29

Please list three things you like best about working with communityworks

1. Staff members are dependable and supportive of consumers' goals
2. It takes a while to find the right staff person to fit with consumers (TLS and PCAs), but once a fit is found, it works wonderfully.
3. Thank you.

Community Reactions

The success of communityworks, inc. has earned a substantial amount of attention in the media in recent years. In 2009, Williams received "**The Dr. Randy Evans North American Brain Injury Society (NABIS) Award for Clinical Services**" for her success with communityworks, inc. and her work as a leading advocate for disability issues across the United States. This award recognizes professionals who develop innovative services for individuals with brain injuries. In the same year, communityworks, inc. was rated as the number one "**Top 20 Women-Owned Businesses in Kansas City**" by the Kansas City Business Journal based on the total number of local employees. The Kansas City

Business Journal ranked communityworks, inc. as number nineteen based on total revenue. In August of 2009, Williams also received an award for her outstanding career in disability services at the "2009 Kansas Disability Caucus." Finally, Williams received the "Women Who Mean Business" award in 2006. This award recognizes influential business women who have made an impact in their communities. The recognition that Williams has received in the media for her work at communityworks, inc. is a testament to the positive impact the agency has had on individuals living with brain injuries.

Experiences of Consumers

The following section presents two follow-up stories from the consumers at communityworks, inc. The stories were written by the consumers themselves and were selected in order to illustrate the unique experiences of the consumers at communityworks, inc.

Giving Back By: Lisa Bailey

When Gerard asked me to write an article for this newsletter, I readily agreed since I've been having fun posting letters to the editor of the Lawrence newspaper. However, the deadline's closing in and I'm still having trouble putting my thoughts together. Maybe it's because this is the first time I've tried to write about the brain injury I sustained in 1992. I suppose this is a record of surviving not only the accident, but the aftermath as well, which most will agree was the hard part.

I was schooling my horse over jumps when he fell, causing us to meet the ground together with tremendous force. I'm still proud of the fact that I wasn't thrown, which is ridiculous since falling free of 1500 pounds of horse would no doubt have lessened the severity of the injury. Anyhow, the horse was fine and I was not. I began coming out of the coma at KU Med and did my rehab time at Kansas Rehab Hospital in Topeka. My earliest memories seem to revolve around being tied to things; apparently for my protection as I was unaware of the damaged connection between brain and body.

I regained most physical function in the first year, but was unable to recognize the pervasive cognitive effects for several years. At the time of the accident I was employed, with good insurance, but was also mired in a contentious divorce involving our two children, ages four and eight. My first clue that something was wrong came from the painful realization that I was no longer their primary caregiver. When granted a weekend pass from the hospital, my dad drove me to "visit" the kids at the house that no longer bore any evidence of my presence. Needless to say, that was rather a setback to the recovery process. My new home was that hospital and they had to almost kick me out when the time came.

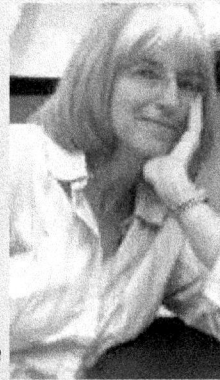

My personal life was in shambles, and returning to work was my lifeline. Throughout this ordeal, ongoing cooperation between rehab specialists, awesome coworkers and company management allowed me to slowly return to the job I loved in an environmental chemistry lab. Continuing to be unaware of any real limitations, I was quite incensed about having my work checked until I had proven myself to be competent and not a safety hazard.

Allowances were made for my new behaviors, and with shared humor and not a few tears, I became the "eccentric" analyst in my section. Everyone was quite aware that moving "my" stuff had dire consequences and would not interrupt work in progress unless the building was on fire. I had my area arranged just right with a large desk calendar to keep track of work deadlines, meetings and projects along with daily notes to track my personal life.

Nothing is as certain as change, and the company closed the Lawrence lab in late 1997. While my buddies found work outside Lawrence, I spent a year looking for something closer to home where at least the addresses made sense. Nothing else did in this newly disorganized and unfamiliar world. I finally talked my way into a job that was an unmitigated disaster, taking less than a month to make it quite clear that I was incapable of learning and using new information. My world had come crashing down and the full consequences of the head injury became harshly real. Simple everyday tasks like getting out of bed were too complicated, and living in a box actually seemed like a viable alternative.

SSDI was awarded before the box thing became a necessity. I was now eligible for the HI Waiver and communityworks, inc. was chosen to administer the services. I clearly recall feeling horrified at the thought of strangers "invading" my small apartment. I cautiously accepted an attendant care who very gently helped me move from cold cereal to more venturous cuisine. I had a lot more trouble accepting help from TLS personnel; no doubt I owe several people an apology for my "less than enthusiastic" participation. I'm glad to see I didn't cause Gerard to find another line of work.

I knew Jean Hetherington from past HI support group meetings as a fellow "survivor" who was quite active with advocacy in Kansas. Jean also had a long-standing connection with Janet Williams of communityworks, inc. and began working with me in 2003. Jean had "been there, done that" for quite some time and was living proof that life can go on. She began by showing me volunteer activities I might enjoy in the library and the annual Science Fair.

Trying out different things that required nothing from me but my physical presence was how I discovered new interests and interacted with people who weren't being paid to talk to me. I was introduced as Jean's friend and could sit like a lump for as long as necessary. When I was ready for more participation, the opportunities were waiting and Jean worked right alongside me until I was ready to branch out on my own. I learned it was not only okay to get lost in the building, but also that the world would not end if I had to ask directions three hundred times. I learned to acknowledge and generally accept limitations; bypassing some with those good old compensatory strategies and finding humor in others.

While every injury is unique, I believe most will agree that stress produces a hasty retreat of cognitive abilities. In my own case, some memories can be retrieved with the right stimulus, but others just don't exist for me any more (which one doesn't know about until they're mentioned). On the other hand, some "truths" persist in my mind only, such as the conviction that my hairdresser's husband is a firefighter, regardless of her good-natured denial. Since it's her life, I guess I'll have to accept her version of the man's existence.

I "graduated" from the waiver late last year. One of my goals was always to find part-time employment and communityworks, inc. offered me just that. As a client, I had become familiar with services, policies, and procedures, so the job hasn't had the steep learning curve that was so disastrous in earlier attempts. It still takes more time to do things, but I don't have any strict deadlines to meet and I can keep my schedule manageable. Detailed planning has to precede action, but that just makes the infamous paperwork easier. I will always have to pay close attention to the signals I now recognize as warnings of overload.

Working with others finding themselves in survivor mode feels right and I'm thoroughly enjoying myself. I like putting these lessons learned the hard way to practical use. Whether it helps or not, when I say to another survivor "I know how you feel", it's most likely true. I feel fortunate to have come through all this with enough brain cells intact to help other survivors find fulfillment in their new lives.

After all, I had some great teachers and a very special role model.

Lost Inside My Head By: John Hoyt

What a difference a few seconds can make. I fell two and a half stories off my roof and hit the crown of my head on a six foot 4x4 wooden post and then landed on a steel "T" post just under my right jaw which broke the jaw, two teeth, fractured the voice box and three vertebrae in my neck and stopped just a micro millimeter short of cutting the secondary vein to my brain, but I still threw a blood clot which caused a mini stroke.

That was October 31, 2000. Now I am 100% disabled with a TBI. The strange thing was that after the fall my family knew that something was wrong but the doc's and everyone else were focusing on the facial and vertebrae damage and not on the brain itself. Consequently it took five years before I started to get some help and only after finding communityworks, inc. by default. The saddest part of all this is that I lost my thirty year marriage and strained or damaged all the relationships and foundations of my life taking all the blame for being lost in my head, never knowing it was a brain injury which was at the core of my problems.

Now is a better world and life than then. Healing is a better direction than lost. Future is a direction I can live with instead of dreading; a peaceful mind and life is a reality I can live with instead of the mental and behavioral chaos that I endured for too many years.

What the support system which I now have in place has provided is first and foremost is confirmation that I can find and achieve the right direction. In short, as I battle the day to day frustrations and setbacks, it is the positive guidance I receive which quite frankly, on my worst days, keeps me going. As I move towards achieving the goals which I have set for myself—some lofty, some mundane, it is this support system which helps me maintain the balance and yes, minimizes the discouragement.

Am I still lost inside my head? At times. The short term memory loss is still the most frustrating, but I am grateful that the long term memory is sharper than ever. Simply put. There's hope after TBI.

Conclusion

Almost 20 years after its commencement, **communityworks, inc.** has emerged as a nationally recognized service provider for individuals living with brain injuries. Its unique focus on social capital and innovative participation strategies has made it a best practice program in community integration. The overarching goal of the agency "to assist individuals to live, work, and play in the community" is achieved through a holistic, individualized approach. The services at communityworks are guided by a series of philosophical principles informed by Williams' research and work experiences. Communityworks, inc. has been well-received by consumers and their families, funding agencies, and the media. Further, annual cost analyses have strongly indicated that the costs of providing services in the home and community are far less than the cost of care provided in TBI institutional facilities. Ultimately, the success of communityworks, inc. highlights the benefits of providing services to individuals with brain injuries using a consumer driven model that promotes community participation.

REFERENCES

Bailey, L. *Giving Back.* Retrieved August 5, 2010 from communityworks, inc. website: www.communityworksinc.com

Hoyt, J. *Lost Inside My Head.* Retrieved August 5, 2010 from communityworks, inc. website:www.communityworksinc.com

Racino, J. A. & Williams, J. M. (1994). **Living in the Community: An Examination of Philosophical and Practical Aspects**. *Journal of Head Trauma Rehabilitation, 9,* 35-48.

State of Kansas Department of Social and Rehabilitation Services. (September 2004). *HCBSMedicaid Waiver for Individuals who have sustained a Traumatic Brain Injury: Policy and Procedure Manual.* Retrieved July 20, 2010 from **http://www.kmap-state-ks.us**

Thorne, D. *The Art of Self Direction.* Retrieved August 5, 2010 from communityworks, inc. website: www.communityworksinc.com

Williams, J. M. (2008). **Building Social Capital: The communityworks, inc. experience.** *Journal of Vocational Rehabilitation, 29,* 157-163.

CHAPTER 3

BRAIN INJURY CLUBHOUSE, CORNERSTONE AND SIDE BY SIDE BRAIN INJURY CLUBHOUSE

By Tanya Morton

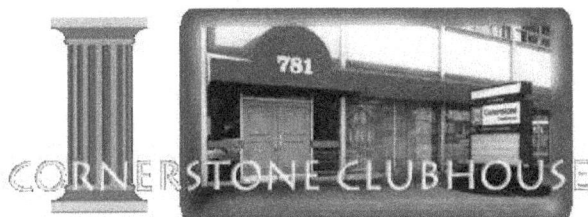

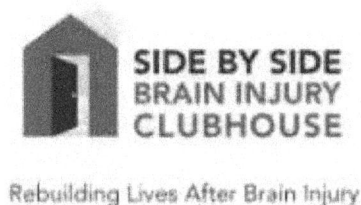

"Life with brain injury rarely makes the news, yet it does continue and we are both changed and grateful for this second chance at life."

Cindi Johnson,
Executive Director, Side by Side Brain Injury
Clubhouse

We would like to dedicate this Best Practices Case Study to Mary Catherine Ann, Executive Director of Cornerstone Clubhouse, who passed away in July 2010 after a long illness. As a key informant for this Case Study, Mary helped tell the story of the program in order to inspire and guide others. As a mentor and worker, her dedication, optimism and courage towards improving the lives of those with ABIs have been an inspiration to us.

Casebook of Exemplary Evidence-Informed Programs that Foster Community Participation After Acquired Brain Injury
Copyright © 2013 by Information Age Publishing

Population Served: Adults	
Contributing Author Contact Information	
Harvey Jacobs Licensed Clinical Psychologist / Behavior Analyst 401-7400 Beaufont Springs Drive, Richmond, VA 23225 Tel: (804) 323-5560; Fax: (804) 323-5562; **harveyjacobs@harveyjacobs.net** Website: **www.harveyjacobs.net**	Deb Wilson-Macleod Facilitator Cornerstone Clubhouse 781 Richmond Street London, Ontario Canada N6A 3H4 **dwm@cornerstoneclubhouse.com** Tel: (519) 679-6809 Fax: (519) 679-6988
Brenda Campeau Executive Director Cornerstone Clubhouse 781 Richmond Street London, Ontario Canada N6A 3H4 **bcampeau@daleservices.on.ca** Tel: (519) 679-6809 Fax: (519) 679-6988	Jamie Fairles Member / Peer Support Coordinator Cornerstone Clubhouse 781 Richmond Street London, Ontario Canada N6A 3H4 **jdfairles@hotmail.com** Tel: (519) 679-6809 Fax: (519) 679-6988
Kevin MacGregor Member Cornerstone Clubhouse 781 Richmond Street London, Ontario Canada N6A 3H4 **kevinMacGregor@sympatico.ca** Tel:. (519) 858-5403 Fax: (519) 679-6988	Andrew Tankus Member Cornerstone Clubhouse 781 Richmond Street London, Ontario Canada N6A 3H4 **alst2010@sympatico.ca** Tel: (519) 679-6809 Fax: (519) 679-6988
Cindi Johnson Executive Director Side by Side Brain Injury Clubhouse 1001 Main Street Stone Mountain, CA 30083 **cindi@sidebysideclubhouse.org** Tel: (770) 469-9355 Fax: (770) 469-9385	Virginia Vaughn Resource Coordinator Side by Side Brian Injury Clubhouse 1001 Main Street Stone Mountain, CA, 30083 **virginia@sidebysideclubhouse.org** Tel: (770) 469-9355 Fax: (770) 469-9385

INTRODUCTION

The Clubhouse Model

Clubhouse models have been identified as a best practice. As a result, two Clubhouse programs are highlighted in this chapter. A Clubhouse represents a specific model for delivering community support to adults living with the effects of an Acquired Brain Injury (ABI; **Cornerstone, n. d.a**; **Jacobs, 1997**). End-users who

> The term "Clubhouse," highlights the message of membership and belonging

participate in the clubhouse community are called members rather than patients or clients, because the program is primarily a club with members having all associated access and decision-making ability (**Macias, Jackson, Schroeder, & Wang, 1999**). Members have responsibilities to their Clubhouse as well as rights; for example, they run their Clubhouse by participating in essential activities that keep it operating (**Macais, Schroeder, Jackson, & Wang, 1999**). As stated by Jacobs, a veteran and developer of the Clubhouse movement (**1997**), "the success or failure of a Clubhouse may depend on how well people work together" (p. 4). The belief that staff and members must work together in a non-hierarchical manner to achieve the members' individual and collective goals is integral to the Clubhouse model.

Community participation in a Clubhouse arises out of the need to serve the members' common cause, similar to what would happen in any other structured organization with an agenda (**Jacobs, 1997**; **Olico-Okui, 2004**; **Sander, Clark, & Pappadis, 2010**). The level and degree of community participation in a Clubhouse is high because it is a member-directed program operated by and for members. In fact, staff are known as "facilitators" at **Cornerstone Clubhouse** (one of the showcased agencies), to highlight the horizontal relationship between them and the members. Community participation has been at the heart of the Clubhouse model since its inception (Jacobs, personal communication, May 10, 2010; **Macias et al., 1999**).

> Within a Clubhouse, **Community Participation** is manifested as members taking responsibility for building their own capacity and that of their community; feeling accepted and regarded as useful contributors by a group of peers; and identifying, accessing and interacting with local resources as necessary to accomplish their goals.[1]

---

[1] See Jacobs, 1997; Olico-Okui, n.d; Sander, Clark, & Pappadis, 2010; Propst, 1987.

Marcias et al. (1999) state, "the basic service offered by every clubhouse is the clubhouse itself" (p. 186). The work of a Clubhouse denotes that in spite of the long-term changes that result from brain injury, people have something meaningful to contribute and must go on with their lives after rehabilitation has aspired to give them functional skills. As stated by Clubhouse member and Peer Support Coordinator Jamie Fairles, "rehab teaches you skills, but now you get to put the skills to use" (personal communication, June 14, 2010). Self-determination and choice are paramount because members access the clubhouse when and how they see fit (K. MacGregor, personal communication, July 9, 2010). Members are provided a safe, unconditional attachment and network of support at a time when other supports may be negatively altered or truncated due to the effects of ABI (Jacobs, personal communication, May 15, 2010; K. MacGregor, personal communication, July 9, 2010).

BACKGROUND

Description of Clubhouses

An efficient albeit introductory way to answer the question "What is a clubhouse?" is to display the ABI Clubhouse Standards. These standards have been developed and endorsed by the **International Brain Injury Clubhouse Alliance** (IBICA) and approved by Consensus at IBICA's 5th Annual Meeting on August 21, 2008. Each IBICA member Clubhouse agrees to follow these Standards. While there is not a system in place for IBICA to certify or accredit Clubhouses, seven ABI Clubhouses in the U.S. are accredited by **CARF**. Cornerstone Clubhouse in London, Ontario, is an exception, being certified by the **International Center for Clubhouse Development** (ICCD). The ICCD Standards, which have been successfully utilized by Clubhouses for people with mental illness, serve as a springboard for the IBICA standards. In addition to serving a quality control role, Standards serve as a "bill of rights" for members and code of ethics for staff and board (**Cornerstone, n.d.a.**). The ABI Clubhouse Standards are summarized as key substantive areas below in Box 1.

Box 1: Key Substantive Areas of the International Standards for Clubhouse Programs IBICA

Memberships, Relationships, and Space: Stresses the non-hierarchical nature of staffs' and members' involvement in all operations and physical spaces of the clubhouse.

The Work-ordered Day: Engages staff and members in the running of the clubhouse through mandating work units, the nature of activities undertaken, and the daily working hours.

Employment and Education: Facilitates employment and educational goals through real-world opportunities, experience, and feedback, as opposed to protected or artificial settings.

Functions of the House: Includes program evaluation, recreation, and social activities as essential components of clubhouse activities.

Funding, Governance, and Administration: Stipulates budgetary and advisory policies and procedures and other venues to engage stakeholders.

History of Clubhouses

The Early Years

The roots of the Clubhouse model go back to the 1930s. **Alcoholics Anonymous** was gaining momentum at that time. The model of alcoholics supporting each other provided some rudimentary impetus for the clubhouse model. The development of the Clubhouse was truly underway with the founding of **Fountain House** in New York in 1948 (**Macais, Jackson, Schroder, & Wang, 1999**). During this time, people with mental illnesses started a We are Not Alone (WANA) group with meetings. Family members became involved and subsequently bought a dilapidated brownstone in Manhattan with a fountain in the foyer—hence the name Fountain House. Members started meeting there and getting support from each other, and realized that jobs and roles naturally developed. For example, someone needed to clean up, prepare food, answer the telephone, and perform other sundry activities in order to keep the house operational (H. Jacobs, personal communication, August 25, 2009).

Expansion

The participatory model of the Clubhouse was facilitated in the 1970s when a multi-year dissemination grant was obtained to train community-based organizations in the Clubhouse model (**Fountain House, n.d**; **Propst, 1987**). Clubhouses began opening all over the United States. However, neophyte clubhouses realized that in spite of the success of the Clubhouse training program, they required more concrete ways to assess the strengths of their outcomes and core program characteristics. This realization invoked further training and consultative channels with established and/or exemplary clubhouses (**ICCD, 2009a**). Evidence began to accumulate that there were distinct fidelity features[2] consistently adhered to by the formalized clubhouses, while informal Clubhouses also

---

[2] For the purposes of this paper, fidelity is a gauge of how well the program is being implemented in comparison with the original program design and validation (i.e., is the program being delivered as intended with all prescribed program components and processes; see **Mihalic, 2002**).

had identifiable program elements and characteristics (**ICCD, 2009a**). By 1987, R. Propst, the director of Training of **Fountain House**, wrote "we were creating Clubhouse communities with enough internal consistency to warrant codification into standards of practice" (ICCD, 2009a). Hence, a stakeholder group known as the **Faculty for Clubhouse Development** spearheaded the **Standards for Clubhouse Programs**. The Standards were ratified in 1989 through a consensus-based consultative process involving the whole Clubhouse community (ICCD, 2009a; **Propst, 1987**). Next, the **ICCD** began in 1994 as a means of quality control (ICCD, 2009a). Specifically, the **ICCD** was "created to provide training in the model, consultation in program development, and certification that a clubhouse is operating in compliance with the Standards for Clubhouse Programs" (**Macias et al., 1999**). Recent research indicates that Clubhouse certification is a valid indicator of program quality (**Macias et al., 2001**).

Facilitated by consumer/family advocacy, low operational costs, and consequent governmental endorsement (**Macias et al., 1999**), Clubhouse programs grew worldwide and are now over 300 strong (C. Johnson, personal communication, April 24, 2009). In comparison with alternative services, there is evidence of reduced costs (Clark et al., 1998; **Mackay, Yates, & Johnsen, 2007**), hospitalization (**Di Masso, Avi-Itzak & Obler, 2001**), incarceration (**Johnson & Hickey, 1999**), increased workforce participation (**Macias, Kinney, & Rodican, 1995**) and social support (**Warner, Huxley, & Berg, 1999**) among Clubhouse members. In sum, Clubhouses changed over the years from grassroots phenomena to best practices programs (Macias et al., 1999).

Adaptation to the ABI Population

About 25 years ago the Clubhouse model began to be adapted to people with brain injuries, with the realization that many of the issues experienced by people with brain injuries are similar to those experienced by people with mental health issues (C. Johnson, personal communication, April 24, 2009; **ICCD/Cornerstone, 2008**, p. 2).[3] In 2004 a group of five ABI Clubhouses, including **SxS** and **Cornerstone**, convened and discussed how they could assist each other with the development of ABI Clubhouses (C. Johnson, personal communication, April 24, 2009; **IBICA, 2010**). Consequently, they laid the groundwork for the formation of the **International Brain Injury Clubhouse Alliance** (IBICA), which was mounted in 2005. (IBICA, 2010). In 2008 IBICA created 33 standards that define what an ABI clubhouse is, with assistance from **ICCD**. Although

---

[3] Although brain injury clubhouses such as SxS and Cornerstone are designed to serve those with ABIs, there can be overlap between mental illness and ABI. For example, amongst the ABI clubhouses listed in the ICCD directory, ~ 50% of their members have mental illness as a secondary diagnosis (ICCD/Cornerstone, 2008, p. 7). However, there are some differences in the characteristics of individuals living with mental illness in comparison with ABI; for example, individuals with ABI may be more consistent in terms of their need for services than individuals with mental health issues (M. Ann, personal communication, June 14, 2010).

IBICA standards have been modeled on the ICCD standards, they were slightly modified with the consent of the ICCD to reflect the differences between mental illness and brain injury (IBICA, 2010). However, by and large the Clubhouse model is "impairment neutral" (H. Jacobs, personal communication, May 12, 2010).

At present, there are 17 ABI member clubhouses who belong to **IBICA (IBICA, 2010)**. Most of the IBICA Clubhouses are located in the US; however, ICCD clubhouses exist all over the world in various communities, with regional variation. The adaptation of the Clubhouse model to different cultures and countries suggests that it is sustainable. The Clubhouses showcased in this paper have been deemed leaders nationally and internationally (**Dale Brain Injury Services, 2006, p. 8;** C. Johnson, personal communication, April 24, 2009), have served as mentors and educators to other Clubhouses (C. Johnson, personal communication, April 24, 2009; Cornerstone, n.d.; Dale Brain Injury Services, 2006; p. 8; M. Ann, personal communication, Jun 14, 2010), and have assisted with policy development and education of the public and professionals (C. Johnson, personal communication, April 24, 2009; **ICCD/Cornerstone, 2008**; Cornerstone, n.d.; K. MacGregor, personal communication, July 9, 2010). These achievements buttress the best practice status of the two showcased clubhouses. The circumstances associated with their best practice status are discussed below.

Cornerstone Clubhouse and Side by Side (SxS) Brain Injury Clubhouse

Side by Side and **Cornerstone** are showcased as best practices programs representing the Clubhouse model with a "two for the price of one" approach. These two exemplary clubhouses are among the first Brain Injury Clubhouses to be fielded and two of the most validated clubhouses in the world. They have forged numerous community partnerships. **SxS** has maintained partnerships with agencies such as the **International Brain Injury Clubhouse Alliance**, The Brain and Spinal Injury Task Force, **Restore Neurobehavioral Center**, the **Shepherd Center**, and **Emory University, Georgia State University, Agnes Scott College, University of Georgia** and **Clark Atlanta University**. Also, a resource coordinator provides supervision to rehabilitation counselling and social work practicum students (C. Johnson, personal communication, August 4, 2009). Cornerstone is the only certified ABI Clubhouse in Canada and maintains relationships with PIE (**Partners in Employment**), a community support group for non-profit organizations in the area of employment, and is part of "Survivors Offering Support," with other local agencies to assist with community supports for Members. Cornerstone also belongs to the local Chamber of Commerce, the local Acquired Brain Injury Association, the Acquired Brain Injury Network, the **London Accessibility Advisory Committee** (L.A.A.C.), the

International Alliance of Acquired Brain Injury Clubhouses, and takes on practicum students (**ICCD/Cornerstone, 2008**).

Although both of these programs adhere to the Clubhouse model, there are differences between them that demonstrate that Clubhouses are the product of communities. The sustainability of these two Clubhouses in their respective settings serves as evidence of the flexibility and adaptability of the Clubhouse model, which can be maintained among different countries, geographical settings, and cultural backgrounds. Key points, similarities and differences of these two exemplary programs are highlighted in Table 1.

Table 1: *Cornerstone and Side by Side Clubhouses: Key points, similarities, and differences*

Cornerstone	Side by Side
Inception: Mounted in late 1990s.	**Inception**: Mounted in late 1990s
Certification: The first and only Acquired Brain Injury Clubhouse to be certified through the ICCD in New York. Has recently received a new three-year certification. Also a member of Accreditation Canada (this used to be called CCHSA,[4] which is the Canadian Equivalent of CARF). Member of IBICA.	**Certification**: Member of the ICCD but not certified by the ICCD. Accredited through CARF.[5] Member of IBICA.
Auspices: Offered under the auspices of Dale Brain Injury Services; hence, has an arms-length parent agency.	**Auspices**: Shepherd Center and Emory Healthcare, two rehabilitation hospitals, agreed to sponsor the start-up of S x S in July 1999. The two hospitals oversaw the Clubhouse for the first two years; since then, SxS has been a free-standing not-for-profit agency. However, staff is still "leased" to SxS by one of the hospitals.
Location: In the heart of London, On., on five bus routes and the Para-Transit route.	**Location:** In an Atlanta suburb (Stone Mountain) that dictates a range of transport options (i.e., bus, family drivers or paid transport providers) and long travel times for some members. About ½ the members come from Dekalb County and 12 other metro Atlanta communities are home to the others.

[4] The Canadian Council on Health Services Accreditation
[5] Commission on Accreditation of Rehabilitation Facilities. SxS is one of seven Brain Injury Clubhouses in the USA accredited by CARF.

Diversity: The ethnic background of facilitators and members is fairly homogenous (reflective of the city). Diversity, when it has arisen, has not been problematic.	**Diversity:** Fourteen different ethnic backgrounds served, Spanish-speaking interpreters and a diverse staff are hired. Different cultures are celebrated in all their forms.
Members: Current active membership of ~79. Served 190 members since opening. ~28 members served per day. Staff of 7 including the director. Members generally aged over 40.	**Numbers:** Current active membership of ~128. Continued contact in some way with ~250 of the ~300 members served since opening. ~25 members served per day. Staff of 10 including the director. Many members over age 40, with modal age of members 40-44 years.

Sources: ICCD/Cornerstone 2008; C. Johnson, personal communication, April 24, 2009; C. Johnson, personal communication, Jun 1, 2010; SxS, 2010a, M. Ann, personal communication, Jun 14, 2010)

RESOURCES

Fiscal Operations

Cornerstone and **SxS** differ in their fiscal operations, largely because of differences between American and Canadian health care delivery. Depending on the funding context, some Clubhouses charge members a fee and some do not. In any event, many individuals who have experienced ABI find their financial resources are drained and their ability to be employed is hampered. Therefore, Clubhouses make efforts to charge little or nothing for their services. A stable funding model facilitates Clubhouse development because the staff and members do not have to allocate many resources towards soliciting funds and can concentrate on the actual Clubhouse programming and operation. Cornerstone is considered lucky by other Clubhouses due to its stable government funding (C. Johnson, personal communication, August 25, 2009). Since the inception of Cornerstone, it has maintained support from the **Ministry of Health** through its auspice agency **Dale Brain Injury services**. However, Cornerstone possesses its own ecology and identity, with the auspice agency being located over 10 km away. Cornerstone is located in a freestanding 3600 square foot facility, which is not rented out to any outside agencies. The Club has a good relationship with the building's owner. The Cornerstone community is pondering the benefits and drawbacks of keeping their space in anticipation of their lease expiring in 2 years (**ICCD/Cornerstone, 2008**). Overall, favourable external socioeconomic and political factors have translated into a consistent level of funding and reliable capacity of human resources for Cornerstone (see **Bourgeois & Noce, 2006, p. 17**).

The financial model of **SxS** is different from **Cornerstone** due to the US context, and SxS is successful in this milieu. Given the recent economic downturn, SxS has been actively soliciting funds to supplement food services and programming (C. Johnson, personal communication, April 24, 2009; January 28, 2009). SxS's director Cindi Johnson explains that in her economic environment she must run a business as well as a social service agency (personal communication, August 25, 2009). SxS is financially viable, being located in a newly renovated freestanding facility that it has owned for about three years, and carries no debt. The facility possesses a new large industrial kitchen that can accommodate twice as many workers as the previous residential-style kitchen. SxS follows best practices for businesses such as having a strategic plan (C. Johnson, Personal communication, June 2, 2010). The board of SxS has planned a conservative approach and is delaying expansion of the program until the economy improves (C. Johnson, personal communication, May 1, 2009). However, there is a demonstrated need for additional SxS programming in Metro Atlanta; for example, SxS is the only Clubhouse resource for people who are no longer in rehabilitation within several hours drive (C. Johnson, personal communication, June 2, 2009).

According to **Bourgeois and Noce (2006)**, adequate and stable resources, including support from a range of community leaders and a strong funding base, increase a program's chances of success. The sustainability of both SxS and Cornerstone and their adherence[6] to similar practice standards, regardless of their differing locales, suggests that the funding models of SxS and Cornerstone fit their respective economic and political contexts. Nuances of the funding models of Cornerstone and SxS are shown in Table 2.

Table 2: *Nuances of Funding models, Cornerstone and SxS*

Cornerstone	Side by Side
• Ontario's Ministry of Health, Long-term Division, funds the Clubhouse through the auspice agency (Dale Brain Injury Services). Members who qualify are funded for life-long membership. • However, if individuals have	• Diverse funding stream. • Offers a sliding scale fee to members. • Charges a per-day fee to cover the cost of providing services • Funds are solicited from local businesses and local governments. • Raises funds to cover between 1/4 and 1/3 expenses from the public.

---

[6] For the purposes of this paper, adherence refers to whether the program service or intervention is being delivered as it was designed and validated, i.e., with all core components and processes implemented (see Mihalic, 2002).

access to insurance money following their injury, Cornerstone must charge a fee for service on a daily basis. • Cornerstone consumes 8.5% of the annual budget of its auspice agency, Dale Brain Injury Services.	• Donations subsidize members who lack external payer sources. • A waiting list is kept of individuals in need who may be subsidized by charitable funds. • Third party payers such as Worker's Compensation or the Independent Care Waiver Program of Medicaid may sponsor qualifying members. • Members may apply to the Brain and Spinal Injury Trust Fund for scholarships to help pay for their membership. • 88% of SxS's expenses are used towards programming. • Staff are "leased" to SxS by one of the founding partners so that staff can have better benefits than what a small employer could offer.

Source: SxS, 2010a, C. Johnson, personal communication, April 24, 2009, August 25, 2009; ICCD/Cornerstone, 2008; D. Wilson-Macleod, personal communication, June 14, 2010

Human Resources

The Clubhouse is about supporting and engaging members through life; hence, there is potentially an abundance of human talent available. Membership in a Clubhouse is life-long and there are not problems accommodating members who return after long absences. Clubhouses can always use additional human resources to accomplish the work. Staff play generalist roles by participating in the various tasks needed to help with the smooth operation of the club. Staff numbers are kept minimal; therefore, staff liaise with and rely on members (**Johnson, 1997**; **ICCD/Cornerstone, 2008**). In sum, the members are the organization's greatest resource.

In addition to the membership, both **Cornerstone** and **SxS** engage volunteers. Cornerstone's volunteers are usually relatives of its members (K. MacGregor, personal communication, July 9, 2010), while SxS actively recruits and engages volunteers for a variety of purposes, such as maintenance facilitator, social activity coordinator, cook, or office helper (**SxS, 2010a**). Similar to the situation with financial resources, as discussed in the Fiscal Resources section, the difference in volunteer characteristics between the two agencies is related to what works in their respective contexts. However, among both agencies, the engagement of volunteers helps the agencies to bridge with the wider community and achieve the Clubhouse objectives as articulated by the Standards.

IMPLEMENTATION

The Domains of the Work-Ordered Day

Clubhouse programs address the personal, social, vocational, and societal challenges faced by its members through a supportive social community. A Clubhouse's spheres of influence generally encompass four main areas: the Work-Ordered Day, Employment, Education, and Evening/Weekend activities. The work-ordered day parallels normal Monday to Friday working hours, indicating that a large amount of work is required from members to sustain their Clubhouse (**Jacobs, 1997**). Hence, it is practical to divide work into discrete units. **SxS** and **Cornerstone** both possess a Kitchen/Culinary Unit, a Clerical/Business Unit, and a Maintenance Unit. Clubhouses are community-based programs and do not have therapists or traditional rehabilitation on-site. However, referrals can be made to such services, and individualized support services such as independent living skills, life skills training, or vocational counselling may be offered in some Clubhouses through their cooperative work environments (e.g., SxS). Member activities promote inner growth such as developing a sense of self-worth and purpose, and more tangible abilities such as interpersonal, cognitive, and work skills through clerical, maintenance, culinary, advocacy, education, and job preparatory tasks (C. Johnson, personal communication, April 24, 2009).

Membership

Membership criteria for a Clubhouse are minimal, with voluntary attendance. All adults (18+) with a history of ABI are eligible, unless they represent a significant threat that would disrupt the Clubhouse community. The ability to independently access the Clubhouse is important, although assistance arranging transportation is provided if necessary. Referrals for **SxS** and **Cornerstone** come from rehab agencies, family physicians, case managers, advertising, and word of mouth (**ICCD/Cornerstone, 2008**). Although there are slight differences between the intake processes of the two showcased Clubhouses, in essence, potential members of both clubhouses receive tours, complete applications, and are assessed and assess themselves as being suitable for the program (**ICCD/Cornerstone, 2008**; V. Vaughn, personal communication, July 2, 2009). The Clubhouse is a self-selecting organization, and those who do not feel a Clubhouse is an appropriate fit can seek other services. There are some individuals who may need more support than what a clubhouse can provide (i.e., a therapist; H. Jacobs, personal communication, May 5, 2010). Applicants are very rarely turned down, although **SxS** has had to limit intakes due to funding constraints at times (C. Johnson, personal communication, June 2, 2010).

Departures from the Model

Overall, **SxS** has had to slightly depart from the original Clubhouse model, as outlined in the **Standards**, more than **Cornerstone**. Although the characteristics of individuals with brain injury vary widely, SxS in particular has a membership with a particularly diverse range of abilities and needs. Therefore, SxS has to have more individualized and tailored programming than the original Clubhouse model envisioned at times. For example, SxS offers follow-up services in the form of individualized assistance (C. Johnson, personal communication, May 1, 2009). SxS also has experienced more safety issues; hence, Executive Director Cindi Johnson has occasionally had to make an independent decision in order to promote the safety of the membership (e.g., call someone to accompany a member home if it appears unsafe for the person to leave alone; personal communication, June 2, 2010). As outlined in the **Clubhouse Standards**, the Executive Directors of both organizations do have veto power if a serious problem requires immediate action and decision-making; fortunately, in true community style they have very rarely had to exercise this power (M. Ann, personal communication, June 14, 2010; C. Johnson, personal communication, June 2, 2010).

If somebody's privacy could be violated in a given situation, both **Cornerstone** and **SxS** have had to depart from the principle that members are involved in every aspect of decision-making. If a confidential issue needs to be discussed, it is respectful that the discussion goes "in camera" (**ICCD/Cornerstone, 2008**; C. Johnson, personal communication, June 2, 2010). In addition, recent changes to confidentiality legislation in Cornerstone's jurisdiction has denoted that members can no longer be involved with agency statistics that represent valuable process evaluation data. Now, facilitators must amass the agency statistics (D. Wilson-McLeod, personal communication, June 14, 2010). Hence, the **Clubhouse Standard** on the inclusion of members in performing research is slightly compromised.

Departures from the model, as outlined in the **Clubhouse Standards**, segue into a discussion of the delicacy and implementation fidelity of the model. According to **Arthur and Blitz (2000)**, pprograms must be implemented with fidelity to the original model to uphold the change mechanisms that produced the original models' effective results. When program participants are embedded in naturalistic settings rather than extracted from their environment in a tightly controlled lab, there is the possibility that program delivery could change over time and inconsistencies between core programmatic components and actual program delivery become apparent (**Jones & Offord, 1991**; **Mihalic, 2002**). For example, some Clubhouse agencies may become increasingly bureaucratic, which could negatively detract from the original model (H. Jacobs, personal communication, August 10, 2009). However, departures from adherence are sometimes necessary in the real world of community-based, voluntary, member-directed programming. In fact, perfect fidelity is practically impossible in a complex and dynamic real-world setting (**Skolits & Richards, 2010**). The evidence suggests that if there is a rationale, such as a practical or clinical reason, to depart from the model and adapt to the nuances of a particular context or situation, some program elements can be modified without compromising the quality of implementation or outcome (**Stern, Alaggia, Watson, & Morton, 2008**).

Relationship of Accreditation to Fidelity Features

Interestingly, when both Executive Directors of the two showcased Clubhouses were asked by the interviewing author about implementation fidelity in an open-ended format, they both cited the Standards and Certification as buttressing and maintaining their programs' core elements. Standards appear to promote accountability, alert the stakeholders to ongoing fidelity issues, and act as a cue for adherence to the original model (see **Stern et al., 2007**). As previously delineated in this paper, the agencies listed in Table 2 provide guidance and consultation in the model and practices of Clubhouses, and accreditation or certification that a Clubhouse is operating in compliance with standards (**Macias et al., 1999**; **IBICA, 2010**). For example, SxS follows a best practices model that is outlined in **CARF** standards for employment in community services, in addition to the more wide-ranging **IBICA standards** (C. Johnson, personal communication, June 2, 2010). The findings of the present paper is consistent with previous findings that suggest that adherence to core programmatic components is associated with strong supervision and monitoring procedures (Schoenwald et al., 2000; Webster-Stratton, 2004) and stakeholders believing in and buying in to the program (Stern et al., 2008).

Implementation Strategies

A look at key implementation strategies, namely, the operationalization of the program, illustrates the activities that occur in the Clubhouse. There is a caveat in regards to the following discussion of implementation strategies: Due to space constraints not all ~35 Clubhouse Standards can be addressed. Therefore, this section cannot profess to discuss the complete operationalization of the program. However, the following non-exhaustive presentation of implementation strategies inform how the program is actually practiced in key areas. Lessons learned and checks on program processes are embedded in the selected strategies. These strategies were designed with a rationale, which can be seen in Table 3.

Table 3 : *Key Implementation Strategies for SxS and Cornerstone: Description and Rationale*

Strategy	Rationale
Long-term participation.	• People need an attachment and a network of support after ABI: A community to count on where return is always possible, even if leaving for a while to pursue other interests or after getting in an argument with someone. • A developmental approach analogous to the unconditional support young people need when trying something new.
All work done in the Clubhouse is for the benefit of the Clubhouse. No outside work or artificial jobs/reward systems are acceptable in the Clubhouse.	• An early Clubhouse failure in the mid-1990s indicated to program developers that the model works when all work done in the Clubhouse is for the benefit of the Clubhouse. • The implicit goal is that the Clubhouse exists to support the members and the members use it voluntarily for the purposes they identify. • Work in the Clubhouse is intended to help members regain self-worth and purpose rather than be job-specific training.
Work is broken down into small manageable pieces to help members reach ultimate goals.	• Members work with a staff member to develop a short-and long-term plan to meet self-defined goals. • The breakdown of goals allows members to have clear benchmarks and cumulatively increase their skill levels.
Transitional Employment (TE) placements are supported and temporary.	• TE enables members to try various job placements, build skills and gain experience. • The employment relationship is between the Clubhouse and the employer, rather than employer and employee. • A high level of support provided to members on placement (e.g., the Clubhouse is responsible for providing work coverage if a member does not attend work). • TE to be available to as many different members as possible, hence their temporary nature. • For TE opportunities to be effective, they must belong to the Clubhouse community as a whole, rather than particular members. • Volunteer work augments paid opportunities and is also valued because it helps people build relationships and employability skills.

Sources: Cornerstone Clubhouse, 2010; K. MacGregor, personal communication, July 9, 2010; C. Johnson, personal communication, June 2, 2010

Feedback

Feedback is structured and given to management, regulatory bodies, and front line staff in on several levels. The guiding principle of fidelity to the Standards is upheld by the application of specific feedback guidelines that are systemically transferred among each level of the Clubhouse Community. As seen below, there are several channels for the Clubhouse community to raise their views and impact change:

➤ Regular house meetings occur among members and staff, where they collectively make decisions pertaining to the Clubhouse (**SxS, 2010b**; K. MacGregor, personal communication, July 9, 2010).

➤ Clear conflict resolution policies exist at the two showcased Clubhouses which assist the community when communicating and resolving problems. (**Cornerstone handbook, n.d.a.**; C. Johnson, personal communication, June 2, 2010).

➤ ICCD and IBICA Standards are living documents that are reviewed every two years by the worldwide Clubhouse community and amended as deemed necessary (**ICCD, 2008**; **IBICA, 2010**).

➤ Members sit on various committees and other feedback forums, which provide venues to regularly address quality control issues in order to maintain accreditation/certification (**Cornerstone, n.d.a.**; **SxS, 2010b**).

➤ Members are regularly surveyed with regard to their satisfaction with the program. They also have annual opportunities to evaluate staff (**ICCD/Cornerstone, 2008**). Families and community also have opportunities to give feedback (**ICCD/Cornerstone, 2008**; **SxS, 2010c**).

Further exploration of member surveys and other means that are conducive to studying program outcomes are discussed in the following section on program outcomes.

OUTCOME

In the 1990s, research on the Clubhouse model was in its infancy; for example, only descriptive studies existed on the effectiveness of the Clubhouses overseen by the **ICCD** (**Macias et al., 1999**). More inferential studies were conducted over time, with the result that measures of Clubhouse performance became more demanding and thorough (**Macias et al., 2001**). This trend is expected to continue given the tendency towards Evidence-based Practice in this age of accountability. However, there are methodological and design challenges in the world of community-based evaluation, where researchers are more focused on external validity than internal validity, and randomized studies are often impossible (**Bourgeois & Noce, 2006, p. 17**; **Jones & Offord, 1991**). Note that some of the evaluative efforts of SxS and Cornerstone are vulnerable to the biases commonly affecting community-based evaluation, namely survey non-response (not all Clubhouse members or family members responded to the survey), and response bias (e.g., respondents want to make a good impression). The following discussion delineates the outcome evaluation efforts of **SxS** and **Cornerstone**.

SxS Outcomes

A strong evaluation capacity is evident by the partnering of **SxS** with individuals from universities, such as that with Debra Berens, Ph.D., at **Georgia State University**. Her doctoral dissertation focused on the vocational outcomes of adults with ABI who participate in the vocational services program, and potential demographic variables associated with the outcomes. Overall, results showed that 89% of the Clubhouse members who participated in the vocational services track of the program either became job ready or obtained a job or volunteer placement (**Berens, 2008**). Generally, males as a gender had a higher rate of positive vocational outcomes, consistent with the higher number of males in the study. Age at time of brain injury was also significant, suggesting the younger the age of the brain injury, the higher the rate of positive vocational outcomes (D. Berens, personal communication, Sept 11, 2010).

The objectives of SxS's programming are also tracked in the Action for Improvement Plan (2010), which helps the agency break down its goals at 6-month intervals and display its outcomes. At SxS, outcomes are attached to individual members meeting their goals; subsequently, these outcome data are aggregated. The non-profit performance management software **Efforts to Outcomes** has been customized to SxS's particular program and population, and helps members track their individual successes (C. Johnson, personal communication, August 4, 2009; August 4, 2010). Overall, the outcome measures indicate that SxS is successful in promoting community participation for its members. Detailed breakdowns of community participation outcomes for the period from January-June 2010 are presented in Table 4.

Table 4 : *Community Participation Outcomes, Side by Side Brain Injury Clubhouse*

Action	Status/Outcome
Community Integration Goal: Improve community integration and achievement of goals through expansion of Employment Program by developing relationships at job sites, exploring volunteer programs, and follow-up of employed members. Effectiveness Goal: 65% of those members with a goal of paid or unpaid work meet that goal.	Goal almost met: 61% of those members who have ever attended Side by Side with a goal of paid or unpaid work met their goal.[7]
Service Delivery Goal: Satisfy stakeholders' suggestions to increase social opportunities and resource identification. Evaluate stakeholders' satisfaction with increase in social opportunities via social outing survey.	12 families out of 50 responded to the survey • 86% of members represented enjoyed the outings they attended very much; • 58% of families would be willing to transport their family member and/or other members; • 73% could pay $20-$35 to help cover costs of the event, 27% could not afford to pay anything; • 58% of families are interested in events that include both members and families; • 50% of families are willing to help organize or host an event.
Outcome Effectiveness Goal: 75% of members will meet at least one goal each 90 days.	Goal met: Quarter 3= 92%; Quarter 4=96%.

Source: SxS, 2010c

Cornerstone Outcomes

Cornerstone tracks process and outcome evaluation data with in-house measures developed by the organization in order to evaluate performance. The organization connects the concepts measured by their open- and closed-ended questions with anticipated program benefits, such

---

[7] Parameters: Attended 30 or more days; Worked or volunteered outside of the Clubhouse; Includes group volunteer activities—this inclusion has encouraged members without a work goal to become involved in community volunteer activities.

as increased "educational and vocational productivity; development of an ongoing network of friends and recreational opportunities; and improved integration skills through regular use in community settings" (**Cornerstone, 2008, p.1**). A 2005 Life, Work, Love, Play Survey (**Cornerstone, n.d.b.**) measured quality of life before and after becoming a Clubhouse member (n=30). The results indicated:

➤ In terms of meaningful relationships, 23% of respondents were satisfied with them before coming to the Clubhouse, while 80% were satisfied after becoming members.

➤ Thirty percent of respondents were happy with work status prior to coming to the Clubhouse, while 80% were satisfied after becoming member.

➤ In terms of leisure/recreation, 31% of members were satisfied in this domain prior to coming to the Clubhouse, after membership, 78% were satisfied.

➤ Prior to coming to the Clubhouse, 30% of respondents were satisfied with their community independence, after membership, 80% were satisfied (Cornerstone, n.d.b).

The Member Satisfaction Survey is administered every 6 months and the Community Partner, Family Satisfaction, and Employment Placement Surveys and are administered annually. Note that due to space constraints the survey results presented in this document are non-exhaustive; however, they are representative of the responses as a whole. In Table 5 community participation outcomes in the form of the survey results are presented.

Table 5: *Community Participation Outcomes, Cornerstone Clubhouse*

Member Satisfaction Survey Items, July 2009, n=23	Response Yes	Response No
1. I now have meaningful relationships since coming to the Cornerstone Clubhouse	22	1
2. My leisure/recreational activities have improved since becoming a member at the Cornerstone Clubhouse	19	4
3. Clubhouse offers enough activities for me	20	3
4. I feel welcomed at Cornerstone Clubhouse	20	1
5. I receive the Support I need at Cornerstone Clubhouse	22	0
6. I am involved in planning my goals at the Clubhouse	19	3
7. Cornerstone Clubhouse is helping me to achieve my goals	16	7
Sample Qualitative answers to the question: "What do you like most about Cornerstone Clubhouse?"		
Friends (5 friend-related responses)		
"Feel good about working at Cornerstone and learning new things, going to events with Members and Saturday socials"		
"Very open atmosphere where things involving the Clubhouse are discussed openly"		
"The support from Members and my favourite staff"		

Sample Qualitative answers to the question: "Why do you come to Cornerstone Clubhouse?"
"To engage in meaningful activities and be with other folks with similar problems"
"I come to have companionship and help other members by tutoring"
"To get out of the house and have friends"
"I love to come help with lunch (now it's more for social reasons) and help with job search and going back to school"
Clubhouse Statistics May 2010 n = 79
10 Cornerstone members spent a total of 232.5 hours volunteering in 11 community agencies.
Cornerstone members participated in giving 2 tours, 3 information sessions, 12 hours external education, and serving 5 non-members.

Source: Cornerstone, 2009; Cornerstone 2010c

Employment Goals

Employment is an important goal for many Clubhouse members (K. MacGregor, personal communication, July 9, 2010). Through access to wages and social networks, employment opens doors to recreation and socialization activities that otherwise would not exist (**Jacobs, 1997**). The fact that members are encouraged to break down challenging long-term employment goals into smaller steps has implications for community participation. For example, the member who wants employment will be supported in this long-term goal by breaking down the requisite job skills into discrete practical tasks to master. These masteries are not only important for an employment goal, but also necessary to be able to manage other community commitments and independent daily living as well. Therefore, the importance of the overriding goal is maintained while working on smaller elements that have relevance to a number of other life domains (**Jacobs, 1997**). According to **Cohen et al. (2007),** striving to meet challenging goals and high expectations gives individuals the opportunity to be contributing citizens in their communities. The individual gains opportunities to be part of the life of the community through meeting the challenge of work or volunteer placements, working with others, and associated venues for ownership and active roles in the community.

Community Participation Goals

Many ABI researchers, practitioners, and rehabilitation consumers make community participation a prime goal of programming (e.g., **Doig, Fleming, & Tooth, 2001**; **McColl, 2005**). This goal is not surprising given that community participation efforts, such as citizens having productive activities to fill the time, taking responsibility for themselves and their community, and being accepted in social relationships, is what keeps us "safe, sane, and secure" (**Condeluci, n.d., p. 3**). Unfortunately, citizens who have experienced an ABI have been found to be more isolated from community than the average (**Sander, Clark, & Pappadis, 2010**; **Willer, Ottenbacher, & Coad, 1994**). Some features of the Clubhouse model that facilitate community participation are shown in Figure 2. As shown in Table 6, SxS and Cornerstone adhere to well-informed definitions of community participation (**Community Participation After Acquired Brain Injury, 2010**; **Condeluci, n.d.**) to help to address the challenges faced by individuals with ABI.

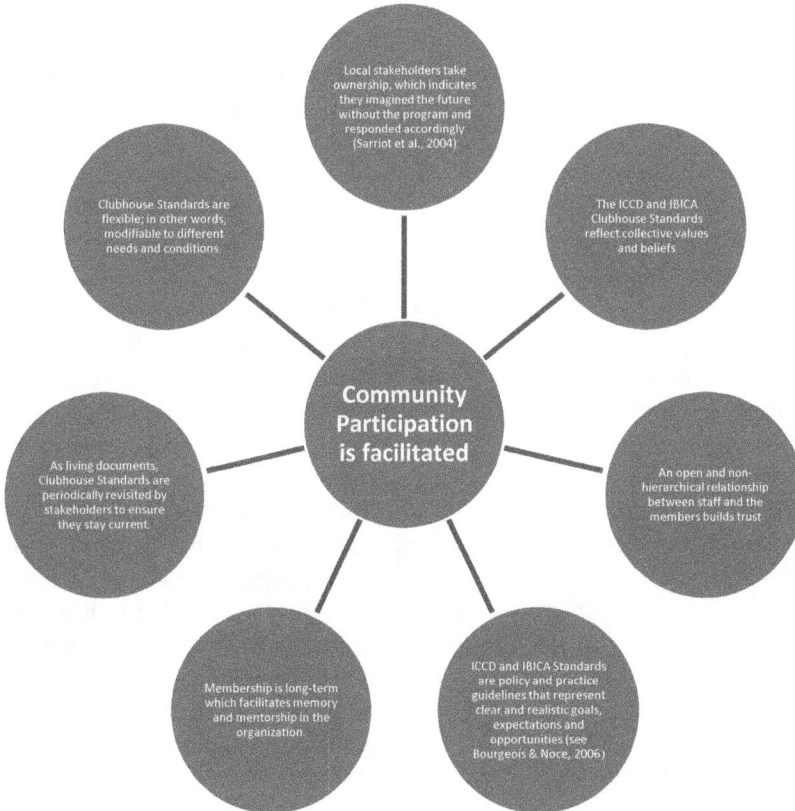

Figure 2: Facilitators of Community Participation

Table 6: *Definition and Examples of Community Participation, SxS and Cornerstone*

Definition of Community Participation	Program Example
Providing a sense of self, giving one a sense of acceptance from "the group" on a level playing field.	• All work in the Clubhouse is designed to help members regain self worth, purpose and confidence; • A consumer-driven model; • Members with special skills are encouraged to share them and/or teach them to others.
An environment where one can gently move beyond one's comfort zone with dignity	• The structure and processes of the program, including repetition and real-world/ immediate corrective feedback, assist members in socially acceptable behaviour.[8] • Mutual support dictates that when disruptive behaviours arise they are addressed in the social community context, not as an isolated clinical issue. • Clear conflict resolution policies with delineation of rights and procedures.
Participating in the ABI community with peers or the larger community.	• Age-appropriate activities such as social nights out; • Adult-oriented program; • Community members take ownership.
A network of people who regularly come together for some common cause or celebrations	• All work done in the Clubhouse is to further the interests of the Clubhouse; • Strong advocacy, education and outreach components[9].
Identifying, accessing and interacting with local resources as necessary to accomplish their goals.	• Paid work, volunteer work, and business is done in partnership with local resources; • Opportunities for members' families and volunteers to contribute while still respecting members' boundaries that the club is "their" space; • Partnered with associated organizations; • Programs designed with community readiness in mind (e.g., when developing TE placements).

Source: Condeluci, n.d.; Cornerstone Clubhouse, n.d.b,; Community Participation after ABI, 2010; SxS, 2010

[8] E.g, if a member does not bring in his or her used plate to the kitchen, a member in the kitchen unit will probably express displeasure. A member who does a considerate act for another member is warmly thanked. In sum, members are responsible for their own behaviours and therefore are subject to the consequences of their actions. Real-world consequences facilitate skill-building generalizable to different settings (for examples see Jacobs, 1997).
[9] For examples see Tankus (2010a), Tankus (2010b) and Ford (2010).

Conclusion

Similarities in essential program characteristics across the two showcased Clubhouses, despite having different member profiles, geographical locations, and socioeconomic contexts, indicate that the Clubhouse model has a "basic resilience" and applicability to diverse community settings (see **Marcais et al., 1999**). Indeed, the **National Institutes of Health** recommended in 1998 that all communities in the United States have brain injury Clubhouses (**Community Clubhouse for Brain Injury, 2010**). The paucity of IBICA-member brain injury Clubhouses in Canada suggests similar sentiments regarding expansion could be echoed in Canada. As medical advancements enable more individuals to survive traumatic injuries than in years past (**Koren, Hemel, & Klein, 2006**), the demand for Clubhouse services can only continue to grow. The challenges of adapting to an increasingly complex and sophisticated global society also suggest a need for flexible and resilient programs that encourage citizens to connect with each other and work collectively to fulfill their human potential.

REFERENCES

Arthur, M. W., & Blitz, C. (2000). **Bridging the gap between science and practice in drug abuse prevention through needs assessment and strategic community planning.** *Journal of Community Psychology 28*(3), 241-255.

Berens, D. E. (2008). Adults with acquired brain injury: an analysis of vocational outcomes from one acquired brain injury Clubhouse [Abstract]. Georgia State University, Atlanta, GA.

Bourgeois, R., & Noce, M. (2006). *Sustainability of community-based health interventions: A literature review.* Prepared for the Ontario Neurotrauma Foundation and Life Span Adaptations Projects, Institute for Child Study, Ontario Institute for Studies in Education.

Cohen, L., Chavez, V., & Chehimi, S. (2007). *Prevention is primary: Strategies for community well-being.* San Francisco: John Wiley.

Community Clubhouse for Brain Injury (2010). About us. Accessed July 30, 2010 from **http://www.commclubhouse.org/AboutUs/Default.aspx -** (http://braininjuryclubhouses.net/about.aspx)

Community Participation After Acquired Brain Injury (Spring 2010). **Neuromatters, Connecting You to the Research, 10, 1-2.** Ontario Neurotrauma Foundation.

Cornerstone Clubhouse (n.d.a). *Cornerstone Clubhouse member handbook*. London, On: Cornerstone Clubhouse.

Cornerstone Clubhouse (n.d.b). Cornerstone Clubhouse: The Clubhouse as a vehicle to recovery. London, ON: Author.

Cornerstone Clubhouse (n.d.c). *Accreditation and affiliation*. Accessed July 16, 2010, from **http://www.cornerstoneclubhouse.com**

Cornerstone Clubhouse (2010a). *Welcome to Cornerstone Clubhouse*. Accessed May 27, 2010 at **http://www.cornerstoneclubhouse.com**

Cornerstone Clubhouse (2010b). [Community volunteer statistics May 2010]. Unpublished raw data.

Cornerstone Clubhouse (2009). *Member satisfaction survey results – July 2009*. London, ON: Author.

Cornerstone Clubhouse (2008). *Who we are and what we do*. London, ON: Author.

Condeluci, A. (n.d.) *Community and cultural shifting*. Unpublished Manuscript, UCP of Pittsburgh.

Dale Brain Injury Services (2006). **2004-2005 Annual report**. London, ON: Author.

Doig, E., Fleming, J. & Tooth, L. (2001). Patterns of community integration 2-5 years post-discharge from brain injury rehabilitation. **Brain Injury,** *15*(9), 747-762.

Di Masso, J., Avi-Itzhak, T., & Obler, D. R. (2001). **The Clubhouse model: An outcome study on attendance, work attainment and status, and hospitalization recidivism**. *Work, 17,* 23-30.

Ford, F. (Speaker) (2010). Frank and Claudia Ford, Storycorps Atlanta [Radio show with archive available through the StoryCorps archive link http://www.pba.org/programming/programs/storycorps_atl/4477/]. Atlanta, GA: Storycorps/Public Broadcasting Atlanta.

Fountain House (n. d.). *Fountain House awarded multi-year grant, 1976*. Accessed Sept 12, 2010, from **http://www.fountainhouse.org/content/history-timeline**

International Brain Injury Clubhouse Alliance [IBICA] (2010). *History of International Brain Injury Clubhouse Alliance*. Accessed September 3, 2010 from **http://www.braininjuryclubhouses.net/history.aspx**

International Center for Clubhouse Development [ICCD] (2009a). *ICCD History*. Accessed September 14, 2010, from **http://www.iccd.org/history.html**

International Center for Clubhouse Development/Cornerstone Clubhouse. (2008). *Self-study certification protocol*. London, ON: Author.

Jacobs, H. E. (1997). **The Clubhouse: Addressing work-related behavioral challenges through a supportive social community**. *Journal of Head Trauma Rehabilitation*, 12(5), 14-27.

Johnson, J. & Hickey, S. (1999). Arrests and incarcerations after psychosocial program involvement: Clubhouse vs. Jailhouse. *Psychiatric Rehabilitation Journal, 23,* 66-70.

Jones, M. B., & Offord, D. R. (1991). *After the demonstration project.* Paper presented at the 1991 annual meeting of the Advancement of Science. Washington, D.C.

Koren, D., Hemel, D., & Klein, E. (2006). Injury increases the risk for PTSD: An examination of potential neurobiological and psychological mediators. *CNS spectrums, 11*(8), 616-624.

McKay, C., Yates, B., & Johnsen, M. (2007). Costs of Clubhouses: An International Perspective. *Administration and Policy in Mental Health and Mental Health Services Research, 34*(1), 62-72.

Macias, C., Barreira, P., Alden, M., & Boyd, J. (2001). **The ICCD Benchmarks for Clubhouses: A practical approach to quality improvement in psychiatric rehabilitation.** *Psychiatric Services 52*(2), 207-213.

Macias, C. Jackson, R., Schroeder C., & Wang, Q. (1999) What is a Clubhouse? Report on the ICCD 1996 Survey of USA Clubhouses. *Community Mental Health Journal, 35*(2), 181-190.

Macias, C., Kinney, R., and Rodican, C. (1995). Transitional Employment: An evaluative description of Fountain House practice. *Journal of Vocational Rehabilitation, 5,* 151-157.

Mihalic, S. (2002). *The importance of implementation fidelity.* Boulder, CO: Blueprints for Violence Prevention Initiative Center for the Study and Prevention of Violence.

Olico-Okui (2004). *Community participation: an abused concept?* Accessed June 12, 2010, from **http://hdl.handle.net/1807/6029**

Ontario Neurotrauma Foundation. (2010). Draft outcomes of ABI programs and services supportive of meaningful community participation. Development and Uses: ONF Community Practice in Community Participation Outcomes Framework.

Propst, R. N. (1987). Standards for Clubhouse Programs: Why and how they were developed. *Psychosocial Rehabilitation Journal*, 11(2), 25-30.

Sander, A. M., Clark, A., & Pappadis, M. R. (2010). **What Is Community integration anyway?: Defining meaning following traumatic brain injury.** *J Head Trauma Rehabil, 25*(2), 121-127.

Sarriot, E.G., Winch, P. J., Ryan, L. J., Bowie, J., Kouletio, M., Swedberg, E. et al. (2004). **A methodological approach and framework for sustainability assessment in NGO- implemented primary health care programs.** *Int J Health Plann Mgmt, 19,* 23-41.

Schoenwald, S. K., Henggeler, S. W., Brondino, M. J., & Rowland, M. D. (2000). **Multisystemic therapy: Monitoring treatment fidelity.** *Family Process, 39,* 83-103.

Side by Side Brain Injury Clubhouse. (2010a). **Welcome to Side by Side Brain Injury Clubhouse! Volunteer opportunities abound!** Accessed June 29, 2010 from **http://www.sidebysideclubhouse.org/GivingandVolunteering/Volunteering/tabid/66/Default.aspx**

Side by Side Brain Injury Clubhouse. (2010b). **Members: A typical day.** Accessed July 2, 2010 from **http://www.sidebysideclubhouse.org/Members/ATypicalDay/tabid/64/Default.aspx**

Side by Side Brain Injury Clubhouse. (2010c). *Action for improvement plan.* Stone Mountain, GA: Author.

Skolits, G. J., & Richards, J. (2010). **Designing and applying project fidelity assessment for a teacher implemented middle school instruction improvement pilot intervention.** *The Canadian Journal of Program Evaluation, 24*(1), 133-156.

Stern, S. B., Alaggia, R., Watson, K., & Morton, T. (2008). **Implementing an evidence-based parenting program with adherence in the real world of community practice.** *Research on Social Work Practice, 18*(6), 543-554.

Tankus, A. (2010a, June). *Editoral report.* Curbside Chronicles, 3-4.

Tankus, A. (2010b, September). *Editorial report.* Curbside Chronicles, 3-4. **http://www.braininjuryclubhouses.net/clubhouse.aspx).**

Volpe, R. (2004). *The conceptualization of injury prevention as change in complex systems.* Unpublished manuscript, University of Toronto, Toronto, ON.

Volpe, R. (2009). Proposal for a review of best practices in programs that foster community participation for survivors of Acquired Brain Injury. Unpublished document, University of Toronto, Toronto, ON.

Willer, B., Ottenbacher, K. J., & Coad, M. L. (1994). **The Community Integration Questionnaire: a comparative examination.** *Am J Phys Med Rehabil, 73*(2), 103-111.

Warner, R., Huxley, P., & Berg, T. (1999). **An Evaluation of the Impact of Clubhouse Membership on Quality of Life and Treatment Utilization.** *International Journal of Social Psychiatry 45*(4), 310-320.

Webster-Stratton, C. (2004). **Quality training, supervision, ongoing monitoring, and agency support: Key ingredients to implementing The Incredible Years programs with fidelity.** Accessed Sept 1, 2010 from www.incredibleyears.com/library

Ylvisaker, M., Hanks, R., & Johnson-Greene, D. (2002). **Perspectives on rehabilitation of individuals with cognitive impairment after brain injury: Rationale for reconsideration of theoretical paradigms.** *J Head Trauma Rehabil, 17*(3), 191-209.

CHAPTER 4

SKILLS TO ENABLE PEOPLE AND COMMUNITIES (STEPS) PROGRAM

By Kelsey Ragan

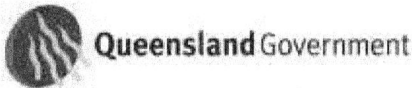

Queensland Government

SKILLS TO ENABLE PEOPLE & COMMUNITIES

Population Served : Young Adults to Older Adults (Age 18- 65)	
Contributing Author Contact Information:	
Areti Kennedy Program Manager Skills to Enable People and Communities Acquired Brain Injury Outreach Service PO Box 6053, Buranda 4102 61 7 3406 2311 STEPS@healh.qld.gov.au	Dr. Heidi Muenchberger Research Centre for Clinical Practice Innovation Griffith University Meadowbook, Australia 4153 61 7 3382 1229 h.muenchberger@griffith.edu.au

INTRODUCTION

Individuals with brain injury are often substantially less integrated into the community than the general population (**Willer, Rosenthal, Kreutzer, et al., 1993**; **Willer & Corrigan, 1994**; **Winkler, Unsworth & Sloan, 2006**). In particular, opportunities to establish meaningful social connections and to engage with the community are limited, leading to an increased risk of social isolation, low self-esteem, poor physical and emotional health, and unemployment (**Engberg & Teasdale, 2004**; **Heinemann, Sokol, Garvin & Bode, 2002**; **Morton & Wehman, 1995**). In addition to the individual with acquired brain injury (ABI), their supporters and caregivers often experience a similar decrease in community participation and engagement, struggling with stress and loneliness (**Leathem, Heath & Woolley, 1996**). It has been convincingly shown that programs aiming to facilitate the development of social networks contribute to positive outcomes in relation to psychological and physical health (**Finset, Dyrnes, Krogstad & Berstad, 1995**; **Morton & Wehman, 1995**; **Hibbard, Cantor, Charatz, Rosenthal, Ashman, Gunderson, et al., 2002**). Increased participation for individuals with ABI in their communities and the formation of peer support reduces social isolation and leads to increased confidence and positive cycles of social contact (**Lord & Hutchinson, 1993**).

Acquired Brain Injury in Queensland, Australia

Individuals who have sustained an acquired brain injury (ABI) and who are now living with ongoing disability are a large and diverse group whose disability service needs are currently not well met in Queensland, Australia. The Australian Bureau of Statistics 2003 Survey of Disability, Ageing and Carers indicated that 432,700 people had an ABI and some activity limitations or participation restrictions (Australia Institute of Health and Welfare, 2007). This equates to 2.2 percent of the total population of Australia, although stroke as a group was not included in these ABI survey results. The national prevalence of stroke in 2004-2005 was 225,800, a number that equates to approximately 1.2 percent of the total population. Of the population with ABI, approximately 110,000 live in Queensland, which represents a significantly higher percentage of the population than any other Australian state (**Australia Institute of Health and Welfare, 2007**).

The challenges faced by individuals with an acquired brain injury in Queensland are complicated by a lack of funding, and are exacerbated by the fact that the majority of services are concentrated with the population in the south-eastern corner of the state, hence it is more difficult for anyone who resides outside of the urban areas to access services (Kennedy, personal communication, 2010). Moreover, service and support opportunities are limited and community attitudes restrictive. The enormous task of family members in caring for a person with brain impairment is compounded by this lack of community awareness and support. This is a notable barrier to overcome, as it is widely accepted that community integration is more difficult to achieve if the community within which ABI individuals live is not able to understand and respond to their needs.

This case example is based on a self-managed support program for people with acquired brain injury that was designed and delivered by a state wide acquired brain injury outreach service and implemented across 85 community sites (to end 2010) in Queensland, Australia. The current report summarizes the development and objectives of the program, provides an overview of the implementation process, and contextualizes the success of "**Skills to Enable People and Communities**" (**STEPS**) in facilitating the creation and restoration of social networks for its participants.

BACKGROUND

The Acquired Brain Injury Outreach Service

The **Acquired Brain Injury Outreach Service** (ABIOS) is a specialist community-based rehabilitation service for people with Acquired Brain Injury and their families. ABIOS offers information, support, and individual programming for individuals with ABI in Queensland, Australia as well as for their caregivers and families; training and consultancy for service providers and family members; and research regarding community outcomes following ABI. **ABIOS** has as a goal community integration and the improvement of quality of life through increased independence, choice, opportunity, and access to appropriate and responsive services.

Skills to Enable People and Communities (STEPS) Program

In 2005, the **Acquired Brain Injury Outreach Service** (ABIOS) applied for and received three-year service initiative funding to develop and implement the Networks of Support Project through the Pathways home initiative of the **Australian Commonwealth Department of Health and Aging**, administered by **Queensland Health**. During this phase of development, data was collected for evaluation purposes. The aim of the Networks of

Support Project was to establish a sustainable model of self-managed support networks for people with acquired brain injury. Networks of Support is now known as the "**Skills to Enable People and Communities**" Program, or STEPS Program, and since mid-2008, the STEPS Program has been permanently funded by the state health department, Queensland Health, and remains a service arm of **Acquired Brain Injury Outreach Service**.

In late 2005, a pilot site was undertaken with the cooperation of a group of individuals with ABI who were already meeting informally in the community, with focus groups and feedback from this original group of individuals influencing program development. The development of the program was also heavily influenced by both the Stanford Chronic Disease Self-Management Program (**Lorig, Holman and Sobel, 1994**) and the **World Health Organization's International Classification of Functioning, Disability, and Health** (ICF) (**World Health Organization, 2001**); ABIOS' community rehabilitation experience; relevant research literature; and knowledge of key community and rehabilitation stakeholders. Over time, the program evolved to be tailored to the circumstances and realities of individuals with ABI in Queensland. These models informed the holistic conceptualization of health, disability, importance of autonomy and independence, as well as the focus on peer and community participation evident in the STEPS Program.

Key Principles of Self-management and Support

The 3 key principles that underpin the STEPS Program are:

1. Self-Management

Stroke or brain injury can mean many changes for the injured individual, but also for their families, friends and caregivers. Some of these changes can have a major, long-term, and permanent impact on all of these individual's lives. In this way, a self-management approach and self-management strategies can be beneficial for both the injured person and also for those around them, fostering independence and promoting new connections.

The **STEPS Skills Program** offers a self-management approach that can be used by people with acquired brain injury as well as their friends, families, and carers. Each of these people is able to adopt the general approach of self-management and use specific strategies for their individual situation. The **STEPS Skills Program** emphasizes the use of self-management strategies to facilitate involvement and connections within communities.

2. Use of Peer and Lay Leaders

The **STEPS Skills Program** is ideally led by both a "peer leader", who is an individual with a lived experience of an ABI or caring for a person with an ABI, alongside a "professional leader", who is an allied health professional with an interest in support or disability work. This peer-professional relationship has proved a meaningful method of program delivery. These trained facilitators deliver the **STEPS Skills Program** in their local communities in Queensland.

By the end of 2010, **STEPS** had 102 peer and professional leaders across the state. The engagement of lay and peer leaders is a critical component for a number of reasons:

➢ STEPS leadership provides a valued participatory role for people with ABI, or their families and friends, particularly when return to the paid workforce is not likely

➢ Peer leaders offer an authentic, lived experience of ABI or caring for a person with ABI

➢ Their commitment is to their local community and facilitates the formation of sustainable social networks, strengthening their ability to support on-going networking activities

➢ Local leaders are aware of the local context including existing networks and available services

In particular, the involvement of peer leaders in peer-professional partnerships (i.e. peer leader co-leading the **STEPS** Program with a health/disability service provider) has emerged as a successful method of program delivery, with each co-leader bringing different strengths and perspectives to the workshops.

3. Network Groups

The **STEPS Skills Program** uses the self-management approach to foster the development of ongoing informal community networks of support, called **STEPS Network Groups**. These groups emerge from the STEPS Skills Program and, as self-determined groups, provide an ongoing source of support for group participants, according to their local group members' preferences and community context.

Program Description

The STEPS Program

The **Skills to Enable People and Communities** (STEPS) Program consists of two distinct yet related phases. The first phase is the **STEPS Skills Program**, an educational program delivered in the local community setting by locally based leaders. Following the Skills Program, individuals typically form **STEPS Network Groups**, which provide sustainable, self directed and ongoing support networks.

To participate in the **STEPS** program, individuals have to have had an adult-onset brain injury (i.e., not a congenital condition, childhood injury or developmental impairment) and be aged between 18-65 years. Their family members and friends are also eligible to participate. A major issue in terms of ability to participate is aphasia; while several people with aphasia do participate, they need to attend with someone who understands their communication and can support them in their participation in the program (Kennedy, personal communication, 2010).

Initial contact with participants is made either through direct contact with existing community support groups or through the local health care services. Demographics for a subset of STEPS participants (as of October 2007) can be found in Table 1. Participants are predominantly male (68 %), with the majority falling in the 21-44 year age group. Thirty-three percent acquired their brain injury as a result of a motor vehicle accident, and thirty-five percent as a result of a stroke. Injuries as a result of falls and assaults accounted for twenty-two percent of injuries. The average time since injury is 7.12 years, ranging between 6 months and 29 years. Fifty-one percent were unemployed while twenty-two percent volunteer their time (**Muenchberger & Kendall, 2007**).

Table 1. *Demographics of STEPS Program Clients and Supporters (as of October 2007). (Source: Muenchberger & Kendall, 2007)*

Demographics	Clients * (%) (n = 31)	Supporters (%) (n=20)
Gender		
Female	32	85
Male	68	15
Age (years)**		
21-44	39	30
45-58	19	35
59-79	6	35
Nature of Brain Injury		
TBI- Motor Vehicle Accident	33	NA
TBI-Fall	11	NA
TBI- Assault	11	NA
Hypoxia	9	NA
Stroke/CVA	35	NA
Other	2	NA
Time Since Injury		
</= 2years	19	NA
> 2- 5 years	19	
> 5years	26	
Carer Commitment		
Full time	NA	55

Part time	NA	5
Marital Status		
Never Married	43	10
Married or Living with Partner	36	70
Separated, divorced or widowed	19	20
Living Arrangements		
Alone	33	10
Partner/children	50	80
Parent	17	5
Friends	0	5
Education		
< 12 years completed	48	50
Year 12 completed	26	15
Apprenticeship, certificate, or diploma	13	30
Completed university	13	5
Financial status		
Pension	80	17
0-500	6	11
501- 1000	6	28
1001-1500	6	28
1501- 2000	0	11
2000 +	0	6
Productive Activity Status ** (more than one role may apply)		
Full time carer	NA	55
Part time carer	NA	5
Full-time paid work	10	20
Volunteer work	20	20
Part-time / Casual paid work	7	10
Full time study	0	0
Part time study	7	0
Not in labour force	57	15

* At initial assessment

**Not all values represent 100 % due to missing data or more than one answer

The STEPS Skills Program

The **STEPS Skills Program** consists of a structured two-hour group session once per week for six consecutive weeks in a small group setting (6-10 people). Participants, who are both individuals with ABI and their carers, friends or family, work through the accompanying workbook with the facilitation of a local leader or team of leaders. The weekly sessions are structured around the three main themes:

1. How I look after myself

2. How I live in the community

3. How I work with services

Discussion is guided around these themes while participants work sequentially through the workbook on topics related to self-management and social skills development (See Table 2 below). Participants engage in reflection and share their experiences of life after brain injury or as a caregiver.

Table 2: *STEPS Weekly Course Outline*

Session 1	Introduction to Program	About Self Management
Session 2	How I Look After Myself	Goal Setting Understanding ABI Changes after Brain Injury
Session 3	How I Look After Myself	Managing Stress Working on specific problems after ABI
Session 4	How I Look After Myself How I Live in the Community	Getting structure and balance in my life Relationships with family and friends Relationships with other people Linking with friends
Session 5	How I Live in the Community How I Work with Services	Common difficulties in the Community Exploring activities and experiences Our group future Risk taking How I work with services
Session 6	Our Group Break up Activity	Break up Activity

STEPS groups are responsible for generating ideas, making necessary plans and working together to ensure a successful Week 6 Group Break-Up Activity. Culminating the program in such a fashion allows of the consolidation of group support, and allows participants to enjoy and engage with their community with their newly formed support group. Typical examples of the Group Break-Up Activity include a picnic in the park, an outing to a beach, playing croquet followed by lunch, or a ferry ride on a river.

STEPS Network Groups

Box 1 below contains an example of how a self-managed group might organize ongoing meetings in the community.

Box 1. Description of how a STEPS group developed a self-managed group

In one community, the STEPS course developed into a self-managed social network. Outcomes for this group post course included:

- Monthly meetings, alternating between centre-based meetings and social outings
- Group schedule developed to send to all members
- Two members coordinating the group consistently
- Contact list of all attendees established
- Donation for tea/coffee and costs for meeting from community
- Informal transport assistance arranged amongst members
- ABIOS received flyer and schedule from group in the mail for inclusion in the STEPS Newsletter

(Source: Muenchberger & Kendall, 2007)

RESOURCES

All resources required to participate in the **STEPS Program Leader Training**, deliver the **STEPS Skills Program** and coordinate a **STEPS Network Group**, are provided by the program. They include brochures, leader manuals, posters, activity planners, STEPS Workbook, referral forms, and attendance records.

Two centralized Program Managers, supported by administrative staff, provide the coordination and training. All program delivery is done at the local level through peer and lay leaders who are not employed by **STEPS**. Leaders are eligible for a stipend, contingent on their completion of **STEPS** training and agreement to **STEPS** principles.

The **STEPS Skills Program** is ideally led by both a 'peer leader', which is an individual with a lived experience of an ABI or caring for a person with an ABI, alongside with a 'professional leader', who is an allied health professional with an interest in community rehabilitation. This peer-professional relationship has proved a meaningful method of program delivery.

A key component of the **STEPS** program is this insistence on the involvement of a peer leader. While it would be possible for health professionals to run the **Skills Program**, an essential component of the workshops is the peer facilitation, and without that the program loses the flavour of peer involvement and support it is meant to develop (Kennedy, personal communication, 2010).

The recruitment and screening of Peer Leaders happens primarily through interested clients and participants contacting **STEPS**. It is critical at this point to ensure that interested individuals understand the role before progressing: potential leaders need to understand that it isn't just about telling their story to the group, but facilitating a dialogue based on a common experience (Kennedy, Personal communication, 2010). Once this understanding is established, there is a self-assessment about their attitude toward community participation in brain injury, work checks, personal interviews and the leader training.

To enhance uptake for peer leaders there is an incentive scheme. Individuals can apply for a stipend to run the program which consists of several hundred dollars to run all of the weekly sessions, participate in the supervision and help the group to set up a sustainable, appropriate future plan.

IMPLEMENTATION

The **STEPS** Program operational model (Figure 1- see below) shows the relationships between community, intervention, the resource building process and community preparation in contributing to sustainable networks.

The process map highlights the complexity of community engagement within three components of the **STEPS** course implementation, namely first contact with the community, leader training and course development. In each component there are cyclical and resource intensive processes that relate to preparation, participation and promotion. The leader training component is identified as the most time-intensive and demanding process relative to the other phases. Given that the leader engagement represents a key strategy in the sustainability of the STEPS course in future, commitment to this aspect of implementation is crucial.

STEPS Program Operational Model

C
O
M
M
U
N
I
T
Y

Resource Building Process
- Supporting Group Processes
- Developing Individual Support Networks
- Fostering Community Inclusion and Partnerships

Community Intervention
- STEPS Skills Program
- STEPS Network Group
- Education
- Capacity building

D
E
V
E
L
O
P
M
E
N
T

Sustainable Networks

Community Preparation
- Link up with community leaders
- Gauge interest/skills
- Foster collective responsibility
- Promote healthy alliances Networks

Community Profiles to Identify Communities

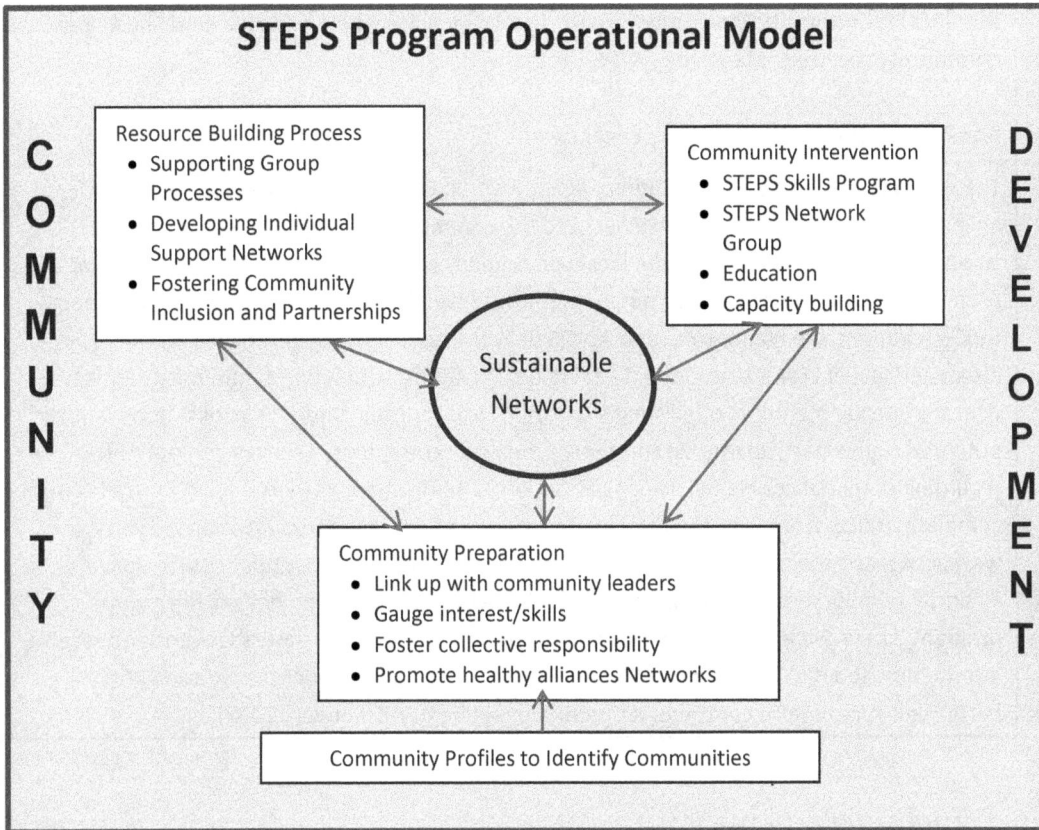

Figure 1. STEPS Program Operational Model (Source: Kennedy, personal communication, 2010)

The Five Phases of Implementation

There are five distinctive phase of **STEPS** Program implementation, as described below:

1. Community Engagement

Local communities are approached to gauge their interest in the program and to explore local solutions for people with brain injury, their families and carers. Collective responsibility is fostered between **STEPS** Program staff and key local stakeholders. From the outset, **STEPS** establishes firm partnerships with its potential local leaders to ensure continued program development occurs in locally responsive ways. As an example of this process, Box 2 describes community engagement by the **STEPS** team. **STEPS** Program staff may engage communities by telephone, email and/or videoconference, or may travel to the local community and meet with local agencies, key people, and host public community meetings about the **STEPS** Program.

Box 2: Description of Community Engagement

The ABIOS team contacts a community agency within Queensland by telephone, and offers an invitation to present the STEPS course to the community. ABIOS arranges for a community forum to be held in the local community, and to travel to that community for a promotional tour. Potential community members (including community services) approach ABIOS regarding the leader role, and ABIOS deliver leader training at the location for interested leaders (at a later time). Leaders begin actively contacting community members who are already members of existing support groups for brain injury or stroke, and identify potential course participants. At the same time, local community services contact ABIOS regarding potential course participants, and ABIOS sends them a referral form for them to complete. ABIOS work with the local leaders to source a local course venue, send workbooks, and maintain regular weekly contact with leaders throughout course delivery. Financial reimbursement is also facilitated by ABIOS for leaders who deliver the group program locally. Meanwhile, other potential community locations across Queensland receive information about STEPS from ABIOS team and the process of leader preparation and participant recruitment continue. (Source: Muenchberger & Kendall, 2007).

---

2. Leader Training

Local people are provided with training to develop and deliver local group interventions. **STEPS** Program staff typically offer **Skills Program Leader Training** in the local community. Often, people from other nearby communities might also attend the training. Leader training is a 2-day training package, with a strong emphasis on interaction and experiential learning. Practical experience of the format for weekly support/supervision is gained in the training. Training is supported by facilitator manuals and resources; supervision and support of facilitators continues through all phases of the program. Leaders must be trained to deliver the **STEPS Skills Program**.

3. Group Intervention- STEPS Skills Program

Ongoing planning and liaison occurs between trained leaders and STEPS Program staff to work towards local **STEPS Skills Program** delivery. Specific topics addressed in the **STEPS** workbook include self-management, goal setting, understanding brain injury, stress-management, relationships, developing a routine, and participating in the community. A STEPS poster, program workbooks and other resources are provided for all group programs, either via email or post. While the original intent was to deliver the workshop using PowerPoint slides as well as a workbook, pilot group feedback indicated that this resulted in difficulties with attending to and retaining information for some participants. It was decided that the workbook alone supplemented with group-driven discussion was a more manageable and effective way of working through the material. In addition, the volume and pacing was adjusted so as to not be overwhelming while still focusing on the important material (Kennedy, Personal communication, 2010).

An important aspect of the **STEPS Skills Program** beyond the benefit to the participants is that community awareness is built through the presence of the group in the community. Particularly in rural Queensland there is a lack of awareness about brain injury, and creating the "network of support" often gives individuals the confidence to get out into the community and advocate for their needs. In addition, when a **STEPS Skills Program** is set up, **STEPS** encourages running stories in the local press about the success of STEPS in the community, further contributing to a heightened profile and awareness (Kennedy, Personal communication, 2010).

The **STEPS** Program actively fosters partnerships amongst local community stakeholders to optimise uptake and delivery of the program. Some examples of partnerships include:

➤ Co-leadership between service providers and peer/lay leaders.

➤ Co-leadership between peer and lay leaders

➤ Incorporation of STEPS Skills Program into standard model of service.

➤ Strategic, sequential offering of STEPS Skills Program to raise local awareness of the STEPS program

➤ Sequential offering of STEPS Skills Program to achieve critical mass for ongoing Network Groups

➤ Formation of service partnerships to deliver STEPS Group Program locally.

➤ Ongoing partnership amongst STEPS, local host service and local peer leader.

Many of these arrangements have been particularly important in uptake in regional and rural settings, due to workforce mix and retention, workload management, service burden, and local cultural issues. Sequential offering of the Skills Program is strategic, with the rationale being that the second session will also be much better attended as word of mouth communication travels in that local community. Notably, the **STEPS** Program eventually decided to accept working with hospitals in some regional/rural areas when there was no other infrastructure (e.g., regular community health services), although the program is still delivered in the community. Although this affiliation does not reflect the community orientation of the program, it was decided that it was better to partner with hospital-based health services than not offer the program at all (Kennedy, Personal communication).

4. Network Groups

STEPS Skills Program facilitators are provided with additional support for their role as coordinators of ongoing **Network Groups** through support, training, manuals, and resources. A significant number of group participants are involved in ongoing **STEPS Network Groups**. Most will meet on a monthly basis, with over 100 people attending regularly throughout Queensland. Many groups are open to new members and connections are made through listing the Network Groups, places where they meet, and the contact person in the quarterly STEPS Newsletter. The Newsletter therefore represents another tool used to facilitate new connections within the community.

5. STEPS Leader Network

A dedicated STEPS Leader Network has been formed to provide ongoing support and developmental opportunities for trained leaders. Its main activities are:

➤ Quarterly newsletter—distributed to trained leaders, and other key stakeholders

➤ Leader Contact List- trained leaders can consent to their contact details being made available to other STEPS leaders in Queensland

➤ Bi-monthly, STEPS-hosted teleconferences for business planning, leader reflection and educational topics

➤ Ongoing availability of STEPS Program staff for consultation and support via telephone, email and videoconference

STEPS Program Leaders

A critical component of the **STEPS Skills Program** is that they are led by local, trained facilitators in their communities around Queensland. As previously mentioned, the geography of Queensland is such that many communities have very poor service provision,

"I wanted to help other people as I had been helped...I felt that I had benefited from attending my first STEPS course and I was hoping that other people would get the same help...it opened my eyes...I felt alive...I felt I wasn't alone anymore...it was a wonderful feeling of belonging...it was like I was with likeminded people that I had known for a long time."
(Peer Leader)

continuum of care, and support services for individuals with ABI. The delivery of the STEPS Program in the local context is invaluable to the sustainability of network development and to the community engagement and awareness.

OUTCOME

Given appropriate supports and resources, evaluation of the **STEPS program** has shown that individuals, leaders, and the community benefit from the STEPS course by building knowledge, establishing peer connections, and engaging in constructive self-reflection (**Muenchberger & Kendall, 2007**). Independent evaluation of the STEPS program has been conducted by Griffith University, of which a subset of results was published in the January 2011 volume of Brain Injury (**Muenchberger, Kendall, Kennedy and Charker, 2011**). This section includes results from both published and unpublished data resulting from Griffith University's study of the STEPS Program, which has been ongoing since 2006.

Client Outcomes

A total of 616 people attended the **STEPS Skills Program** from 2006-2010. As of 2010, there were 18 STEPS network groups that met regularly and were open to new members. A further four groups continued to maintain connections but had decided not to be open to new members. Notably, the majority of clients reported that their STEPS groups were still meeting following completion of the course. Of all participants, 71% of clients were still meeting with their groups at three months post-course completion, with 67% still meeting at six months.

A recently published study of the STEPS program by **Muenchberger et al. (2011)**, surveyed participants to measure the impact of the program on their "self" and "social" resources (**Muenchberger, Kendall, Kennedy & Charker, 2011**). Using a longitudinal study design, 51 participants were surveyed across three consecutive time points. Time 1 was within one month of course commencement, Time 2 (T2) was at three months following course completion and Time 3 (T3) was at six months following course completion (Muenchberger et al., 2010). Outcome measures were examined using the following previously validated scales.

Self resources

Emotional health was measured using the short-form version of the **Depression Anxiety Stress Scales** (DASS-21) (**Lovibond & Lovibond, 1995**). The DASS-21 is a self-report questionnaire consisting of 21 items that together measure general psychological distress. Goal setting was measured using an 11-item scale, with 5 goal commitment items and 6 future orientation questions (**Klein, Wesson, Hollenbeck, et al., 2001**). Self-efficacy was measured according to a 5-item scale.

Social resources

Social support was measured using an 11 item multidimensional scale of perceived social support (**Zimet, Dahlem, Zimet, et al., 1988**). Three factors were measured: family support, friend's support, and significant other support. Services and information use was measured using an 8-item scale developed by **Somerset, Peters, Sharp and Campbell (2003)** and was used to describe an individual's sense of control and autonomy in the service environment.

Non-parametric (mixed-model) analysis of the most recent study results showed significant client outcomes in the areas of self-management, goal commitment, and stress management (n=51) (**Muenchberger et al., 2011**). Outcomes for male participants were stable across time after program participation, an outcome which the study authors attribute to the protective effects of the STEPS course. However, female participants showed increased levels of stress and decreased levels of goal commitment over time, possibly as a result of increased awareness of personal limitations following program completion. The authors found no change over time with respect to self-efficacy, general health, use of services, or social support.

Study limitations stated by the authors include the lack of a comparison or control group, as well as loss to follow-up over time (n=51 at T1, n=32 at T2, n=28 at T3). However, given that the study group was predominately male with acquired brain injury, this loss to follow up is not unexpected, and the authors completed a "completer" versus "non-completer" analysis and found no difference between the groups. **Muenchberger et al. (2011)** also put forth the possibility that social support was not an adequate measure of social resources in the current study as it is likely that individuals who participated in the program may have already had increased support relative to non-participants. Overall, the authors conclude that the program may prove more beneficial for males in the short-term, with females requiring more sustained interventions to foster participation (**Muenchberger et al., 2011**). Further details of the evaluation have been recently published and are available online (**Muenchberger, Kendall, Kennedy & Charker, 2011**).

Previous analysis by the same research group reported that the STEPS course contributes to community competence (i.e., capacity for future course delivery). At a broad level, the data indicated **ABIOS** had been successful in promoting the STEPS course in Queensland communities and establishing it as a service in the community. For instance, one community group had voluntarily incorporated the STEPS course into their formal rehabilitation program and was supportive of their health professionals attending the leader training associated with the STEPS course. At the individual group level, there was confirmation that some STEPS groups were active in developing a longer-term social agenda and leadership structure within their local area (**Muenchberger & Kendall, 2007**). Clients surveyed in this unpublished report expressed a decrease in their dependence on others, a stronger sense of autonomy, as well as enhanced perceptions of coping effectiveness.

Carer outcomes

Supporters (caregivers/friends) surveyed were less likely to report stress and feelings of depression. Supporter outcomes were measured using the same scales as clients' with the exception of goal setting and self-efficacy, which were replaced with items to measure carer support and carer stress modified from the Carers Assessment of Difficulties Index (CADI) and Carer Assessment of Satisfaction Index (CASI) (**Grant & Nolan, 1993**).

Of the supporters surveyed (n=20), 67% regularly attended the STEPS Program. Stated reasons for non-attendance of supporters at the STEPS course were difficulties with transport arrangements and work commitments. Supporters who did not attend the STEPS course (non-attendees) were more likely to report experiencing stressful aspects of caring than attendees. Results showed that the majority of non-attendees might have believed that professional health workers did not appreciate the problems faced by carers, which contributed to their feelings of stress. However, supporters who attended the STEPS course were more likely to report feelings of depression than non-attendees. This finding supports the possibility that the

STEPS course represented an opportunity for carers to seek support from others in response to their emotional difficulties related to the caring role (**Muenchberger & Kendall, 2007**).

Conclusion

The **Skills to Enable People and Communities (STEPS) Program** is designed to empower participants and to promote self-reflection, facilitate community participation and provide participants with insights into their ability to self-manage. STEPS implementation in any community is time, resource and relationship intensive and without this input, programs are less likely to occur or sustain themselves. In the Canadian context, the fact that the program does not require centralized delivery and can be facilitated wherever local leader interest is generated, is beneficial and makes program delivery in rural or remote areas feasible. Moreover, as ongoing network groups are self-sustaining, the continued input of financial resources is unnecessary. Evaluation shows that positive group functioning and emerging self-managed networks did occur after STEPS programming, and the program therefore built capacity and met objectives to foster participation and peer connections.

The process of community participation is complex and multi-faceted, requiring ongoing and committed personnel both within the community and to oversee the engagement and training of new communities and leaders. The STEPS model provides an example of a participant- centred, community-directed initiative to facilitate community engagement and increase independence and self-management through participant focused workshops. This positive cycle represents a sustainable and effective mechanism of program delivery to the acquired brain injury community, contributing to positive participants outcomes.

REFERENCES

Australia Institute of Health and Welfare. (2007). **Disability in Australia: Acquired Brain Injury. Bulletin 55.** Australian Government: Canberra, Australia.

Engberg, A., & Teasdale, T. (2004). Psychosocial outcome following traumatic brain injury in adults a long-term follow-up. **Brain Injury,** *18*(6), 533-545.

Finset, A., Dyrnes, S., Krogstad, J., & Berstand, J. (1995). Self-reported social networks and interpersonal support 2 years after severe traumatic brain injury. **Brain Injury,** *9*(2), 141-150.

Grant, G., & Nolan, M. (1993). **Informal carers: sources and concomitants of satisfaction.** *Health Soc Care, 1*(3), 147-159.

Heinemann, A. W., Sokol, S., Garvin, L., & Bode, R. K. (2002). **Measuring unmet needs and services among persons with traumatic brain injury.** *Arch Phys Med Rehabil, 83,* 1052-1059.

Hibbard, M. R., Cantor, J., Charatz, H., Rosenthal, R., Ashman, T., Gundersen, N., et al. (2002). **Peer support in the community: Initial findings of a monitoring program for individuals with traumatic brain injury and their families.** *J Head Trauma Rehabil, 17,* 112-131.

Klein, H., Wesson, M., et al. (2001). The assessment of goal commitment: A measurement model meta-analysis. *Organ Behav Hum Dec, 85*(1), 32-55.

Leathem, J., Heath, E., & Woolley, C. (1996). **Relative's perceptions of role change, social support and stress after traumatic brain injury.** *Brain Inj, 10*(1), 27-38.

Lord, J., & Hutchinson, P. (1993). The process of empowerment: Implications for theory and practice. *Can J Commun Ment Health, 12,* 5-22.

Lorig K., Holman, H., & Sobel, D. (1994). *Living a Healthy Life with Chronic Conditions.* Palo Alto, California: Bull Publishing Company

Lovibond, S. & Lovibond, P. (1995). Manual for the Depression Anxiety Stress Scales. (2nd. Ed.) Sydney: Psychology Foundation. ISBN 7334-1423-0.

Morton, M. V., & Wehman, P. (1995). **Psychosocial and emotional sequelae of individuals with traumatic brain injury: a literature review and recommendations.** *Brain Inj, 9*(1), 81-92.

Muenchberger, H., Kendall, E., Kennedy, A. & Charker, J. (2011). **Living with brain injury in the community: Outcomes from a community-based self-management support (CB-SMS) programme in Australia.** *Brain Inj,* 25(1), 23-34.

Muenchberger, H., & Kendall, E. (2007). *Progress Report- October 2007: Skills to Enable People & Communities (STEPS) Program Participant Experiences and Community Engagement.* [Unpublished].

Paterson, B. L. (2001). **The shifting perspectives model of chronic illness.** *J Nurse Scholarsh, 33*(1), 21-26.

Somerset, M., Peters, T., et al. (2003). **Factors that contribute to quality of life outcomes prioritised by people with multiple sclerosis.** *Qual Life Res, 12,* 21-29.

Stanford Patient Education Research Center. (2010). *Chronic disease self-management program.* Retrieved at **http://patienteducation.stanford.edu/programs/cdsmp.html**.

Willer, B., & Corrigan, J. (1994). Whatever it takes: a model for community-based services. **Brain Inj,** *8*(7), 647-659.

Willer, B., Rosenthal, M., Kreutzer, J. et al. (1993). **Assessment of community integration following rehabilitation for TBI.** *J Head Trauma Rehabil, 8,* 75-87.

Winkler, D., Unsworth, C., Sloan, S. (2006). **Factors that lead to successful community integration following severe traumatic brain injury.** *J Head Trauma Rehabil, 1*(1), 8-21.

World Health Organization. (2010). *International Classification of Functioning, Disability and Health (ICF).* Retrieved at **http://www.who.int/classifications/icf/en/**.

Zimet, G., Dahlem, N., et al. (1988). **The multidimensional scale of perceived social support.** *J Pers Assess, 52*(1), 30-4.

CHAPTER 5

A SIMPLY SELF-SUSTAINING SYSTEM, COMMUNITY BASED REINTEGRATION POST ACUTE BRAIN INJURY PROGRAM

A Promising Practice

By Natasha Jamal

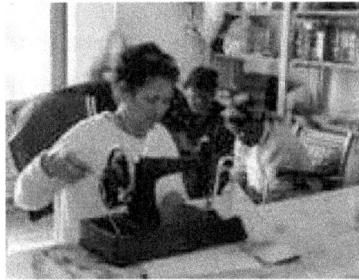

Population Served : Life Span
Contributing Author Contact Information
Alison Madden Program Founder A Simply Self Sustaining System, Community Based Reintegration Post Acute Brain Injury Program Riversdale, South Africa **almadden@mweb.co.za**

BACKGROUND

History & Program Development

The Simply Sustaining System is a promising community reintegration practice that serves survivors of acquired brain injury (ABI) with the philosophy of focusing on clients' capacities as opposed to their deficits. The program is run predominantly in the rural areas of Riversdale in South Africa as an Adult Day Service Program. Dr. Alison Madden, the program founder, initiated the program after her experience in medical legal work after recognizing that there is a shortage of rehabilitation services that focus on community reintegration. This is especially the case after a person has left acute care in the period of hospitalization after a brain injury. Government care currently provides hospitalization during the acute phase of injury where medical treatment, neuro-surgery, and physical therapy are available. Occupational therapy and speech therapy are given only if the injured person has very obvious gait, upper limb, speech, and swallowing difficulties. The period of hospitalization is usually less than three weeks, with little transitional support for the person from the hospital to the home and community. Furthermore not only are survivors of ABI or traumatic brain injury (TBI) unable to receive services for their injuries, many also become highly passive, inactive, and lonely in their daily lives—disheartening characteristics that have been found in research among people with ABI (**Ashley, Persel, & Krych, 1997**; **Dikmen, Machamer, & Temkin, 1993**; **Doig, Fleming, & Tooth, 2001**). From an ethical and moral consideration of the circumstances of people with ABI, Alison wondered whether she could improve the anxiety and apathy that people with brain injury experience in order for them to take on tasks that have value to themselves and to their communities.

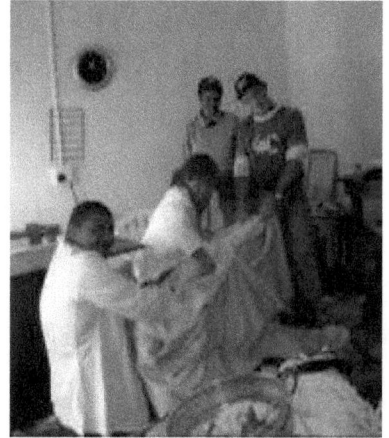

The ultimate aim is to have people with ABI become motivated so that they can *and want* to reintegrate back into their communities. This program was developed to provide a model of rehabilitation different from the traditional medical models that may not take into consideration the clients' needs for social reintegration and community participation. This program aims to find meaningful roles not only for survivors of ABI, but also for local rural community members who are highly skilled yet underemployed. Thus the program is housed and sustained in a rural community setting, benefitting and supporting the needs of people with brain injury as well as community members without brain injury.

The Riversdale Community

The Simply Sustaining project is intentionally situated in a small agriculture community called **Riversdale**. This close community environment benefits clients by allowing easier access and a greater connectivity to the local population and businesses that surround them. In return the clients are able to serve the local population through the program's activities.

The culture of such a small rural community fosters co-operation, interdependence and sharing, where small farmers and local people are encouraged and permitted to have horses and crops on communal strips of land. The environment is conducive to reciprocity, and there is less emphasis on private, individualized lands and crops. The community culture is traditional, where hierarchies exist among families and in the local society. Older people are respected, despite any disabilities. The program encourages accessibility to one's family members, such as children, if clients are mothers or fathers. Visitors are also encouraged to take part when seeing their friends and loved ones participating in the program. For example, many visitors, including children, play and read to the clients, help cook meals, and take on non-medical tasks. The philosophy of respect is a paramount feature of the program; it is required of all participants (for instance, Alison notices a predetermined understanding , especially among children, that there is no laughing at clients who have sustained a brain injury). The importance of this philosophy is echoed in **Willer and Corrigan's** *Whatever it takes* model, which is been highly esteemed and valued among community-based programs and practitioners (1994).

Adapting the program to its local context

The strategies of the program have been modeled by a successful community reintegration program called **Foyer du Handicap** in Geneva Switzerland. The Simply Sustaining System uses a similar approach with the same principles, but has adapted it to fit the differing context of the local community it serves with respect to culture and socio-economic needs. The guiding principles for this program include:

1. Focusing on clients' abilities as opposed to their deficits in program work and social interaction

2. Fostering living conditions which promote independence in one's personal and social life while feeling integrated and accepted into the larger able-bodied community of people

3. Ensuring clients with ABI are involved in professional activities that contribute to their functional, social, and emotional development for participation in their local and personal communities

4. Ensuring that the client's functional, cognitive, and emotional abilities are strengthened in order to foster self-sufficiency

5. Creating opportunities for socializing with other clients, staff and family in order to foster mutual respect, caring, and community.

The small town of Riversdale has a large number of highly skilled local community members who are either underemployed or unemployed. The program provides a mutually beneficial arrangement for these community members as well as the ABI clients: ABI survivors are able to learn and develop an artisan skill or trade, while the non-ABI partner finds a more meaningful contribution to the community while showcasing his or her skill. Both partners interact, problem solve, and apply social reintegration techniques in a real-world setting. The resulting merchandise and/or product is then sold, which in return supports the program financially and provides a means of income for participants. Furthermore, traditional skills that have been passed down through generations—i.e., sewing, nursing, carpentry, caring for cattle, making cheese, tapping aloe plants for aloe vera products—become revived and valued once again. These skills become a form of therapy and pride for both the client (who may already possess some of these skills prior to their accident) and the mentor. Thus local communities become sustainable resources that the program draws from in order to better help clients reintegrate into their societies and communities. Involving the local community within community-based rehabilitation is found to be essential to successfully integrate the client into their communities and for the program's success (Mitchell, 1999).

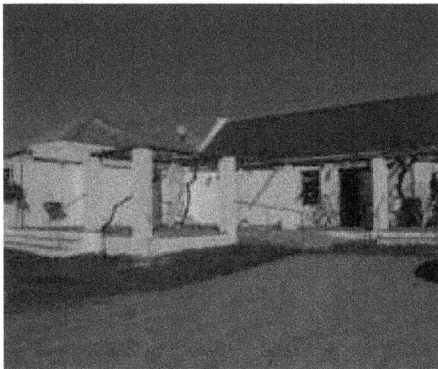

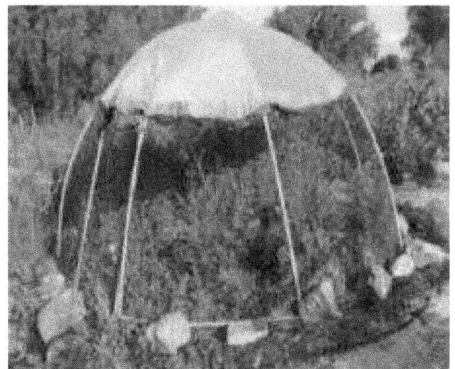

RESOURCES

The initial investment to develop the Simply Sustaining project was made by program founder Dr. Alison Madden, who saw the importance and need for post-acute therapy for people who are survivors of ABI. The current program has the capacity to take on eight to ten clients at a time and runs on farm land that was acquired for the purpose of this project. Workshops that teach or re-teach skills and trades for the ABI clients take place within old stables of the country town that have been renovated by the local people. Local townspeople build some of the furniture and donate environmentally friendly fabric and raw materials. A *flatlit* or residential space is attached to the workshops for overnights guests, such as family members of clients. A renovated farm house has eight rooms, where four are used by therapists for physiotherapy, and the other four rooms are available for clients' short term stay. Showers and baths are wheelchair friendly. The kitchen is an industrial sized facility for cooking meals and which also provides an area for clients to produce baked goods, including jams and other types of preserves. A future plan is to run a tea garden out of these facilities where clients learn hospitality skills while providing a service to the community. There is also a sustainable garden and chicken coup; chickens till the soil enabling local produce to develop. It is also been found that chickens are wonderful pets for people with head

Client enrollment and roles

The clients who require short term therapy usually stay between six weeks to six months. Other clients attend the day program but do not live on the premises. These clients usually have a higher degree of integration within their communities, have acquired a skill from going through the program, and are now participating in the capacity of working with the community coordinators or mentoring new clients. Clients with higher capacities serve as mentors and can work fairly independently on the production line, producing goods for the market. Clients who assist in running the program are also paid for their services with a percentage of the sales from the products and merchandise. The payment percentage also depends on other factors such as the speed of production, the amount of independence to sustain performance in producing items, and whether clients can improvise and ask for assistance.

As outlined in Figure 2, the staff structure consists of a program manager who oversees and coordinates the production line and the clinical care/program, community coordinators who are required to have a trade or skill, seek out contracts for work orders (in order to sell the products made), create awareness in the community, offer assistance to others, alert the founder to people in need, encourage other community members to get involved as volunteers in the program, liaise with business and tourism, and involve themselves as mentors with the clients in the program. Mentors, unlike community coordinators, do not have the tasks of managing the administrative aspects of the program, but rather usually work only with the clients to help support the skill or trade being learned or re-learned. Mentors usually have three or four clients to work with. Established clients who have higher capacities can also serve as mentors to other clients who are still developing their capacities.

Medical consulting staff work in partnership with the program, such as the neuropsychologist and program founder, registered nursing sisters, and a back up doctor. The program predominately runs without the need for an external medical team; however, when required, a medical consultation is sought out as a safety net.

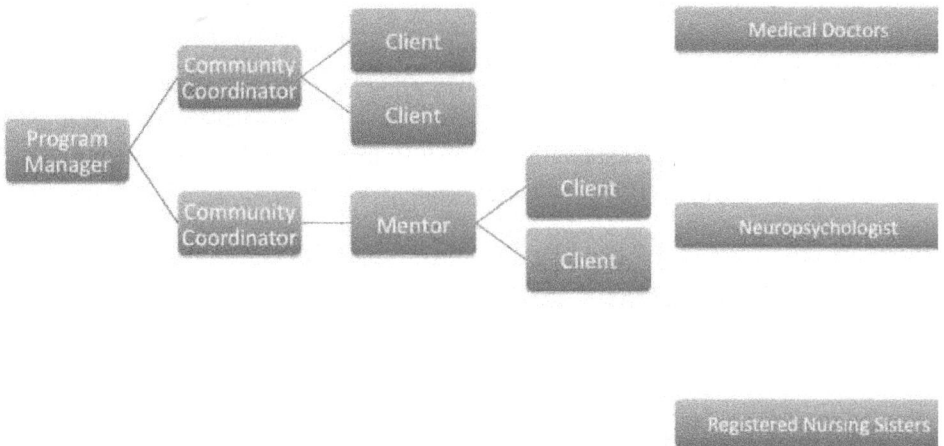

Figure 2 :Rehabilitation Staff Structure for Simply Sustaining project

Geographical Requirements

The program itself has been purposely set up in a rural area of South Africa in order to help create jobs among community locals who are educated but have little employment opportunities. The town, which includes a small hospital, is a comfortable farming community where people have been found to be more willing to create partnerships between the program and community organizations, unlike a more impersonal, busy urban environment. The program founder strongly upholds that such a model would be difficult to run in a city because of the associated increase in cost, community danger, and the lack of generosity of emotion and time by the urban locals. Thus the rural location is fundamental and a pre-requisite to the success of the program. Although the client's environment, which may support or hinder their community reintegration, has been acknowledged to be an important factor to consider (**Sloan, Winkler, & Callaway, 2004**), the urban/rural setting has yet to be seriously considered when looking at rehabilitation programs that utilize and simultaneously serve local community members as resources and partners within a program.

The Simply Self-Sustaining project has been developed using a grassroots approach in which various community members have come forward to support the program as volunteers –with donations of raw materials, of skills, and of time. For instance, local farmers have dropped off food, and the generosity and empathy from local community members have helped provide free services such as carpentry and construction. Many of the workshops are led by the community coordinators who volunteer their time to work with mentors and to teach or work with ABI clients. Together they create goods and products that are sellable in their local markets. Thus the program tries to harness the resources of the local community by incorporating the skills and services of its community members, in turn empowering them to take on the responsibility of the ABI survivors in the community. The program creates partnerships in order to sustain and share ownership (**Arnstein, 1969**). In a way, the model is seen as a microcosm of the family network and is expanded to include the rest of the local community.

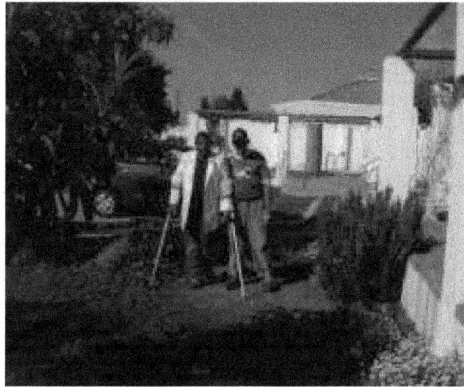

Community Coordinators

The community coordinators are sympathetic, yet non-professional therapy facilitators. Training is provided to allow community coordinators to become expert in a specific skill (sewing, design, cooking, baking, woodwork, nursery, forestry work, chocolate making, shell polishing and creating recycled carrier bags among others) in which they teach, support, and guide clients, who ultimately produce items for sale in the local markets. Many townspeople who have been recruited as community coordinators initially have less confidence in their skills and in the belief that they can contribute to the program. Due to lower levels of formal education, less opportunity, and less exposure to technology, the local people benefit enormously in the involvement in a more formal program, making this a positive experience for them as well. The program founder maintains that it is imperative that they continue to be involved. This can only be made possible if the structure is flexible enough to consider their domestic chores, their limited earning capacity, their cultural characteristics, and the strong awareness of improving the destinies of their descendants in the recently emerging democratic structure of the South African system.

The initial collaborators of the program are still involved, and their roles and have become more powerful over time. The emphasis of the program has now incorporated the necessity for each person to fulfill a "business function. This is based on time lines, producing items which are acceptable in quality, completing tasks, and taking on jobs which are perhaps not pleasant but needed for the sake of the survival of the business to support both the community and the program. For instance, a home industry feature has started within the program, whereby clients are now making jams, selling fresh vegetables, and making organic compost. Clients may be required to work with chicken manure and dig in the garden; thus the importance of "being part of a team" is emphasized, especially when participants show signs of disinterest or defensiveness by not taking part in the work-related activities. Sometimes members of the program feel that such tasks are beneath them, and so the program emphasizes the team component as its driving force and motivational tool to get work done.

Funding

The auto insurance (Road Accident) fund receives its funds from the governmental taxes on all fuel. In other words the funds are acquired at source, and there are sufficient funds as long as there are vehicles on the road. The issue that many survivors with Acquired or Traumatic Brain Injury have is that the funds from this source are difficult to obtain, and if they are acquired, it's usually after the critical time period when rehabilitation is found to be most effective. Thus there is a concern that the funds from this source are neither distributed in the benefit of the survivor, nor distributed appropriately. Alison has noted that, in her extensive experience, primary health care institutions have tended to focus on symptomatic relief for survivors—a practice in local health care that makes it difficult for people with ABI or any other disability to be cared for since they can be seen as on-going burdens to the society and no longer economically viable citizens. The attitude towards rehabilitation is that it is "not cost-effective", a culture that predominately believes disabled persons will never be able to overcome their disabilities or be gainfully (re)employed. Although there is provision in labour law that a certain number of disabled persons should be part of the workforce, the implementation of this provision by the locals has been difficult, and so people with disabilities are rarely seen in the workforce. Hence therapy in South Africa is usually practiced as the provision of basic nursing services and wound care rather than the reduction of the impact on functional abilities through interventions and the strengthening of existing skills, or of compensation strategies in order to facilitate independent living.

Self-Sustaining program

Given the challenges in receiving federal funding and the lack of other external funding, this program is different from other models in that it is financially self-sustaining. Survivors of ABI take on the necessary tasks within their capacities, and with mentors and community coordinators, produce items for sale in their local markets. Each member who is involved within the program understands his or her role in sustaining the current program, which is tied to their own means of employment. One of the drawbacks of running this type of program in a small town is the difficulty in finding contracts for selling the items produced by the clients/community coordinators. Since selling the goods is the main source of income, the program's survival relies on finding purchasing outlets. The Simply Self-Sustaining System is in its infancy, and thus administrators continue to seek ways to market its items in the city, and ideally to find feasible ways to export its goods.

Government Interest

The **South African Government** has recently shown interest in the program by requesting an opportunity to fund the program and implement a protective workshop for the entire area. This request however has come with a condition of re-managing the program with the aim to offer 25 disabled persons per day the opportunity to be part of the current workshops that are run. The request is being opposed by the program founder on the principle that the service is for persons who have acquired brain injuries and not for all disabilities. The hesitation from letting the South African government manage the program is that the program's philosophy may not continue to be carried through. Specifically the current program's philosophy may be misinterpreted by those who run the agency if they utilize a deficit approach when working with the clients instead of encouraging survivors of ABI to maximize their capacities.

IMPLEMENTATION

Therapy approach

The Simply Self-Sustaining System aims at providing an opportunity for people with ABI (both traumatic and non-traumatic) to re-learn skills, re-access social groups, and modify behaviour in order to contribute to their communities in meaningful and sufficient ways. This approach steers away from the medical model that is currently prevalent with rehabilitation services (**Condeluci, 2002**). Rather, the program has been initiated using a grassroots approach that involves educating and empowering not only ABI survivors, but also their local community members. Mentors and community partnerships have been created using this approach since the program is supported by community volunteers, donations of raw materials, and of skills and time. The ABI survivor is trained to work and contribute to small business ventures by producing items or providing services for their local community market in collaboration with their local community members. The small business ventures and items made for market help sustain the project and fund employment for the local community members who serve as mentors and project coordinators, as well as for the clients themselves if they have the capacity and seek to offer their newly developed services and skills.

The Simply Self-Sustaining Philosophy

The program is based on the principal to provide a simple, non-medical, social re-integration service so that ABI survivors who have traditionally been marginalized by their disabilities can be part of a working organization. A concern with a traditional medical rehabilitation approach is that it endorses a philosophy that may not take into consideration the clients' needs or personal requirements for social and emotional integration (**Willer & Corrigan, 1994**). Rather medical rehabilitation approaches are found to have a greater focus on the functional rehabilitation of clients, without ensuring that clients are emotionally and socially supported and reintegrated into their communities (**Condeluci, 2002**).

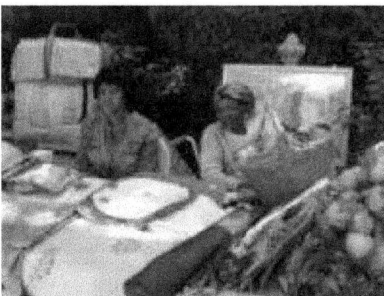

This program espouses and practices the importance of individualizing the therapy (**Willer & Corrigan, 1994**). A comprehensive pre-screening process is undertaken to provide an outcomes-based program that is relevant and applicable to the client. The founder feels that the program is a dynamic project as opposed to a service "to keep disabled persons busy". It is a program of inclusiveness; thus there is the expectation that the ABI survivors maximize their capacities, not their deficits.

The underlying philosophy is to have clients become self-sufficient. This is done by encouraging clients to reintegrate themselves slowly to their community of origin and their family through a re-engineered environment and while taking on an identity of value such as feeling good, loved, and of value. Self-sufficiency may be best expressed in a re-developed environment since it is safe way for clients to experiment with their newly acquired social skills and receive feedback in a non-threatening situation (**Sloan, Winkler, & Callaway, 2004**).

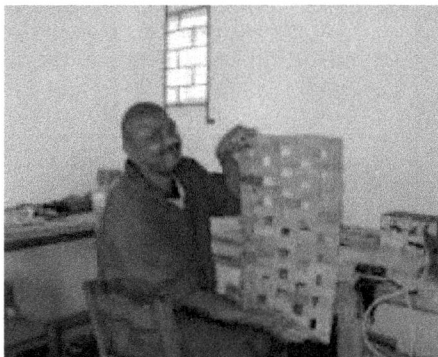

The Simply Sustaining program's goals are:

➤ To be able to produce items for sale which could finance the mentors and community coordinators.

➤ To create a workable option for the state-based auto insurance fund to use for survivors of motor vehicle accidents. Short term rehabilitation is offered within the state hospital system as part of the insurance claim, however it is less than 3 weeks. For ABI there is no state based rehabilitation. Only the private sector currently offers rehabilitation services within privately funded hospitals.

➤ To modify ABI survivors' behaviours and neuro-psychological function through real-life interpersonal situations in order to facilitate their integration into the group

➤ To teach novel skills and to remediate learned skills in ABI survivors through 'real life' activities/tasks/projects

➤ To educate both the survivors and families of the survivors that post-acute rehabilitation is within the capacity of non-medical people.

➤ To provide a workable model for duplication in other rural areas where there are plenty of skills, many ABI survivors and little formal employment opportunities among locals.

Sustainability has been successful by slowly training and incorporating responsibility of running the program to local members of the community. These individuals become community coordinators and mentors (mentors have less responsibility than community coordinators)—an arrangement which has been found to be most effective in developing community participation strategies. Local community members once trained as mentors, and who then move up to become community coordinators, are found to be able to successfully manage and confidently serve members of their community who are survivors of ABI.

Since the program espouses a non-medical rehabilitation service, the criteria for admission requires potential clients to be medically stable. The structure of the rehabilitation is to provide opportunities for:

A transitional facility to bridge the gap between the hospital bed and home

Living in an environment with reduced stimulation
and maximum space

Experiencing consistency of management with graded exposure to new
stimuli through one care-giver and / or primary rehabilitation therapist

A gradual shift in responsibility for rehabilitation from the medical model
to the client / family as the primary caregiver

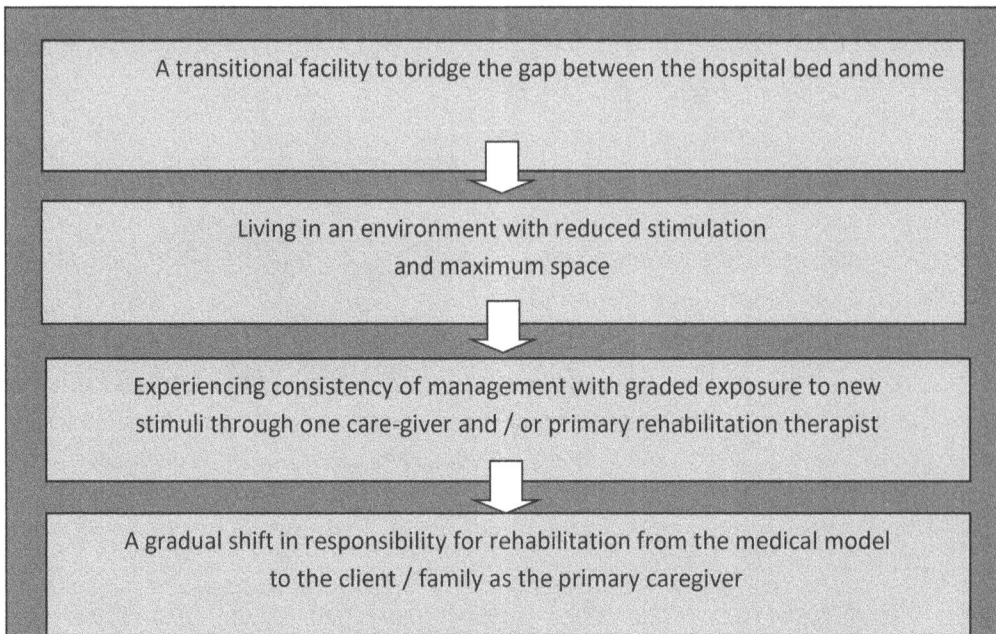

Figure 1 : Goals of the Simply Sustaining rehabilitation project

Community and Social Reintegration

Adaptability. The social reintegration component, in addition to the workshops provided, is fostered by extending therapy to the clients in their own homes (or an elder care facility, if they are placed in one). In this way the clients are able to re-learn, problem solve, and take on the skills within their own contexts and environment. The program also tries to make connections with other social programs that the client may also be associated with in order to build partnerships and mutual support.

Business Training. Locally skilled but non-professional community co-ordinators begin to take a larger responsibility within the program after receiving therapy training. The aim is to have community coordinators take over the responsibilities of bridging the client to their working communities by creating an actual business structure with a focus on encouraging punctuality and task completion. Throughout thisis approach lies

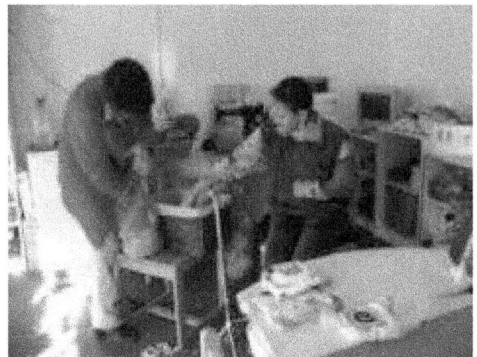

the principle of improving the clients' functional abilities and the development of client capacity –different from the traditional rehabilitation approach which may focus on the clients' deficits as opposed to strengths.

Redeveloping socially acceptable skills. The therapy itself is tailored to the clients' interests and functional capacity with lots of opportunity to meet other clients and work in a buddy system overseen by a community mentor/coordinator. Since the program is small and has approximately ten clients at any given time, there is more opportunity for community bonding and forming of relationships. Through these working relationships, social interactions, and team work clients are able to go through real-life interpersonal situations, find supportive and safe avenues to learn socially acceptable skills when encountering social conflict, and are better facilitated by their mentors to integrate into the group. Furthermore, the development and learning of problem-solving strategies becomes more successful when clients are placed in relevant and applicable contexts of everyday situations and functional activities (see Box 1).

Box 1

Sam* is a 38-year-old client of the Simply Self-Sustaining program. He was injured at 32 years of age in a motorcycle crash and has been wheelchair bound since injury, incontinent and neglected by his caregivers. His injury also left him with a non-functional right upper limb, athetoid (a stream of slow, sinuous, writhing movements), and telegraphic speech (shorter than 5 words in a sentence). Sam was aggressive and oppositional, and since he had been lying in bed most of the time, he did not want to be mobilized.

Interventions were prioiritized according to the Sam's functional needs and capabilities. Knowing that he was a jazz musician and a qualified motor mechanic, goals were developed for Sam so he could eventually play his instruments, use the computer, have a sense of autonomy, develop continence, use his right arm again, have more upright posture, establish respect among his peers, and eventually walk.

A local community member first worked on helping Sam re-learn continence. Knowing he was fond of music, Sam was allowed to listen to music on the computer, which is in the computer room, next to the seamstress. The toilet is also equally close. At first, a timer was set every hour for toilet visits. When the seamstress heard the timer, she assisted Sam to 'walk' to the toilet and then back to the computer. She also took Sam to her family for the evening meal, where he played chess with her adult son. Through this mentorship relationship, it took 4 weeks for Sam to discontinue using diapers during the day. He now calls to go to the toilet, is continent of bowel movements and walks (with some assistance, using the railing and at times with the help of the seamstress) between the computer room and toilet. On the weekend, a local 75-year-old who plays the mouthorgan and the guitar comes to play music with him. Sam will start to learn to re-experience music using the mouthorgan using his left hand first. As there is a tradition in the small community of respecting the elders, Sam will not refuse to do what the older man asks. In time the program coordinator will try to teach Sam how to pluck the guitar using his left hand. It is hoped that Sam will eventually be part of a music group.

(*name has been changed)

Extending problem-solving strategies to everyday circumstances and in authentic settings is recommended as an effective intervention in community reintegration and functional skill development among a meta analysis of 17 studies assessing intervention strategies (**Cicerone et al., 2005**). In her practice, Alison finds that the most effective way to develop community participation is for clients to feel acknowledged as part of a group and to have an opportunity for learning which gives them the chance of improving their positions in the community.

Production of goods

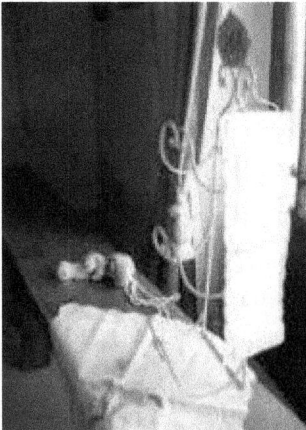

Workshops led by community coordinators are held to help clients learn a valuable skill, as both a vehicle for the reintegration of the client into society and as a vehicle for behaviour modification. The workshops also run along business lines in order to run efficiently. For instance a specific task may be required for making a soccer ball, such as sewing the final flap of the ball after being stuffed. This task is performed by one individual, as repetition improves functional capacity, confidence in performance, and efficiently creates the soccer balls that will be sold in the market. The goods produced need to be able to compete in the market (of items produced by able-bodied individuals) and make a profit, thereby feeding funds back into program and continuing the cycle of purchasing material to make more goods, employing the community coordinators, and maintaining the facilities to sustain the program.

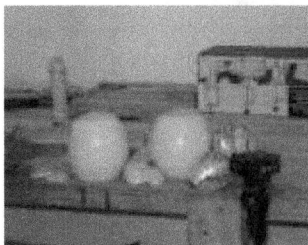

The most successful way to have clients learn a skill is to find a service and match it with the clients' capacities (**Sloan, Winkler, & Callaway, 2004**; **Willer & Corrigan, 1994**). Rather than trying to fit the client to the product, the product's tasks are matched with the client's abilities. Understanding the disability is an important aspect in matching the work to individual. Simply Self-Sustaining tries to market its items with a label to promote the production value of the item. This is done by outlining the uniqueness of an item created by people with an acquired brain injury. Not only can this help sell the items, it also highlights the remarkable capacities of survivors of ABI within societies (see Box 2).

Box 2

Condom demonstrators are distributed throughout sub-saharan Africa for education about AIDS. Community coordinators with woodworking skills cut these condom demonstrators at the sawmill using a lathe and a template; clients then finish each piece by sanding, varnishing, and apply a stamp to each one. In order for clients to perform the work safely, the condom demonstrators are drilled down with a guard and a support to hold them upright. The finishing tasks are repetitive, safe, and physically manageable. The men who are responsible for fulfilling these orders are vigilant about quality; they regulate their work to accommodate the time line, and they are able to explain to the community and visitors the importance of this item in healthcare.

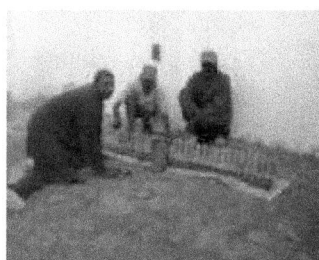

Underlying the premise of producing marketable goods, the program is able to meet its aims by being able to:

➢ Teach clients what constitutes socially appropriate behaviour

➢ Help clients facilitate and increase of self awareness

➢ Develop an appropriate skill for the client which may be transferred back to their community of origin

➢ Better facilitate the re-integration of the client into their family and society

➢ Assist families and caregivers by providing the clients with a raison d'être

One of the ways the program tries to establish a respectful environment is by helping clients recognize appropriate behaviours for their employment and work placements. This is encouraged by mandating a contract for employment for both the clients and community co-coordinators that includes:

➢ A clear set of expectations for acceptable behaviour

➢ A clear set of expectations for task completion

➢ Dichotomous choices of tasks to be offered for the clients

➢ Upholdment of the equality of gender, race, creed and language

➢ Respect for the equipment, peers, staff and oneself

➢ Confidentiality

➢ Opportunity for discussion/arbitration during times of conflict resolution

Although clients are required to participate within a certain amount of imposed structure—such as the respect for other people, controlling his or her temper, having a tea break at a given certain time—these structural constraints are seen as ways to help the client learn about and respect organizational behaviour rules in order to ensure that all of the clients are able to benefit from the program. Community reintegration programs that understand the importance of providing respectful practices and services are recommended to explicitly communicate and post the clients' and staff rights and expectations (Willer & Corrigan, 1994).

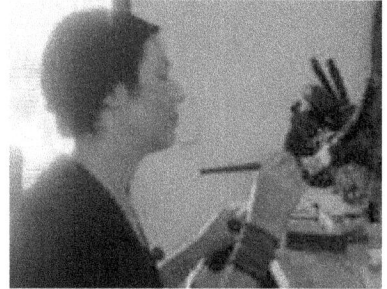

Program Challenges

The program founder currently feels that there are two important items lacking in the Simply Sustaining project. One is regular contracts for work in the rural areas and the other is having a person who can market the products. Furthermore, although community coordinators are found to be equipped to manage the integration process for the clients into their communities, they also need to develop the confidence to take on the management of the small businesses from the goods that they create with the client.

Possible Expansion

Despite these challenges, the program has shown promise and a beneficial impact for the people with ABI as well as local community members who volunteer or are employed with the program. The founder has a proposal underway to duplicate the program in other rural areas where there is high unemployment yet a large number of skilled individuals.

Program model within a Canadian context

There is some interest in being able to replicate this model within Ontario for January 2012, however, the founder is adamant that for such a program to work successfully, it can only be run and operated within a rural community. A small town close to Niagara Falls is being considered as a possible site since the town is large enough to have resources for its local community. These resources include a hospital, a grocery store, and a local market. The town is also small enough that local community members interact with each other on a continuing basis and may be more willing to support and collaborate with a small, post-acute program. One of the conditions for such a program to work successfully is investment from the local community. This would entail helping build, run, and maintain the facilities since most of the resources would have to come from the local community members themselves. The program in return helps the local community members by providing skilled training, jobs, and meaningful roles for both themselves and clients with ABI. Also clients can only feel genuinely part of their local communities if the local towns people are sympathetic individuals who are willing to absorb the responsibility of including and supporting these members into their community activities.

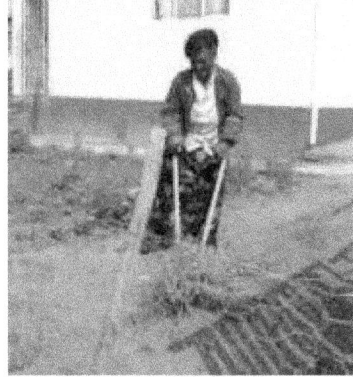

OUTCOME

The Simply Self-Sustaining System has made a substantial, positive impact on the lives of those who have participated in the program. This is noticed from qualitative accounts by survivors of ABI and from the testimonials of the community coordinators. There have also been a noticeable improvements in the behavioural restructuring of the clients, the development of skills, and greater reports of satisfaction from clients in terms of community integration and participation. Evidence for this has been documented in a short video clip that has been created to give a glimpse of the work the Simply Self-Sustaining project does from the perspective of its clients. The theme song is written by a former client and features members who are current mentors and/or former clients of the program.

Currently, formal outcome measures have not been developed and employed to be able to systematically assess the success of the program. Alison feels that rehabilitation, especially in the acute care of some of the private hospitals in South Africa, has too commonly been understood to require the use of measurable outcomes, such the **Functional Independence Measure** (FIM). She feels a limitation with the over reliance of using such measurable outcome instruments is that such scales do not take into consideration the cognitive, social, and emotional aspects of therapy for people with ABI. There is also some debate whether systemic assessment measures can accurately capture whether clients are adequately reintegrated into their communities given that many measures are found to be culturally irrelevant and/or insensitive (**Sander, Clark, & Pappadis, 2010**). Since no two individuals with ABI or TBI are equivalent, there is debate whether standardized measures are authentically able to measure the effectiveness of such rehabilitation programs (**Gordon, et al., 2006**). Nonetheless measures assessing outcomes of the program are currently being explored. The program founder is available for contact for more information as the program continues to develop and further integrate into the community it largely serves. A case study of a client who had sustained a severe brain injury is available in Box 3.

Box 3: Case Study of Mrs. McDillon

Mrs. McDillon was involved in a motor vehicle crash in May of 2009 in which she sustained a severe head injury requiring extensive rehabilitation. She was first hospitalized and then transferred for rehabilitation. It was evident that Mrs. McDillon was handled in an aggressive manner, since it was difficult to prompt and initiate reaction from her. There were also signs of neglect and exploitation. At the time of the assessment she had not yet established continuous recall of events and was only intermittently aware of the fact that she had been involved in an accident. She remained passive during social interactions, and the quality of her attention was varied and deteriorated markedly with increased fatigue, strain, and length of task. Mobility was also limited and she required assistance to walk. Communication was not spontaneous and she needed prompting to offer an opinion or a response. It was difficult for Mrs. McDillon to perform complex tasks, and she would become confused and frustrated quite easily. She had relatively little functional use of the left hand and arm and did not use it supportively unless requested to do so. She was not independent as far as bowel and bladder management were concerned, and this was felt to be due to her impaired immediate memory function.

Mrs. McDillon had been a teacher for most of her working life, which was estimated to be about 35 years. Interests that were immediately noted were that during the day she practised writing and calculations, watched TV, read and visited friends. At the time of assessment she was medicated to reduce agitation and to facilitate sleep. After performing some psychometric data and neuro-psychological batteries, it was noticed that the best way to support Mrs. McDillon was to have tasks that were relatively brief in order to not stress her. Pre-trauma personality characteristics such as discipline, high expectations, accuracy and politeness were evident in the assessment and it was difficult to interrupt her thought processes when she was busy with a task. She remained determined and motivated throughout the assessment.

After participating in the Simply Self- Sustaining project working alongside the community coordinators, she has shown a remarkable improvement in her functional as well as her social and emotional well being. Modifying behaviour was the first approach taken with Mrs.

McDillon in order to encourage socially preferred behaviour and change behaviour that was socially destructive. This was done through creating a daily social integrated routine for her while she received physiotheraphy to help with better functional mobility. Her carers also recieved training on her capacities and on strategies to better integrate her within her social settings. Specific scripts for taking instruction and eating were also used to help Mrs. McDillon target the priority of the behaviour problems that hindered her social reintegration. Once Mrs. McDillon was more receptive to the community coordinators and the people around her, she was introduced to the workshops that not only helped with creating goods for the market, but also with social reintegration and the strengthening of her functional abilities.

Still currently a client twelve months into the program, Mrs. McDillon now uses a quadrapod (a stick with 4 legs) instead of being bound to a wheelchair, is continent and needs only occasional assistance with dressing. Mrs. McDillon can dress independently, read topical items such as the bible and magazines, and enjoys singing, playing cards and drafts. And although she responds very well to familiar tasks, people, and prompts, she still finds it difficult to initiate conversation (but proudly gave a speech at her son's wedding). She responds very well to routine, which serves to generate more activities. She is now initiates tasks independently without prompts and offers to help others.

Mrs. McDillon's independent living skills include washing and drying dishes, cooking simple foods under supervision, shopping, using cutlery to eat independently, cleaning up the table, having greater independent mobility, having a greater sense of hygiene and sewing using a manual sewing machine. Her emotional well being also has improved greatly as she is now able to communicate emotions, effectively express herself, shows more positive emotion and general well being, and is not passive as she initially was. She enjoys socializing with the local community members, staff,and clients at the program, and is a regular contributing member of the program, spending everyday from 9:00 am to 5:00 pm participating in the workshops for unilateral tasks. She has begun to mentor some clients based on her familiarity of the program and workshop tasks. Her future plans is to purchase a home near the facility and live with a community of 3 to 4 people who are able to supervise her in her daily living activities, and to continue contributing the program.

Conclusion

The Simply Self-Sustaining System program is designed to help survivors of ABI develop their capacity and strengths, and steering away from the deficit hypothesis of traditional rehabilitation programs that focus on lifelong dependency. Although clients may not be able to fully recover, the philosophy of this program would maintain that clients with brain injury do not have brain "damage" but rather a slightly different brain and way of thinking. The program involves providing workshops delivered by local community members who simultaneously are able to help with strengthening the functional abilities of the clients while socially integrating them by testing and learning problem-solving strategies in relevant settings. Clients also learn new skills and develop their capabilities and confidence while the local community members are given employment opportunities by teaching clients new skills, appreciating their roles and values within their communities, and becoming partners in the therapy program. Clients develop autonomy in their lives and find meaningful roles in their local communities. The program was briefly featured in a national television program called Carteblanche in South Africa (2nd clip of the episode).

References

Ashley, M. J., Persel, C. S., & Krych, D. K. (1997). Longterm outcome follow-up of post acute traumatic brain injury rehabilitation: An assessment of functional and behavioural measures of daily living. *Journal of Rehabilitation Outcomes Measurement, 1,* 40-47.

Arnstein, S. R. (1969). **A ladder of citizen participation**. *Journal of the American Planning Association, 35*(4), 216-224.

Cicerone, K. D., Dahlberg, C., Malec, J. F., Langenbahn, D. M., Felicetti, T., Kneipp, S., Catanese, J. (2005). **Evidence-based cognitive rehabilitation: Updated review of the literature from 1998 through 2002**. *Archives of Physical Medicine and Rehabilitation,* 86, 1681-1692.

Condeluci, A. (2002). **The Process of Cultural Shifting. Cultural Shifting: Community, Leadership and Change.** Florida: Training Resource Network Press.

Dikmen, S., Machamer, J., & Temkin, N. (1993). Psychosocial outcome in patients with moderate to severe head injury: 2 year follow-up. **Brain Injury,** *7*(2), 113-124.

Doig, E., Fleming, J., & Tooth, L. (2001). Patterns of community integration 2-5 years post-discharge from brain injury rehabilitation. **Brain Injury,** *15*, 747-762.

Gordon, W. A., Zafonte, R., Cicerone, K., Cantor, J., Brown, M., Lombard, L., Chandna, T. (2006**). Traumatic brain injury rehabilitation**. *American Journal of Physical Medicine & Rehabilitation, 85(*4), 343-382.

Mitchell, R., (1999). The research base of community-based rehabilitation. *Disability and Research, 21*(10), 459-468.

Sander, A. M., Clark, A., & Pappadis, M. R. (2010). **What Is Community integration anyway?: Defining meaning following traumatic brain injury**. *Journal of Head Trauma Rehabilitation, 25*(2), 121-127.

Sloan, S., Winkler, D., & Callaway, L. (2004). **Community integration following severe traumatic brain injury: Outcomes and best practice**. *Brain Impairment, 5*(1), 12-29.

Volpe, R. (2010). *An outcomes framework for the ABI community of practice: Development and uses.* Centre for Community Based Research for the Ontario Neurotrauma Foundation.

Willer, B., & Corrigan, J. (1994). Whatever it takes: A model for community-based services. **Brain Injury**, *8*(7), 647-659.

CHAPTER 6

COMMUNITY HEAD INJURY RESOURCE SERVICES (CHIRS)

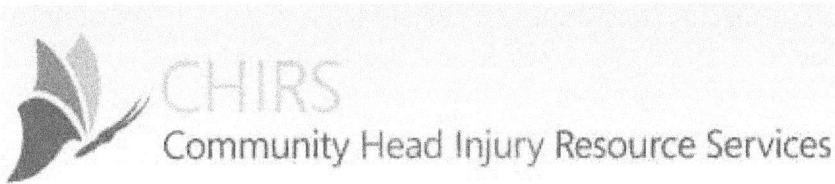

By Danielle Hryniewicz

Population Served : Life Span	
Contributing Author Contact Information	
Hedy Chandler	Carolyn Lemsky
Executive Director	Clinical Director
CHIRS	CHIRS
62 Finch Avenue West	62 Finch Avenue West
Toronto, Ontario M2N 7G1	Toronto, Ontario M2N 7G1
416-240-8000	416-240-8000
416-240-1149 (fax)	416-240-1149 (fax)
hedyc@chirs.com	**clemsky@chirs.com**

BACKGROUND

Community Head Injury Resource Services (CHIRS), formerly known as Ashby House, was founded in 1978 as the first community-based brain injury rehabilitation program in North America. Dr. Mira Ashby, a hospital social worker whose "pioneering efforts" (H. Chandler, personal communication, March 18, 2010) contributed to the foundation of the Ashby House, recognized a need for continued community support for persons with acquired brain injuries (ABI) discharged from the hospital. Prior to the foundation of the Ashby House (CHIRS), few resources for people with ABI existed (H. Chandler, personal communication, March 18, 2010).

From its origins as a transitional group home, **CHIRS** has evolved into a multi-service agency that provides a broad range of supports to an adult clientele (aged 18-60) with diverse and complex needs (H. Chandler, personal communication, March 18, 2010). Both adults with ABI and their families are included within CHIRS' target population.

Guiding Philosophy

CHIRS provides services for persons who have sustained an acquired brain injury (ABI), based on the following principles: 1) All individuals have a right to education, a secure home life of their own choosing, and opportunities for meaningful work and recreation; 2) All individuals have the right to be supported on the basis of their own unique needs and abilities; 3) Services must be sufficiently flexible, adaptable and secure in terms of adjusting to the individual's personal choice and need for learning and adaptation; 4) Services, supports, and life opportunities must be provided to correspond as much as possible with the individual's community environment and in a manner which enhances the individual's well-being, dignity, self-respect, and physical and emotional security; 5) Individuals should have access to the full range of experiences offered by their community; and, 6) Individuals develop as full citizens and responsible community members only when supported to direct their lives and destinies through their own interests, aspirations, and links with the community (**CHIRS, n.d.**).

CHIRS Staff

CHIRS staff members receive intensive on-site training where they learn about client support, community-based participation, agency systems, and procedures. Within the first three months, CHIRS employees attend an orientation training session where they are introduced to the agency's philosophy and approach to service. They also receive training in brain injury anatomy, brain functions, sexuality and brain injury, crisis prevention and intervention, infectious diseases, First Aid and CPR, **Workplace Hazardous Materials Information System** (WHMIS), family-centred service, and clinical-based skills such as "Collaboration, Communication, Brain and Behaviour" (**CHIRS, n.d.**).

Decision making and planning

Clients and their families play a large role in the planning of services and supports. Clients who receive community support services participate in an annual service plan meeting—attended by the client, his/her significant others, and **CHIRS** support staff—in which goals for the next year are discussed and an individual plan of service is created.

Service planning is built into each step of the referral process. The formal process of creating a "Service Plan" involves a comprehensive assessment of the client's goals and needs. Service Plan teams may include any or all of the following: the individual, family members, friends, employers, volunteers, case managers, funders, attorney, **CHIRS** staff (Service Coordinator, Primary Worker and any other staff member deemed appropriate—e.g., Behaviour Therapist, Social Worker, Program Director, and Employment Specialist), partnering or consulting agencies or individuals—e.g., Home Care, Corbrook, Neuropsychiatric Clinic). Service Plan meetings review past progress or recent assessments, and establish long-term rehabilitation and support goals for the next few years of service. For a new client, the content of the initial Service Plan documents the recommendations made in the CHIRS Assessment Report. Subsequent Service Plan Meetings take place on an annual basis (unless a request to meet more frequently is made by **CHIRS**, the individual, or the family). The format for these meetings follows a process similar to the initial Service Plan Meeting, in which the recommendations of the **CHIRS** assessment report are reviewed. Sources of information may include the individual, participants, update reports, and additional assessments.

Every client that accesses services through **CHIRS** has a different set of goals, as well as different strengths and needs, that direct the nature of the support he/she receives. Consequently, the process of service planning and goal documenting is critical to ensuring that support services are appropriate and beneficial.

Services

Several community-based services and supports are provided by **CHIRS. Ashby Community Support Services (ACSS)** offers support to clients within the community. Staff support is provided to clients on a one-to-one or group basis, as ACSS staff work with clients, their families, and many other community partners. Assistance is provided in the areas of home management, personal management, education, and employment (H. Chandler, personal communication, March 18, 2010).

Adult Day Services (ADS) affords a wide variety of social, recreation and skill-building programs to meet the needs and interests of its participants. These programs are developed and planned in collaboration with program participants and staff. Programs are run in accessible locations across the city in order to minimize travel and assist clients in getting to know the resources within their local communities. Many of the programs are run in partnership with local organizations and private businesses. These relationships are mutually beneficial in allowing participants to try new programs and in helping to create a profile for brain injury within the greater community. One of the unique components of the service is the **CHIRS** "Club", which provides both structured activities and a drop-in centre housed at one central location. Members are encouraged to stay for lunch and socialize with peers and community members in a less structured setting (H. Chandler, personal communication, March 18, 2010).

Education Support Services (ESS) assists clients in participating in a variety of work and learning opportunities. Education supports include the following activities: working with clients to research educational resources in the community, interviewing potential instructors, providing information and education regarding acquired brain injury, conducting in-class assessments and recommendations for accommodations, and providing both in-class and tutorial support (H. Chandler, personal communication, March 18, 2010).

Family Centered Services provide services to **CHIRS** clients and their families. Both **Individual and Family Counselling** (social work counselling and support to assist the client and family with adjustments related to the brain injury) and **Family Support Group** (an informal group for family members to share experiences and resources, problem solve together, and give and receive support) are offered. With respect to the latter, guest speakers occasionally join the Family Support Group to facilitate discussion of topics relevant to family members. A variety of topics are discussed including adjusting to role changes, understanding the cognitive changes of brain injury, and balancing family member needs with the needs of the individual with the ABI. The Family Support Group meets monthly (H. Chandler, personal communication, March 18, 2010).

Aging at Home directly addresses the needs of seniors who are caregivers in their own homes of adults with ABI. It is an innovative approach to providing a menu of support, respite, information, and education to aging caregivers of adult children with an ABI, while offering highly specialized ABI support services to adults with an ABI. The goal of these services is to prevent caregiver and patient morbidity, and preserve the integrity of the families served (H. Chandler, personal communication, March 18, 2010).

Residential Services, or long-term, supportive housing options, are provided by **CHIRS**. The Residential Team works collaboratively with the client, his/her family, clinical consultants, and Adult Day Services to deliver comprehensive, individualized programs and support. Residential Services are provided at three Toronto sites, each site offering different degrees of support (H. Chandler, personal communication, March 18, 2010).

Clinical Services are offered by CHIRS' consulting Neuropsychiatrist, Neuropsychologist, and occupational therapist. **CHIRS** clinicians provide internal consultations to address the needs of clients (as they arise), and to provide leadership to support teams.

CHIRS' **Substance Use and Brain Injury Program (SUBI)** is supervised by the neuropsychologist and co-led by a trained substance abuse counsellor (provided by the Centre for Addictions and Mental Health) and a CHIRS community support worker. SUBI aims to develop initial treatment alternatives for clients of **CHIRS**, whose cognitive impairments precluded their treatment in mainstream substance use programs. SUBI's cost-effective case-management model facilitates early substance use interventions by ABI network agencies (CHIRS, n.d.). Participation within each service is often ongoing (C. Lemsky, personal communication, June 30, 2011).

RESOURCES

Financial Resources

In 1978, at the time the Ashby House was founded, an operating budget of approximately $78,000 supported program operations. Under the leadership of Hedy Chandler, CHIRS' current Executive Director, funding was sought and received from the Province of Ontario. **CHIRS** now operates on an annual budget of approximately $7,500,000. A strategic planning exercise, renewed every 5 years, assists in guiding and sustaining growth (H. Chandler, personal communication, March 18, 2010).

Over the years, CHIRS' funding has moved from the **Ministry of Community and Social Services** to the **Ministry of Health and Long-Term Care**. Although the "provincial players" (H. Chandler, personal communication, March 18, 2010) have changed, a few of the same families that were instrumental in the development of Ashby House continue to provide input into the current services. A close partnership with the **Toronto ABI Network** also helps **CHIRS** collaborators and stakeholders to respond to the needs of the community (H. Chandler, personal communication, March 18, 2010). From a sociocultural standpoint, CHIRS collaborators and stakeholders are provided with educational and practical resources by which to address sociocultural considerations (relevant to their clients) across the lifespan.

Presently, the **Ministry of Health and Long-Term Care**and the **Central Local Health Integration Network** (LHIN) provide financial support and a base budget that limits the number of clients **CHIRS** is able to support (H. Chandler, personal communication, March 18, 2010). The **Ontario Neurotrauma Foundation** (ONF) has provided direct support to the **Substance Use and Brain Injury Program** (SUBI), enabling the development of the SUBI materials and a provincial Community of Practice. Likewise, the Ontario Disabilities Support program provides support to CHIRS' vocational program.

CHIRS has recently expanded its service to include specialized **Adult Day Programs**, **Residential** options, Outreach Support, employment opportunities, **recreation and leisure programs**, as well as and neuropsychological services.

Human Resources

The stakeholders of the program include individuals with an ABI and their families, the Ontario **Ministry of Health and Long-Term Care**, and the five Greater Toronto Area **Local Health Integration Networks**. At the time of program development and implementation, stakeholders faced several issues. Central to these issues was an observed lack of community programs and supports for individuals who had sustained an ABI in the Toronto area (H. Chandler, personal communication, March 18, 2010).

Similarly, the **Substance Use and Brain Injury Program** (SUBI) was formed by Dr. Carolyn Lemsky, CHIRS clinical director, in collaboration with Dr. Dennis James (deputy clinical director, addictions program) and Dr. Tim Godden (advanced practice clinician, addictions program) of the **Centre for Addiction and Mental Health** (CAMH). Prior to SUBI, clients with ongoing detrimental substance use were not optimally served by either CAMH or CHIRS (H. Chandler, personal communication, March 18, 2010).

CHIRS provides leadership in the development of brain injury services across the province and participates in regional and provincial planning for government-funded ABI services. Through its involvement and partnerships within the larger community, CHIRS strives to provide productive and meaningful activities for all participants. CHIRS is affiliated with a number of organizations, which include The Directors' Network, The Ontario **Association of Community-based Boards for Acquired Brain Injury Services** (OACBABIS),

Provincial ABI Advisory Committee (PABIAC), **Toronto ABI Network** and its many subcommittees, **Scarborough Chamber of Commerce**, North York Chamber of Commerce, **Ontario Non-Profit Housing Association**, **Brain Injury Society of Toronto**, **Ontario Brain Injury Association**, Neurological Services Planning Group, **Active Living Alliance for Canadians with a Disability**, **Parks and Recreation Ontario**, Ontario Rehabilitation and Work Council, **Toronto Board of Trade**, **JOIN**, Ontario Alliance for Action on Brain Injury, and **Bloorview Kids ABI Program**.

IMPLEMENTATION

In addressing the perceived lack of community programs, a grass roots movement, led by Dr. Mira Ashby, designed individual **CHIRS** programs which fostered community participation and support (H. Chandler, personal communication, March 18, 2010). For example, the Continuum of Vocational Placements was developed by CHIRS program managers. This program has resulted in numerous community collaborations, including charitable groups and commercial enterprises (e.g., IKEA and Sheridan nurseries).

Program Registration and Intake

An application to **CHIRS** can be made through the **Toronto Acquired Brain Injury Network** (TABIN). TABIN offers a single point referral service to publicly funded member agencies, including hospital-based brain injury rehabilitation, long-term care facilities, and community-based services in Toronto (**CHIRS, n.d.**).

A recent neuropsychological assessment and/or rehabilitation team report such as occupational therapy, physiotherapy, and speech pathology, are required as part of the intake process. Any other reports relevant to the service requested are also valued in order to help determine support needs. Once the completed application and supporting documentation have been provided to **CHIRS**, an Intake staff arranges a meeting with the individual requesting service and their support network (professionals and/or family members). This meeting provides an opportunity for information sharing (**CHIRS, n.d.**).

The request for participation is then presented to the Intake Committee to determine whether CHIRS has the appropriate resources to meet the individual's needs. The Committee may also suggest alternative resources and/or make appropriate referrals, if necessary (**CHIRS, n.d.**).

CHIRS offers subsidized services, funded through the Ministry of Health and Long-Term Care, to eligible individuals. Given CHIRS' limited resources, there may be a waiting period depending on the service requested. **CHIRS** also offers services on a Fee for Service basis to individuals with access to private funding. A proposal outlining services and cost is submitted to the payer for authorization prior to services commencing (CHIRS, n.d.).

Ashby Community Support Services

The **Ashby Community Support Services** (ACSS) program provides highly specialized Employment and Education Services, assisting clients to participate in a variety of work and learning opportunities which challenge their unique abilities. An Employment Preparation Workshop is offered to clients interested in exploring job readiness skills and competitive employment potential in an interactive, group setting. The workshop focuses on educating clients on CHIRS' supported employment model, practical interviewing techniques, resume preparation, presentation skills, work site behaviours, and compensation strategies.

In conjunction with the Supported Employment Program, a CHIRS' Job Developer works with clients to determine their areas of interest and to design individualized work assessments enabling the client, his/her family, and CHIRS staff to assess their vocational skills. The Job Developer also undertakes an extensive job search, partnering with interested community employers (H. Chandler, personal communication, March 18, 2010). Positions are individually designed to ensure a match between a client's strengths and the employer's needs. Once a client obtains a placement, a trained Job Coach provides a variety of work site supports to assist the client in learning his/her job and maintaining employment. Work site supports can include travel training, job-site and task analyses, ongoing assessment, the development of individualized strategies, employer education, social skills training, and other such supports relevant to human development within the physical environment. "Fading of supervision" at the job site is initiated when individuals, employers, and CHIRS agree that a person has demonstrated the ability to perform the job over a consistent period of time (CHIRS, n.d.)

Adult Day Service

The **Adult Day Services (ADS)** program is an offshoot of the residential program. It provides productive adult employment through mentorship and volunteer opportunities, and offsite opportunities to clients who have expressed an interest in working within the community (though may not be able to secure and maintain regular employment within the community).

Mentorship

Clients are able to volunteer their time around the **ADS** Club to see what strengths and interests they have. Having volunteered, they are invited to become mentors, and may assist with the lunch preparation, club coverage (i.e., greeting new members of the Club, helping others to feel welcome, assisting with the gardening) and operations of the Club. Supervisors help to review goals and determine what each mentor would like to do, on an ongoing basis (C. Lemsky, personal communication, June 30, 2011).

The **ADS** model is loosely based on the **Clubhouse Model**. It differs from the Clubhouse Model in that it has been adapted to promote autonomy and ownership without a vocational end point. Purposeful activity, inside of pension restraints, is facilitated by ADS (C. Lemsky, personal communication, June 30, 2011).

Offsite Programming

Offsite programming is designed to launch clients into the community—(individual) participation within adapted programs promotes community participation through the building of community connections and autonomy (C. Lemsky, personal communication, June 30, 2011).

The **ADS** program started organically; staff responded to client requests for community participation by forming/introducing programs and activities (such as CardSharks [a work-alternative craft program] and bowling), first within the organization and then outside of the organization. Community participants (e.g., IKEA) were invited to become involved in community-based programs developed by staff and clients, alike (C. Lemsky, personal communication, June 30, 2011). Within the years 1998-2000, additional office space became available and subsequent programs were developed. At this time, the "Club" was formed (where a small number of clients,15-20, attended 5-6 programs a week at the Etobicoke head office). Gradually, additional programs were added as interest was generated.

Using existing community partner relationships, the program expanded further in later years. Eventually, the majority of programs occurred offsite, in the community. The staff compliment present at **CHIRS** continued to develop and coordinate programs, as additional programs were added by service coordinators in charge of ADS (C. Lemsky, personal communication, June 30, 2011). As the entire CHIRS staff evolved, CHIRS (subsequently) expanded its ADS program to meet needs identified in the community. For example, clients asked for work programs and a partnership with IKEA soon developed. In the case of IKEA, CHIRS' practice of 'job carving'—in which a job is created to the stated specifications of an individual client—requires a job coach and a period of supervision (in some cases). A recycling job, for instance, was carved out for a former **CHIRS** client (C. Lemsky, personal communication, June 30, 2011).

Over the years, partnerships with other companies, including Sheridan Nurseries and Canadian Tire, have developed as the program's operating model has been expanded and adapted to different industries and sites. In forging community partnerships with companies, willing employers were identified and business models considered, in accordance with Wehmen et al.'s work on supported employment (1992, 1999).

Obstacles

The process of finding willing employers can be a challenging task. Perceptions of **CHIRS** as a palliative service create a significant obstacle for CHIRS staff to overcome. Stigmas related to ABI have proven to be obstacles in building partnerships with employers, community service agencies, and medical professions. To this end, staff members who seek to find willing employers must provide information regarding past clients and their successes within the employment sector (C. Lemsky, personal communication, June 30, 2011).

A significant barrier to program operations relates to WSIB regulations: insurance is required for a client who is working on an ongoing basis, yet WSIB is not willing to insure such clients. A second barrier pertains to restrictions placed on wage earning. At IKEA, for instance, clients are able to earn a maximum of $120 a month. Clients who wish to extend their participation within the community and earn more than $120 a month are unable to do so (C. Lemsky, personal communication, June 30, 2011).

Currently, **CHIRS** staff are looking at social enterprises and prospective partnerships within mental health to get around the **WSIB** and insurance issues previously noted. Although the program is no longer in operation, it has proven successful from the point of view that clients were able to achieve their personal goals, as outlined in client satisfaction surveys (C. Lemsky, personal communication, June 30, 2011).

Cultural and Diversity Issues

CHIRS has staff representation from many of the main cultural communities served. While clients are not matched based on culture, staff and community-based culture agencies are often called on to provide education and to help in assessing agency cultural competence. In the words of Hedy Chandler, "...our primary strategy is to partner with advocacy and cultural agencies" (H. Chandler, personal communication, March 18, 2010).

Toronto ABI Network

CHIRS maintains a waiting list and works with other service providers, networks, and associations to keep abreast of changes in policy, practice, and funding (H. Chandler, personal communication, March 18, 2010). In determining needs and gaps in service, and developing proposals to meet identified needs in the community, a close collaboration exists between **CHIRS** and various other members of the **Toronto Acquired Brain Injury Network**. The Toronto Acquired Brain Injury (ABI) Network, an umbrella organization of 17 partners in the city of Toronto, Ontario, attempts to create a cost-effective, seamless, efficient, and effective integrated system of service. The ABI Network includes a diverse array of organizations and agencies, from acute care inpatient to long-term care reintegration. The recent development of Network-wide best practices related to assessment and outcomes, and rooted in empirical evidence and current research, has resulted in enhanced consistency across programs, ensuring universal access to community-based efforts and interventions following brain injury (**Laan et al., 2001**). Sociocultural obstacles and barriers influenced by social class, ethnic membership, age, sex, and personal contacts are minimized through a network-based approach to service delivery.

CHIRS and PHABIS: Members of the Toronto ABI Network

A strong collaboration has been established between **CHIRS** and **PHABIS** (another non-profit charitable Ontario corporation providing community-based rehabilitation and re-integration services to people living with the effects of acquired brain injury). CHIRS and PHABIS are members of the Toronto ABI Network, Director's Network, and the Ontario Association of Community-Based Boards for ABI Services. The Executive Directors and Program Directors of both CHIRS and PHABIS meet a minimum of four times a year and sit on a number of common committees. Information regarding community-based initiatives and community participation is shared freely between each organization (H. Chandler, personal communication, Jul. 8, 2010).

OUTCOME

Data Collection and Evaluation

Client satisfaction surveys, constructed of five to seven questions, are disseminated (via email) once a year to clients of the **ADS** program. Clients are approached by persons who are not members of their care team and asked to complete the surveys by a scheduled date. A 50-70% response rate is typically yielded (C. Lemsky, personal communication, June 30, 2011).

Assessments are carried out by a staff member who is not involved in care and does not know the respondents. Once the results of the surveys are analyzed, internal reports are written. The results are communicated to staff by way of report cards. Previous surveys have indicated that clients wanted more employment opportunities. To this end, offsite opportunities were introduced and onsite work opportunities, including program management, development and implementation, were established (C. Lemsky, personal communication, June 30, 2011).

Measurement Criteria

Previous attempts to measure outcome have been unsuccessful in capturing client satisfaction and community integration. Previous attempts to measure outcome have been largely unsuccessful in capturing client satisfaction and community integration, as clients tend not to change once scoring on the standard community integration measures incorporated within 5-point scales. Given this fact, client satisfaction with services is the best measure of outcome. Client satisfaction is operationalized in terms of "respect", "community participation", "contentment with programming" and "client-centered care", among other things. Practical questions pertaining to cleanliness and fee structures are also included in the client satisfaction survey (C. Lemsky, personal communication, June 30, 2011).

Clinical statistics are collected on client goal attainment, use of ethical framework, and client complaints. Client safety data pertaining to falls, medication errors, incidents of choking, adverse events, and infectious diseases are also assessed.

Accreditation Status

CHIRS has successfully achieved and maintained full accreditation status for the past 12 years. CHIRS is evaluated against national standards in the areas of ABI Injury services, infection prevention and control, medication management, governance and effective leadership. Clinical services use goal attainment scaling to measure the effectiveness of service provision to clients (H. Chandler, personal communication, Jul. 8, 2010).

Short- and Long-term Outcomes

In the short-term, client outcomes are reviewed and compared against performance indicators on a quarterly basis. Targets are adjusted as required (H. Chandler, personal communication, Jul. 8, 2010).

Long-term outcomes, articulated in **CHIRS'** strategic plan, are operationalized and reflected in annual operational plans. Plans remain flexible in order to adjust priorities based on funding initiatives and directives from the Ministry. Current strategic plans include the following: supporting more clients and families, becoming a Centre of Excellence in Community-Based ABI Services, and building a capacity of external partners.

"Enabling foundations", or mechanisms by which to achieve strategic goals, include inspired teamwork, optimal environments to meet client needs, a safety and wellness culture, enhanced information and management systems, financial sustainability, and sound governance (H. Chandler, personal communication, Jul. 8, 2010).

Strategic Changes to Service Delivery

Within the satisfaction surveys, clients have noted that vocational services are especially important to them. In addressing this need, **CHIRS** has placed an increased emphasis on the provision of vocational services. ESS has recently received a funding increase to meet the needs of CHIRS' client base (H. Chandler, personal communication, March 18, 2010).

Unanticipated Positive or Negative Outcomes

Since CHIRS' inception, the manner of funding allocation has changed. At times, the **Ministry of Health and Long-term Care** (MOHLTC) provides individualized funding to prospective clientele. As a result, CHIRS must create spaces and individualized services for clients who are referred by MOHLTC. It has been observed that the allocation of funds might be better spent if it were spread across a range of people (instead of a concentrated few) (H. Chandler, personal communication, March 18, 2010).

Conclusion

CHIRS is a registered not-for-profit charitable organization in Toronto, Canada, primarily funded by the **Central Local Health Integration Network** (LHIN) through the Ontario **Ministry of Health and Long-term Care**. Formerly known as Ashby House, CHIRS started in 1978 as the first community-based brain injury rehabilitation program in North America. From its origins as a transitional group home, **CHIRS** has evolved into a multi-service agency that provides a broad range of supports to a clientele with diverse and complex needs. CHIRS' services are designed to form the basis of a comprehensive model of service delivery.

Two fundamental practices have been identified by **CHIRS** collaborators and stakeholders as best and/or effective practices. "Developing community participation strategies" and "measuring community participation" have proven effective in soliciting and representing the views of a diverse clientele. Individual goal attainment has proven to be the best outcome assessment by which to measure community participation. Client satisfaction surveys allow for individualized goals to be tracked in an objective fashion.

An emphasis on collaboration with clients in goal setting is placed upon client-staff interactions. **CHIRS** staff strive to find opportunities for clients to address their current goals in the community, while providing a structured environment where individual and interpersonal skills and supports can be "learned" or "honed" (H. Chandler, personal communication, March 18, 2010). Community supports and participation include working with individuals to research education resources in the community, interviewing potential instructors, providing information and education regarding acquired brain injury, conducting in-class assessments and recommendations for accommodations, and providing both in-class and tutorial support (**CHIRS, n.d.**).

REFERENCES

CHIRS. (n.d.). **CHIRS Client & Family Handbook**.

Laan, R. V., Brandy, C., Sullivan, I., & Lemsky, C. (2001). **Integration through a city-wide brain injury network and best practices project**. *NeuroRehabilitation*, 16, 17-26.

Wehman, P., Bricout, J. (1999). Supported employment: Critical issues and new directions. In G. Revell, K. J. Inge, D. Mank, & P. Wehman (Eds.), *The impact of supported employment for people with significant disabilities: preliminary findings from the National Supported Employment Consortium* (1-24). Richmond (VA): VCU-RRTC on workplace supports.

Wehman, P., & Kregel, J. (1992). Supported employment: Growth and impact. In P. Wehman, P. Sale & W. Parent (Eds.), *Supported employment. Strategies for integration of workers with disabilities*. Boston: Andover Medical Publishers.

CHAPTER 7

THE COMMUNITY APPROACH TO PARTICIPATION (CAP) MODEL FOR COMMUNITY INTEGRATION IN PEOPLE WITH ACQUIRED BRAIN INJURY

By Helen Looker

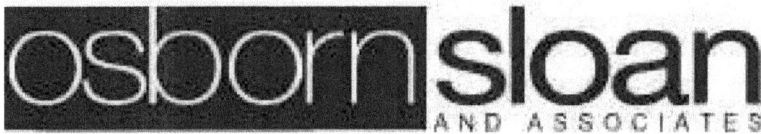

Population Served : Children & Adults with ABI	
Contributing Author Contact Information	
Sue Sloan Osborn, Sloan & Assoc. 97, Princess St., Kew, Victoria, 3101, Australia Phone: 03 9853 2638 Fax: 03 9855 1435 Email: **sue@osbornsloan.com.au** **http://www.osbornsloan.com.au** Libby Callaway Neuroskills Pty Ltd PO Box 310, Sandringham 3191 Phone: 9598 5122 Fax: 9598 5122 **libbycallaway@neuroskills.com.au**	Diane Winkler Summer Foundation PO Box 208, Blackburn, VIC 3130 Australia Phone:03 9894 7006 Fax: 03 8456 6325 **http://www.summerfoundation.org.au**

INTRODUCTION

In Australia, disability services have largely been developed to meet the needs of people with congenital disabilities. Policy and funding of services needed by the ABI population has been slow to align with the reality that many people with various forms of ABI live long lives and require disability support due to medical advances over the last 20 years. Complex care involving many different health care professional services may be needed by individuals for many decades. Once discharged from a hospital, ABI survivors must navigate the disability services system that is separate from the health care system (Winkler, personal communication, January 12, 2010). While 66% of resources for non-compensable disability funding in the State of Victoria, Australia is allocated for intellectual disability and 4% to ABI services, numbers of individuals with intellectual disability and ABI are similar, being 20% and 14%, respectively (**Kelly & Parry, 2008**).

A report published in 1991 by the **Transport Accident Commission** (TAC) found that the incidence of public hospital admissions for traumatic brain injury (TBI) in people aged less than 65 years-of-age was approximately 5,000 annually and that two thirds were aged less than 25 years, half of which were under 15 years-of-age, and that 71% were male. At this time, most needed services for people with ABI were inadequate, creating hardship, marginalization, and limiting opportunities for recovery for the ABI population (**Southern Health, July 2009**).

Insurance Policy

The **Transport Accident Commission** (TAC), governed by the *Transport Commission Act, 1986* to ensure that people who sustained transportation-related injuries get effective rehabilitation, is a scheme providing medical, rehabilitation, and disability service benefits on a no fault, needs-based basis. These benefits were expanded in 2002 moving to a comprehensive lifetime model that included additional elements to rebuild personal lives to the extent possible through inclusion of training, therapy, and supported long-term living that would be life-long, if necessary. This new model from TAC was person-centred and introduced a focus on community integration, outcomes for clients, and flexible community supports (**Transport Accident Commission, 2010; Sloan, 2008**).

Causes of ABI

There are multiple sources of brain injury across the life span attributable to trauma, disease such as encephalitis and meningitis, a result of surgery, instrumental birth, and medical pathology, for instance. Trauma includes accidents, falls, and assault. Brain injury can also be the result of substance abuse, near drowning, and attempted suicide. Oxygen starvation to the brain as a consequence of anaphylactic shock in reaction to a bee sting will also cause brain damage (**Southern Health, 2009**). In Australia, brain injury at, or acquired at birth generally falls under an intellectual disability status and any other cause post birth is defined within the "National community services data dictionary as:

> Multiple disabilities arising from damage to the brain acquired after birth. It results in deterioration in cognitive, physical, emotional or independent functioning. It can be as a result of accidents, stroke, brain tumours, infection, poisoning, lack of oxygen, degenerative neurological disease etc. (**AIHW 2009**)."

More than fifty-five percent of ABI cases in Australia, however, are caused as a result of traffic accidents at a ratio of somewhat greater than 2:1 for males and females, respectively (**Australian Institute of Health and Welfare, 2009**).

Health Effects

Although brain injury alters a person's life, life expectancy is relatively normal once acute trauma to the brain has subsided (**Lippert-Grüner, Maegele, Haverkamp, Klug & Wedekind, 2007**). ABI may result in new medical problems such as dementia, epilepsy, possible paralysis, heightened levels of fatigue, and impairment to senses such as hearing and vision. Cognitive changes can be profound, with concentration, memory, and executive functions often significantly impaired. Speech and the ability to use and comprehend language also present difficulties and emotional repercussions may be manifested in depression, anxiety, and mood instabilities (**Gordon, 2004: Southern Health, 2009**). Behavioural outcomes from ABI such as physical and verbal aggression, repetitiveness, loss of initiative/inhibition, and inappropriate social behaviour further complicate recovery (**Kelly & Parry, 2008**).

Challenging Behaviour

As a direct result of brain injury, or secondary sequelae, behaviour patterns may change dramatically and create problems in a person's life, altering the quality of life for an individual and those who interact with the person on a frequent basis. Many organizations providing services or care for the ABI population will not accept a client displaying high levels of challenging behaviour. Such behaviours that may benefit from a targeted intervention in a community setting include verbal outbursts, screaming, unwelcome sexual advances, and acting in an overtly familiar way to others. Violent behaviours, perhaps comorbid with pre-existing or secondary neuropsychiatric illness, may need intervention within a restrictive setting such as a specialized institution or neurobehavioural unit. The fact that in Victoria, Australia, 16% of all referrals to one behavioural consultancy service are clients who are an average of 20 years post injury shows the persistence of such problems and the chronic need for suitable therapy. Such clients also need repeat therapy to control behaviour as there is no evidence it can be eradicated (**Kelly & Parry, 2008**).

BACKGROUND

Sue Sloan has been working with people who have sustained traumatic brain injury (TBI) or acquired brain injury (ABI) for over thirty years. Sloan worked initially in traditional clinical practice in a range of institutions specializing in the care and treatment of patients with TBI/ABI within the State of Victoria's health care system as both an occupational therapist and a neuropsychologist (Sloan, personal communication, December 28, 2009). Sloan's private practice, **Osborn Sloan & Associates** in Melbourne provides specialist services to people with ABI within their communities throughout Victoria. Case management is used to bring specialists, the client, and family and friends together in the process of rebuilding the client's life (**Osborn Sloan, 2010**). In the early 1990's Di Winkler, Libby Callaway and Sue Sloan all worked at Ivanhoe Manor, a slow stream rehabilitation centre in Melbourne, and this was the start of their long-term collaborative relationship (Winkler, personal communication, January 12, 2010).

Sue Sloan, Di Winkler, and Libby Callaway practiced and extended the philosophy espoused by **Willer & Corrigan (1994)** who published on long-term rehabilitative possibilities for ABI populations, aptly titled "Whatever it Takes" (Sloan, personal communication, December 28, 2009). The work of Sloan, Winkler, and Callaway has been recognized as part of the body of empirical evidence that demonstrates successful community integration through targeted intervention is possible in the acute phase of ABI and many years post injury (**Kelly & Parry, 2008**).

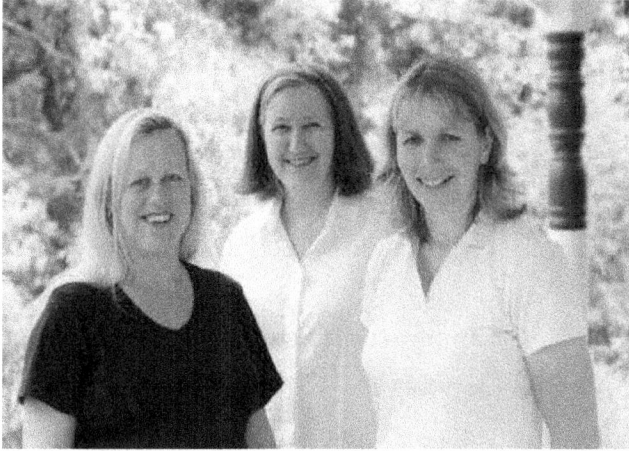

Figure 1. Practitioners of The Community Approach to Participation (CAP) : From left to right: Libby Callaway, Sue Sloan, Di Winkler

The Community Approach to Participation (CAP) Model

The CAP model was devised within the framework of the **World Health Organization's International Classification of Functioning, Disability, and Health (ICF)** for those with ABI and is participation-driven, rather than impairment-driven (**World Health Organization, 2002**; Sloan, personal communication, December 28, 2009). The Rehabilitation Research and Training Center on Community Integration of people with TBI at **Mount Sinai School of Medicine** in New York, USA also stresses Participatory Action in their research framework; the CAP model included Participatory Action in assessments before interventions are customized to the individual (**Gordon, 2004, Sloan et al, 2004**). Client-centred assessments and evaluations are the basis of a relationship between the person with ABI and the therapist as they reveal complex needs over time, providing flexibility to adapt interventions aligned with client goals and needs. An initial semi-structured interview may involve a variety of formal assessment tools examining occupation, community integration, and satisfaction with life. Observation of task performance, preferably in a client's environment, is critical to harmonizing client goals with any limiting factors (**Sloan et al, 2004**).

The CAP's six foundational principles make participation a focus and support meaningful occupation and therapeutic relationships. Therapy is collaborative and integrated to meet as many of the client's needs as possible, and the long-term view is taken for individually customized life goals and flexible support. A positive feedback loop is sought to be created so that limitations on activities are minimized through skill development that prepares a client and enhances successful participation. Client-preferred life roles provide the road map for skill development and add context to a customized intervention plan. Gradual success in participation then facilitates greater scope for further development of skills (Sloan, personal communication, December 28, 2009).

The CAP Principles:

➢ Maximize level of participation in life roles valued by client and inclusion within home & community life

➢ Assist client to develop or maintain network of social relationships & supports

➢ Facilitate engagement in meaningful occupation

➢ Support development of specific activities that underpin role performance

➢ Promote self-confidence and empower client to make everyday decisions and life choices

➢ Enhance adjustment and satisfaction with circumstances of changed life

Role Development Pivotal to The CAP

Using the roles of friendship and hobbyist as examples of client goals, Sloan reported that the creative part of therapy is to identify activities to support such roles which may differ for each individual. Existing skills that underpin role performance are assessed, and then rapport is built with a client to understand the boundaries of their abilities and discuss and plan incremental steps to achieve desired role participation. Charting a person's social contacts and their frequency provides therapists important signposts for ways to reconnect a person socially and to ask questions that inform case management and build understanding of each client. Various roles reveal the underpinning of abilities and skills needed to achieve proficiency levels within roles. Friendship networks are usually depleted in people with ABI, but a new hobby may open new avenues for social contact, structure the use of time, and add or enhance leisure routines which may or may not lead to friendship development in addition to providing a host of other positive qualities for those with ABI (Sloan, personal communication, December 28, 2009).

Sloan stressed that there is much trial and error for clients regaining life roles and self-identity and in working toward life satisfaction; clients are always encouraged to "have a go" no matter how daunting desired goals may be. Sloan added that most clients with profound brain injuries she has worked with do not return to a worker role and much time is taken by clients to rebuild their lives. When Sloan begins working with a client, they are often at a very low baseline in terms of quality of life that is impoverished on many fronts. Poor quality of life may equate to a passive, home-based existence heavily reliant on television for stimulation, and the client in this state can be socially disconnected and a burden for family members assuming the care-giving role (Sloan, personal communication, December 28, 2009). The CAP model has been documented through a case study of one of Sloan's first clients, "Sarah" who, as a young woman had goals similar to all young people who seek independence and gratifying pursuits in their lives (**Sloan et al, 2004**).

Through the case study for Sarah, the collaborative approach involving the client's family, friends, and other people of significance in the client's life, such as a gym instructor, is demonstrated. Negotiating goal achievement was done through tailored support and enhancing already supportive relationships useful to the client to detract from a sense of dependency. Closely monitoring independent functioning built awareness in Sarah who then developed insight into her abilities and chose when to ask for practical support. The sense of control gained by Sarah over her daily destinies built self-esteem and resulted in significantly fewer incidents of challenging behaviour (**Sloan et al, 2004**).

Sloan describes the Community Approach to Participation as dynamic since each client presents a different profile and combination of needs and issues. The delivery of services within the individual's home or community setting gives clients more control in the process of adjustment, learning, and therapy. Having transitioned from a hospital workplace setting, Sloan commented that although institutional care programs strive to adopt a client-centred approach, this focus is not always easy to achieve given the potential for institutional, funding, insurer and time restrictions. Adhering to the CAP model demands flexibility, tolerance, humility, creativity, and the ability to relinquish control, Sloan asserts. Adopting this stance brings many advantages to the client/therapist relationship and generally in the context of real life. Sloan added that from her experience and research, ABI rehabilitation in hospitals, which is centred on internalized learning within patients then generalizing skills and concepts to a new setting such as the patient's own home or community, does not work for participation-focused goals. Following the CAP model, a client's home environment and life context is central so that the interdisciplinary team meets the client's family, friends, neighbours, and other relevant community members (e.g., local shopkeepers). Systemic to the CAP model are policies that recognize the potential of clients (Sloan, personal communication, December 28, 2009).

Resources

Professional Networks

Sloan, Winkler, and Callaway have maintained contact with each other and professional colleagues and actively pursued professional development by attending and presenting at conferences to share ideas, connect with other professionals, and stay abreast of new research and evolving philosophy in ABI (Sloan, personal communication, December 28, 2009).

Funding

One of the main funders for the CAP services is the **Transport Accident Commission**, which requires a report outlining goals, achievements, and progress for each client every six months while clients are receiving services. Continued funding of therapy, however, hinges on the demonstration of progress by clients individually. Many other clients, some of whom may require twenty-four hour support, are funded by government schemes such as the *Slow To Recover* program for those with catastrophic injury (Sloan, personal communication, December 28, 2009). Direct purchase of therapy services is also often considered by people with ABI and their families, in an environment where compensation is not always available for the injury sustained (Sloan, Callaway, & Winkler, personal communication, October 10, 2010).

Private Practice

Office equipment was gradually acquired in Sloan's practice as most of her work was done in the homes of clients throughout the state of Victoria. The office environment did not convey the nature of the practice as there were no props or posters. Sloan's sister helped by keeping the books for the business and is now the Business Manager at Osborn Sloan & Associates. After a few years in private practice, Sloan wrote an actual business plan and won a 2004 Business Award for the plan and went on to write a book to help Occupational Therapists to set up private practice (Sloan, personal communication, December 28, 2009).

Interdisciplinary Teamwork

At Osborn, Sloan, & Associates, two occupational therapists are employed and Sue Sloan's neuropsychology skills are needed as clients may have significant cognitive deficits resulting from injury. Sloan performs an informal analysis of strengths, weaknesses, opportunities, and threats (SWOT) for each client at the outset as part of the baseline assessment. Client assessment is an ongoing, collaborative process, but begins with a semi-structured interview to gather information about routines, roles, activities before injury, and impairments that present barriers to desired role performance. The assessment tools that may be utilized are summarized in Table 1.

Within the Osborn, Sloan & Associates practice, a speech pathologist takes a broad approach to help clients with social communication skills to develop their capacity to express themselves, rather than act out emotions. Other staff members may include a physiotherapist, an M.D. or G.P. as needed, to prescribe medications, a family therapist, dietician, and sometimes a team member who acts as the case manager. The role of the case manager is to take care of administration and to be the clinical coordinator of the team approach to care for a client. The team has a common direction to work constructively with clients and address all items of care; designated case managers are often the occupational therapists within the interdisciplinary team (Sloan, personal communication, December 28, 2009).

Kelly and Parry (2008) described key factors to promote success of an ABI management service (which are all found at Osborn Sloan & Associates Pty Ltd. and Neuroskills Pty Ltd.) Staff are qualified specialists and provide a hub of expertise in teams allowing for brainstorming and creative problem solving. As professionals, the staff has working relationships with local agencies and can coordinate external services, if necessary. Staff liaise closely with a client's support network and know the client's home environment firsthand from site visits. Sue Sloan and colleagues Libby Callaway, and Di Winkler are scientist-practitioners, all active in the ABI community adding the evidence base to the practice. Sloan teaches at **Monash** and **La Trobe** Universities and Winkler founded the **Summer Foundation**, a not for profit organization which aims to resolve the issue of young people in nursing homes, and is completing a PhD; Callaway specializes in OT, teaches at Monash University, conducts research, and co-authors journal articles. Research is one defining feature of best practice (**Kelly & Parry, 2008**).

Table 1. *Measurement for Community Integration.: Summary of Tools Used to Measure Community Integration*

Tool	Aim	Items	Scoring	Approx Admin Time	Key References
Community Integration Questionnaire	To measure an individual's level of integration into the home and community	15 items	Three subscales: home integration, social integration, and productivity. Total score with a range of 0-29.	15 minutes	(Willer et al., 1993)
Community Integration Measure (CIM)	To measure community integration from the perspective of people with ABI	10 items, each with 5 response items	Single summary score with a range of 10-50	5 minutes	(McColl et al., 2001)
Sydney Psychosocial Reintegration Scale (SPRS)	To measure psychosocial integration. Forms for the person with TBI and family	12 items	Three domains: vocational-avocational, interpersonal relationships, and independent living. Total score ranges from 0-72	15 minutes	(Tate, Hodgkinson et al., 1999)
Role Checklist	Role participation and value attached to roles	18 items	Part I—role identification Part II—value designation No.	10 minutes	(Oakley et al., 1986)
Canadian Occupational Performance Measure (COPM)	To measure change in a client's self-perception of occupational performance over time	Individual identifies up to 5 problems with occupational performance	Self-evaluation of current performance and satisfaction with current performance. Following intervention, performance is reassessed	30-40 minutes	(Law et al., 1990)

Tool	Aim	Items	Scoring	Approx Admin Time	Key References
Occupational Questionnaire Interest Checklist	Elicits information about occupation over the course of a typical day.	Records information in half hour intervals throughout the day	Produces scores that represent the amount of value, interest, personal causation, pain, and fatigue experienced in a day	40 minutes over the course of a day	(Smith, Kielhofner, & Watts, 1986)
Interest Checklist	Leisure Inventory appropriate for adolescents. Focuses on avocational interests that influence activity choices	Asks about current interests, how interests have changed, and whether one participates or wishes to participate in an interest in the future	Reveals each individual's unique pattern of interest	20-30 minutes	(Kielhofner, 2002)
Life Satisfaction Questionnaire	Measures the levels of satisfaction in nine domains of life	Nine items	Each item is checked along a six-point ordinal scale ranging from 1 (very dissatisfied) to 6 (very satisfied)	5 minutes	(Fugel-Meyer, 1991)
Satisfaction with Life Scale	Global measure of life satisfaction	Five items	Each item is scored on a 7-point Likert-type scale, the range of possible scores is 5 (low satisfaction) to 35 (high satisfaction). A score of 20 represents a neutral point at which the respondent is equally satisfied and dissatisfied (Pavot, 1991)	5 minutes	(Diener, 1985)

Source: Reproduced from Sloan, Winkler & Callaway, 2004

IMPLEMENTATION

Impact of Health Policy

Sloan had worked in a hospital which specialized in ABI rehabilitation with Libby Callaway and Diane Winkler for many years before choosing to move to private practice. With changes in the health care system around 1995 in Australia when hospital stays were shortened, Sloan found herself at an important crossroads realizing that community integration for people with TBI was more achievable working with clients in their home settings rather than at an institution where institutional culture, rules and regulations imposed constraints because clients could not practise skills in familiar, comforting surroundings in a real life context. Policy change in the health care system resulted in a shortfall in the continuity of care as there were limited services planned for patients discharged from clinical settings much sooner than the time prior to health care reforms. Initially, referrals from the institution Sloan had worked at became a steady stream and Callaway and Winkler also ventured into private practice, research, and teaching (Sloan, personal communication, December 28, 2009). As experienced professionals in the ABI field, Sloan, Callaway, and Winkler advocate to influence public policy through the dissemination of knowledge concerning service and support for the ABI population.

The first six clients Sloan saw did not fit into a hospital setting due to their very challenging behaviour. For another group of clients, traditional therapy in the formal rehabilitation setting was a waste of time as the clients were resistant. Within one year, Sloan had a full-time caseload at home and used a spare room in her own home as an office and worked with clients in their own home or community settings. After two years of working alone, Sloan gave a placement to a 4th year occupational therapy student for ten weeks. With the assistance of the student, Sloan was able to help a client from a secure hospital psychiatry ward return to life within the community. Business snowballed and in five years, Sloan moved into a local office space. The larger premises had eight rooms and Sloan had a staff of twelve people giving two annual 6 month placements to students involved in the Monash University Neuropsychology program (Sloan, personal communication, December 28, 2009). Although the CAP was originally developed to guide occupational therapy practice, the framework has been adopted by the neuropsychologists at Osborn Sloan & Associates.

The Community Approach to Participation (CAP) Applied

The CAP involves working in a collaborative manner with the person with ABI and their family, where available or appropriate, to identify interests and develop skills in those life role areas that the person wishes to return to or explore within community living. The CAP involves developing support models with clients to establish community connectedness and access to environments which are important to the individual with a focus on important relationships. Support structures are designed to guide what happens, when, how, and at what intensity it happens to direct workers delivering the CAP and provide clients with the assistance necessary to participate in those life roles that they identify as being personally meaningful (Figure 2) (Sloan, Callaway & Winkler personal communication, October 10, 2010).

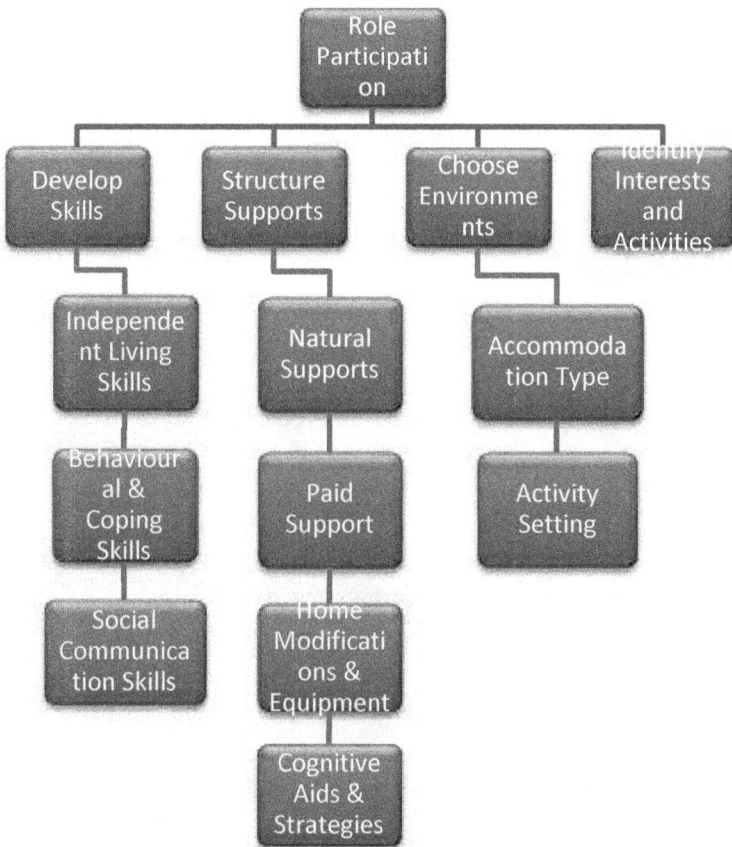

Figure 2. The CAP Support System   underpinning Role Participation
Source: Reproduced from Sloan et al (a) 2009

Workers are trained to use an open approach and actively listen to clients to find what will and will not work for individuals, accepting that the process may be time-consuming. Sloan noted that small steps and gains can, over time, lead to substantial changes in participation for the person with ABI. Clients are encouraged to set achievable goals; a series of small steps may form an indirect path to a larger goal. Goal-setting is a dynamic process because it may involve many small progressions and the pathway or the prime goal itself may be modified, as decided by the client at any point. The incremental steps help clients to experience positive results quickly, for the most part, and may also serve to bring realistic expectations to bear on their desires and decision making (Sloan, personal communication, December 28, 2009).

The journal article by **Sloan et al, (2004)** describes the process of implementation of the CAP approach as well as a single case study of its application. More recent publications of longitudinal studies using the CAP provide detail of the evidence upon which the model is based (**Sloan et al, 2009a** & **2009b**). Strategies used depend on the client's needs and the strengths or weaknesses they may have. In the case study of Sarah, for instance, counselling was an ineffective strategy to help Sarah deal with frustration that led to challenging behaviour, since memory deficits cancelled out any potential benefit of receiving input from a counsellor; access to a therapist by telephone was effective, however, for this client (**Sloan et al, 2004**).

Empowerment

The CAP's prime directive is to empower clients by involving and consulting them in plans for role development and decisions for therapy. **WHO ICF** standards are certainly reflected in all aspects of ABI management (**WHO, 2002**).

Education

Not only does Osborn Sloan & Associates and Neuroskills train accredited professionals to deliver the CAP within its holistic framework respecting the WHO ICF and a *Whatever It Takes* philosophy, but training is available to external organizations and ABI workers so that the CAP is disseminated beyond the practice, raising professional standards and helping a best practice to become widespread (**WHO, 2002**; **Willer & Corrigan, 1994**).

OUTCOME

Sloan's initial referrals were clients with very challenging behaviours. In private practice, Sloan was able to work in a way that was different from a hospital environment, allowing for attention to client-centred goals for independent living skills and various life roles in natural environments for each client. Results were "amazing". (Sloan, personal communication, December 28, 2009).

Sloan, Callaway, and Winkler met with Mary Ann McColl at a conference in Australia to discuss the model of client care to "take it to a higher level and articulate it more formally". Evaluation of outcomes was needed since evidence had to be captured and quantified. A research project was undertaken as a case series design (Sloan, personal communication, December 28, 2009).

Sloan recalled that earlier studies of ABI focused on the injurious event and the plateau of progress that occurred in the rehabilitation of ABI patients several years after the "event". The plateau in impairment levels was accepted as the marker for the limit of productive rehabilitation, so there was no "push" for ongoing rehabilitation; the assumed futility of further rehabilitative therapy was communicated to ABI patients by hospitals in earlier years. In turn, people with ABI held no anticipation of helpful therapy in their futures—supplementary services were geared to helping families to cope as caregivers. Sloan stressed that building participation opportunities and a new self-identity in ABI clients was a foundation in helping to alleviate psychological distress and challenging behaviours while also improving the capacity of each person (Sloan, personal communication, December 28, 2009).

Following client assessment and discussion with the person with ABI and family or supporting friends, a report draft is typically given to the client and family to sign off on the plan for therapy and to provide feedback. The feedback received is then incorporated into the initial plan for the client and recommended goals. Following a course of therapy, families are informally checked on later when a decision can be made by the family and client to continue according to the client's plan or scale back or re-evaluate goals and expectations (Sloan, personal communication, December 28, 2009).

Sarah, in the case study from **Sloan et al. (2004)**, now lives independently needing help with financial management, some everyday problem-solving, and psychological support, but can shop, cook, do the laundry and other housework and drives a scooter. Sarah's score on the Community Integration Questionnaire has improved from 7/29 to 16/29 following the CAP intervention. Sloan found that some environmental modification helped Sarah to increase her independence, such as substituting an induction stovetop instead of a gas range to avoid burns, "spot" telephone counselling as needed for a coping strategy, and facilitating skill development, through task simplification, where possible. Sarah currently participates in valued life roles such as being a family member, gym user, friend, community group member, home owner and pet owner (Sloan et al, 2004).

Evidence

Within the ABI research community, there is acknowledgement that important questions about community-based interventions for ABI may not be answerable by Randomized Control Trials (RCT). Determining outcomes over long periods, for example, is not a characteristic of trialled research. Using waiting lists to provide a "control" group may not be helpful if the wait is not as long as the period required for the effects of community-based rehabilitation to become observable (**Turner-Stokes, 2008**). Turner-Stokes (2008) suggests that a breadth of evidence from experiential, qualitative techniques and clinical experience, in addition to quantitative methods as found in the evaluation standards for the UK National Service Framework (NSF), would be more appropriate than RCTs to determine Grade "A" evidence for community-based ABI interventions. Studies on the CAP model outcomes have shown meaningful and cost-effective results of therapy, even though it is delivered over the long-term and it benefits the clients years after injury (**Sloan et al, 2009a** & **2009b**).

Cost-effectiveness

The most recently published study of the CAP has demonstrated "care and support needs of participants who had sustained a severe ABI, significantly reduced over three years of CAP OT intervention" (**Sloan et al, 2009b**). Although a causal relationship could not be established due to study design, the study analysis concluded there were potential savings for paid care. Since conventional evaluations by funding agencies are over short intervals, typically three, six, or twelve months, the positive results that emerged over the three-year study suggests that funding timelines should be longer before decisions are made to ration resources. Furthermore, the burden to care givers who are family or friends is be reduced, not simply transferred when paid attendant care may be reduced.

Evaluation

First Study of the CAP Intervention

The first evaluative study of the CAP model involved 85 participants admitted consecutively over three years, receiving up to one year of therapy. Seven occupational therapists (OT) were involved in delivering an average of 51.02 OT hours per participant across two private practices, Osborn Sloan & Associates and Neuroskills Pty Ltd. Measured were the Care & Needs Scale, the number of hours of paid and freely given support, Functional Independence Measure (FIM), Role Checklist (RC) and Community Integration Questionnaire (CIQ). For assessment and comparison, the participants were sorted into acute and chronic groups. Positive changes were seen in FIM, CIQ, and RC for both groups, and hours of total care per week and scores on the Care & Needs Scale were reduced for both groups. Overall, changes were greater in the acute group who had more recently sustained the ABI (average of 343 days versus average 3,732 days in the chronic group). Study limitations prevented establishment of a causal relationship between the CAP interventions and successful outcomes as the participants varied on many dimensions not controlled for. Beneficial effects are indirectly legitimated, however, by studies from 1994 & 1996 that showed deterioration of role participation over the long term in the absence of a targeted intervention (**Sloan et al., 2009a**).

Second Study of the CAP Intervention

A second intervention study consisted of 43 participants, who were, on average, over six years post injury and had received three years of community-based intervention. The 43 study participants showed similar positive changes as seen in the first study and an overall reduction of 15.64 hours of total care per person, per week, over the course of the three-year CAP intervention. Aggregated group data, however, masked important distinctions in the variability of data for total hours of care. Refined statistical analysis revealed no change in support hours for 41.86% of participants, an increase of 7.14 hours of total care per person, per week, in 16.28% of participants, and an average decrease of 40.14 hours of total care per person, per week, in the remaining 41.86% of participants. With the CAP intervention, community integration, role participation, and functional independence significantly increased and were undiminished with regard to injury severity and time post injury (**Sloan et al., 2009b**).

Reductions in care hours were greater over time, indicating that funding decisions based on short-term interventions may be short-sighted and undervalue slow-stream interventions such as the three-year period in this study. Causal relationships between outcomes and the CAP interventions were not established largely due to participant variations and the crude measure of support hours by number obscuring the impact of frequency, type of provider, and intensity of the care provided, for instance. The study did affirm that reduced support hours and greater participation are possible for severely brain injured individuals and that customized, targeted, community-based intervention is needed for an extended period of time (**Sloan et al., 2009b**).

Although the second intervention study results reflected no change in total hours of care for participants needing 24 hour care to begin with and a small increase in 16.28% of participants, the significant decrease in 41.86% of participants saving more than an estimated AUS$725,000 shows the potential of the CAP to be cost effective. More importantly, community integration and changes in life roles were positive across the three annual measure points and also statistically significant (**Sloan, 2009**).

Future Research

Di Winkler, who has worked with Sue Sloan in ABI rehabilitation at Ivanhoe Manor in Victoria and is CEO of the **Summer Foundation**, has collaborated with Sloan in research to evaluate the CAP. Winkler suggests that the next phase of research will involve a series of single case designs (Winkler, personal communication, January 12, 2010). A randomised control trial is not ideally suited to an intervention that involves a tailored approach that takes individual preferences and goals into account. An observational trial of a larger sample, however, has the potential to provide a similar level of evidence as a randomised control trial and be more generalizable than the studies of the CAP conducted so far (Winkler, personal communication, October 10, 2010).

Canadian Context

Due to similarities in evolving health care systems, the CAP model is highly transferable to the Canadian setting. The fact that interventions appear to result in less of a burden to care givers close to the client is also encouraging and a desirable element of community-based care. Health professionals may also derive greater autonomy and satisfaction in providing useful interventions to ABI clients from the philosophical culture of the CAP. The model is useful in urban and rural settings without program modifications and service delivery can be tailored to each client using the team approach.

Although the CAP model is delivered through private practice, it can certainly be implemented within a public health care system. In the State of Victoria, considerable political effort was needed to create a Consultancy to serve uninsured ABI individuals with behavioural issues, so the relative ease of private enterprise fulfilling critical service needs should not be scorned. Providing ABI services, however, is not truly part of the public marketplace. Government policies in Victoria determine how services are funded and on what terms which impinges on business cash flow and expense control, for instance, when funding rates for services are static for a few years at a time because of agreements in place while demand for ABI services may increase within the same time frame. Since 2001, the Victorian government has also favoured funding generalist services rather than specialist-based ones (**Kelly & Parry, 2008**).

Conclusion

Due to the prevailing trend in developed countries to reduce institutional care, community-based interventions for ABI that are successful, beneficial to individuals, and cost-effective are urgently needed (**McColl, Carlson, Johnston, Minnes, Shue, Davies et al, 1998**). Meeting the demand for individuals with ABI and challenging behaviour to receive timely therapeutic intervention must be a priority. In Australia, community-based programs such as the CAP model at **Osborn Sloan & Associates** and Neuroskills gained enhanced sustainability due to policies in government and the Transport Accident Commission supporting community-based care and acknowledging long-term commitment to the ABI population. Scarcity of resources coupled with rising demand for ABI services calls for collaborative effort from all stakeholders to allow community-based models such as the CAP to be implemented and funded in a way that makes service continuity possible and integrated with complementary health and social services regardless of whether operation is in the public or private sector. The CAP model of community integration has proven to be effective in practice and meets the goals of many health care systems where ABI interventions are a high priority on the public health agenda.

REFERENCES

Access Economics Pty. Ltd. Report for The Victorian Neurotrauma Initiative .(2009). *The economic cost of spinal cord injury and traumatic brain injury in Australia.* June accessed May 23, 2010 at: http://www.accesseconomics.com.au/

Australian Institute of Health and Welfare, **Disability in Australia: acquired brain injury. Bulletin 55**, December, 2007 accessed October 29, 2010 at: http://www.aihw.gov.au/publications/index.cfm

Gordon, W. A. (2004, April). **Community integration of people with traumatic brain injury: Introduction.** *Archives of Physical Medicine Rehabilitation* (85) Suppl 2:S1.

Kelly, G., & Parry, A. (2008, December). **Managing challenging behaviour of people with acquired brain injury in community settings: The first 7 years of a specialist clinical service.** *Brain Impairment,* 9(3): 293-304.

Lippert-Grüner, M., Maegele, M., Haverkamp, H., Klug, N., & Wedekind, C. (2007). Health-related quality of life during the first year after severe brain trauma with and without polytraum. **Brain Injury** 21(5):451-455.

McColl, M. A., Carlson, P., Johnston, J., Minnes, P., Shue, K., Davies, D., & Karlovits, T. (1998). The definition of community integration; Perspectives of people with brain injuries. **Brain Injury,** 12: 15-30.

Osborn Sloan & Associates Pty Ltd. Retrieved July 23, 2009, Sep. 12, 2010 from: **http://www.osbornsloan.com.au**

Southern Health Acquired brain injury: **Slow to Recover program (ABI:STR)** Retrieved July 23, 2009 from: http://www.southernhealth.org.au/acquired_brain/acquired_brain_injury.htm

Sloan, S., Winkler, D., & Callaway, L. (2004, May). **Community integration following severe traumatic brain injury: Outcomes and best practice.** *Brain Impairment,* 5(1):12-29.

Sloan, S. (2008, April). ABI:Slow To Recover Program. Report of the Therapy Review Project.

Sloan, S. (2009). Rebuilding Lives, Improving long-term participation outcomes following severe brain injury. Powerpoint Presentation for Keynote Address, ASSBI.

Sloan, S., Callaway, L., Winkler, D., McKinley, K., Ziino, C., & Anson, K. (2009a). **The Community Approach to Participation: Outcomes following acquired brain injury intervention.** *Brain Impairment,* 10(3):282-294, December.

Sloan, S., Callaway, L., Winkler, D., McKinley, K., Ziino, C., & Anson, K. (2009b). **Changes in care and support needs following community-based intervention for individuals with acquired brain injury.** *Brain Impairment,* 10(3):295-306.

Transport Accident Commission accessed October 21, 2010. **http://www.tac.vic.gov.au**

Turner-Stokes, L. (2008). **Evidence for the effectiveness of multi-disciplinary rehabilitation following acquired brain injury: A synthesis of two systematic approaches.** *Journal of Rehabilitation Medicine,* 40:691-701

World Health Organization (WHO), Geneva. (2002). Towards a Common Language for Functioning, Disability and Health. ICF Beginner's guide. Publication Ref. WHO/EIP/GPE/CAS/01.3 accessed June 7, 2010 at: **http://www.who.int/classifications/icf/training/icfbeginnersguide.pdf**

Willer, B., & Corrigan, J. D. (1994). Whatever It Takes: a model for community-based services. **Brain Injury,** 8(7): 647-659.

CHAPTER 8

ABI PARTNERSHIP PROJECT

Highlighting Aboriginal ABI Community Support Program & Outreach Teams

By Heather Finch

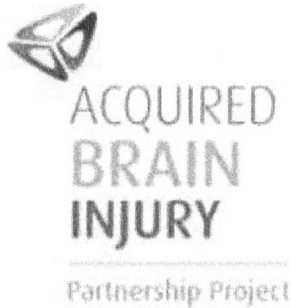

ACQUIRED
BRAIN
INJURY

Partnership Project

Population Served: Survivors of ABI of all ages and their families	
Contributing Author Contact Information	
Michele Cairns Provincial ABI Coordinator ABI Partnership Project Saskatchewan Ministry of Health 3475 Albert Street, Regina, SK S4S 6X6 Phone: (306) 787-6949 Fax: (306) 787-7095 Email: **mcairns@health.gov.sk.ca**	Blaine Katzberg Outreach Team Manager (Sask South) ABI Partnership Project Wascana Rehabilitation Centre 2180 23rd Avenue, Regina, SK S4S 0A5 Phone: (306) 766-5617 Fax: (306) 766 - 5144 Email: **blaine.katzberg@rqhealth.ca**
Janine Baumann Program Manager, Saskatoon Branch Saskatchewan Abilities Council 1410 Kilburn Avenue, Saskatoon, SK,S7M 0J8 Phone: (306) 653-1694 Fax: (306) 652-8886 Email: **jbaumann@abilitiescouncil.sk.ca**	Sandy Millar ABI Community Support Supervisor Saskatchewan Abilities Council 1410 Kilburn Avenue, Saskatoon, SK,S7M 0J8 Phone: (306) 653 - 1694 Fax: (306) 652 - 8886 **abicommunitysupport@abilitiescouncil.sk.ca**

BACKGROUND

Each year in Saskatchewan, approximately 2,200 people sustain an acquired brain injury (ABI). **Saskatchewan Ministry of Health** estimates 150 of these survivors will need multiple services and lifetime support. The **ABI Partnership Project** is a coordinated and integrated continuum of community-based services for survivors of ABI and their families. The Partnership is comprised of 36 programs that are offered by non-profit, community-based organizations and **Regional Health Authorities** throughout the province of Saskatchewan. The Partnership enables clients, families, and caregivers throughout the province to receive therapy, education, life enrichment, respite, residential, and vocational services as close to home as possible. Highlighted here are two of the 36 programs offered: **Outreach Teams** and the **Aboriginal Community Support Program**.

The Partnership was established in response to gaps in services for survivors of ABI and their families. In the mid-1990's in Saskatchewan, these gaps included a poor coordination between existing ABI programs and services, a lack of support for family members of survivors of ABI, inadequate education for ABI survivors, service providers, and caregivers, and a lack of general public awareness regarding ABI. In 1995, an ABI Working Group was formed among ABI survivors, family members of people with ABI, and professionals from diverse backgrounds: physical therapy, case management, occupational therapy, neuropsychology, home care, community services, physical medicine and rehabilitation, recreational therapy, mental health, **Saskatchewan Health**, **Saskatchewan Abilities Council**, Saskatchewan Head Injury Association (SHIA), **Saskatchewan Education, Training, and Employment**, and **Saskatchewan Government Insurance** (SGI).

The Working Group drafted *Acquired Brain Injury—A Strategy for Services* that articulated a vision and mission and outlined recommendations for a three-year ABI pilot program, funded by **SGI** and managed by the **Saskatchewan Ministry of Health**. Following the three-year pilot program and a process evaluation (1996-1998), SGI renewed their commitment for a five-year period (1999 – 2003) at which point the ABI Pilot Project became the **ABI Partnership Project**.

The document developed by the Working Group, *Acquired Brain Injury: A Strategy for Services, September 25, 1995*, put forward six recommendations:

1. The working group recommends that there be an ongoing Advisory Council that will provide direction to the project and will review the progress of the pilot project.

2. The working group recommends actively pursuing First Nations and Métis consultation as well as membership on the Advisory Council.

3. The working group recognizes that each person with acquired brain injury (ABI) is unique and requires an individualized service response. The group recommends that appropriate services and resources be available to all individuals with ABI on the basis of need, regardless of age, the severity of injury or other characteristics.

4. A comprehensive inventory of services broken down by health districts be developed and maintained on a regular basis. The inventory must be available to individuals with ABI, their families, professionals and other caregivers.

5. Outcome and quality of life indicators for individuals with ABI should be reviewed and appropriate tools incorporated for program evaluation. Evaluation tools should be consistent with National and International recommendations.

6. Evaluation tools consistent with National and International recommendations should be adopted.

The **ABI Partnership Project**'s mandate is to assist survivors of ABI in setting and achieving goals that help them develop their functional ability, independence, and community participation to the best of their capabilities. The Partnership recognizes the unique nature of the needs of ABI survivors and their significant others and thus centers programs and services on individual client's goals. Putting this directive into practice rests in the hands of many.

RESOURCES

SGI has funded the Partnership since its beginning and continues their financial commitment to the present day. SGI provides the main source of funding, and other agencies within the Partnership supply additional funding through grants, fundraising, and in-kind contributions. The annual budget was $3.1 million for the initial three-year pilot, and the average annual funding is $4.9 million for the current three-year contract (2010–2013). The Partnership has provided and continues to provide professional development and training opportunities for the staff of programs within the Partnership as well as other ABI service providers.

The **Partnership** currently consists of 36 programs throughout the province, designed and integrated to bridge the gap between acute care, therapy, and community participation, and to meet the individual needs of clients, family members, and communities. The services are broad in scope and include:

- assessment
- case management
- consultation
- support
- education for individuals, families and service providers

- life enrichment programming
- vocational and avocational programming
- crisis management services
- rehabilitation (direct therapy and therapeutic aid/assistance (*Program Evaluation 2004 – 2006*

Instead of duplicating services that were already in place prior to the partnership, the ABI Partnership Project supplements and partners with already existing human service providers to holistically contribute to clients' community integration and improved quality of life.

The *Program Evaluation 2004 – 2006*, along with other reference documents available on the Partnership's website, provides a description of the support services and programs offered through the ABI Partnership Program.

Outreach Teams

Saskatchewan is divided into three service areas: Sask North, Sask Central, and Sask South. There are three **Outreach Teams** that coordinate and provide services through **health regions** and are based in Prince Albert (Sask North), Saskatoon (Sask Central), and Regina (Sask South). Each team is made up of a variety of professionals who provide multidisciplinary assessment, case management/coordination, consultation, and sometimes provide direct services to clients within their respective regions. The members of the **Outreach Teams** help clients and families navigate ABI support services and programs (*Program Evaluation 2004 – 2006*).

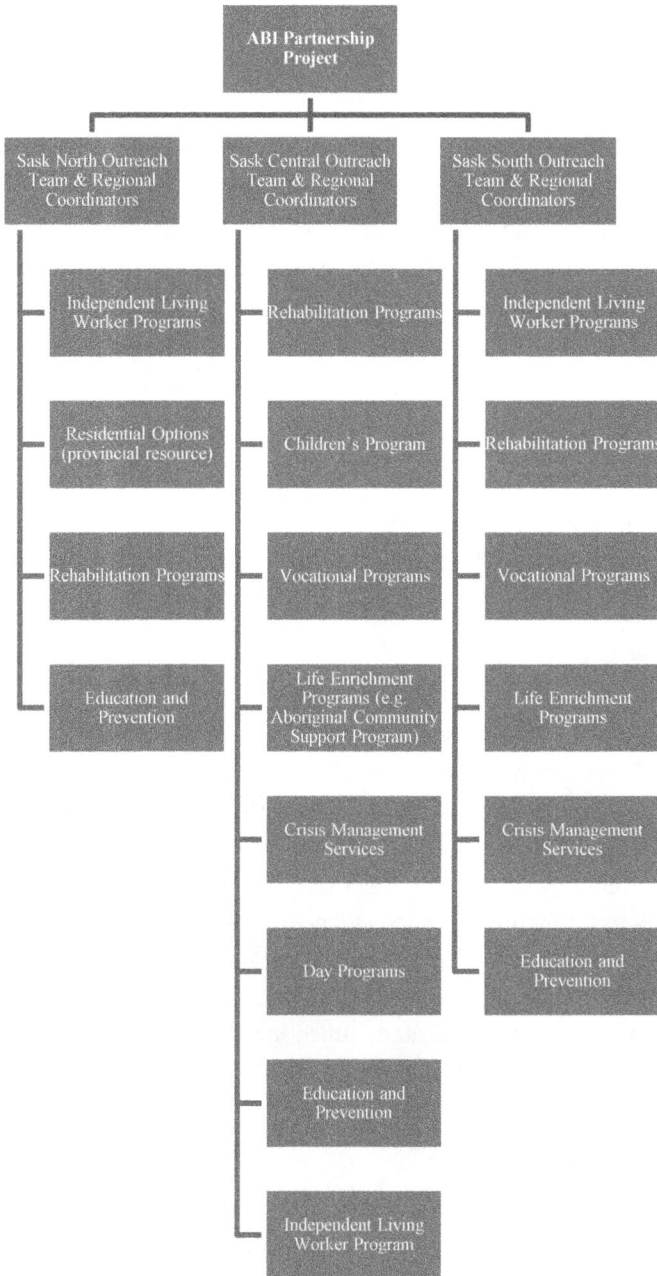

Regional Coordinators

There are five **regional coordinators** located in Swift Current, North Battleford, Weyburn, Yorkton and Moose Jaw who wear several hats for their respective **health regions**. They identify, coordinate, and support programs and resources for individual needs of ABI survivors; provide family support and education; and identify and support appropriate residential options. Community development is also a central role of **Regional Coordinators** in following through with individual care plans. In addition, Regional Coordinators also train other human service providers.

Independent Living Worker Programs (ILWP)

Three **ILWP**s contribute to the coordination of services for clients as well as provide direct services such as life skills, therapy, recreational activities, and vocational and avocational support. They collaborate with **Regional Coordinators**, survivors, families, and caregivers to help the survivor attain the most appropriate level of independent living.

Residential Options

Two transitional supported living options are in place to help clients learn how to live more independently by helping clients restore functional abilities. **Phoenix Residential Society—PEARL** is located in Regina and is mandated to act as a provincial resource. **Sask North Independent Living Program** serves the northern region.

Rehabilitation Programs

There are three main rehabilitation programs: the **Saskatchewan Association for the Rehabilitation of the Brain Injured** (SARBI) is located in Regina, Saskatoon, and Kelvington; a Speech and Language Pathologist (SLP) is located in Melfort; and PA **Parkland Health Region** provides rehabilitation services to Keewatin Yatthé and Mamawetan Churchill River Health Regions. The SARBI programs are provided by volunteers and focus on increasing independence through slow-stream rehabilitation. The SLP assesses and works to help improve communication skills of ABI survivors. The two northern rehabilitation programs work with survivors who live in the most remote areas of the province to restore and maintain functional skills and enhance quality of life. Services provided include community development, case management, and education and prevention activities.

Children's Program

The **Community Integration Program (CIP) at Radius Community Centre** in Saskatoon offers community integration programs exclusively for children and adolescents with ABI. CIP provides age appropriate programming for children and youth who live or go to school in the Saskatoon area. With a community support worker, children and youth participate in social and recreational activities and have the opportunity to work on personal management skills and get work experience and pre-vocational training as well. Support services are available after school, in the evenings, weekends, and during the summer.

Vocational Programs

Through skill development and therapy, three vocational programs help survivors of ABI work toward their individual goals of obtaining or maintaining employment: **Partners in Employment**, a branch of the Saskatchewan Abilities Council, in Regina and Saskatoon, and Multiworks in Meadow Lake.

Life Enrichment Programs

Three **ABI Life Enrichment Programs** operate out of the Regina, Saskatoon, and Yorkton branches of the **Saskatchewan Abilities Council**. These programs help ABI survivors develop social skills through leisure and recreational activities that are based on client interests and organized individually or for a group.

Crisis Management Services

Mobile Crisis Services located in Regina and **Crisis Intervention Services** located in Saskatoon, both provide crisis management services when mainstream services been unsuccessful as well as crisis intervention services that are available 24-hours per day.

Day Programs

Two day programs, **Lloydminster Acquired Brain Injury Society** (LABIS) and **Sherbrooke Community Centre "Moving On" program** (Saskatoon), offer programs that include physical and cognitive exercises and life skills that contribute to independence and community integration.

Education and Prevention

This program includes three **Regional Education and Prevention Coordinators** (Regina, Saskatoon, and Prince Albert), the **Saskatchewan Prevention Institute** (SPI), **Saskatchewan Brain Injury Association** (SBIA) and the **Provincial Education and Prevention Coordinator**. The Regional Education and Prevention Coordinators work with communities to develop injury prevention strategies and education initiatives that raise awareness of the effects of ABI. SPI, a provincial program located in Saskatoon, creates educational materials about injury prevention in children that are user friendly and accessible to professionals and the public. SBIA is a provincial grassroots organization that provides support to survivors and families through support groups, education events, and resource development.

IMPLEMENTATION

The goal of the **ABI Partnership Project** is "to provide individual and family support to people with acquired brain injury so that they may live successfully in their communities with improved quality of life" (**ABI Partnership Project, n.d.**).

An Advisory Group has been guiding program development of the **Partnership** since its beginning. It is made up of survivors, family members, professionals, and agency representatives. The ABI Provincial Office handles day-to-day project management, consulting **SGI** in certain decisions as required, and seeks advice from and reports to the Advisory Group at face-to-face meetings three times per year. The **ABI Partnership Project** contracts with individual funded agencies to provide services and support. These agencies are responsible for following the **Program Guidelines** of the Partnership as well as establishing policies and procedures with the non-profit agency, individual health regions, and the departments to whom they report. The funded agencies also provide input to the ABI Provincial Office through various committees, such as the Outcomes Working Group and the ABI Information System User Group (ABIIS). The ABIIS became operational in January 2000 and was developed to gather demographic and service utilization data of ABI registered clients. Service events include direct therapeutic services to clients as well as education and community development activities undertaken by funded agencies within the Partnership.

At the Partnership's inception, there was a call for program proposals, of which 23 were funded. Calls for additional program proposals continue, and with recommendations from the ABI Provincial Office (managed by **Saskatchewan Health**), final advice and decisions are made by the ABI Provincial Advisory Group, which includes **SGI**.

Ongoing proposals are made to the **ABI Partnership Project** when gaps in services within the community are found. An example of one such proposal is the **ABI Community Support Program**. In 1999, the **Saskatchewan Abilities Council** recognized the need to offer a program to ABI survivors whose needs went beyond the scope of a vocational service. An application was made to the **ABI Partnership Project** to offer a life enrichment program to adults with an ABI in Saskatoon. In 2000, the **ABI Community Support Program** was approved and began to be offered by the **Saskatchewan Abilities Council**. The goal of the Community Support program is to "enhance the quality of life of adults with an ABI by assisting them in engaging in meaningful activity, becoming more independent, and becoming more integrated in the community" (Saskatchewan Abilities Council). The ABI Community Support Program is designed to serve individual needs and promote active participation of people with varying abilities. It promotes optimal independence, provides respite for caregivers, and provides opportunity to build and practice a range of skills as well as develop meaningful relationships.

Aboriginal ABI Community Support Program (Saskatchewan Abilities Council—Saskatoon Branch)

In response to the lack of insurance and funding for Aboriginal people with ABI to receive support, and in keeping with the recommendations set out by the Working Group, the **Saskatchewan Abilities Council** began offering the Aboriginal ABI Community Support Program. The ABI Community Support Program and the **Aboriginal ABI Community Support Program** promote the same goals. The main difference is that the Aboriginal ABI Group provides client-centered services designed specifically for Aboriginal adults with moderate to severe ABI, providing group activities as opposed to the one-on-one outings of the ABI Community Support Program . This program makes new connections in the community with elders, ceremonial groups from various reserves, cultural centres, urban services, Aboriginal agencies, and Aboriginal community programs. These connections with their communities help decrease feelings of isolation; strengthen spirituality by participating in traditional practices; and help Aboriginal survivors of ABI feel more part of their communities. Groups of participants are formed based on similarities and interests, and support workers for each group are Aboriginal. Services are of no cost to Aboriginal clients, as the program makes annual applications for funding through the **City of Saskatoon**, **Saskatchewan Lotteries**, **Community Initiatives Fund**, and **Saskatchewan Indian and Gaming Association**. Both the ABI Community Support Program and the Aboriginal Community Support Program are housed in the same building in Saskatoon, often using the large meeting room for groups to meet with elders as well as provide a space for traditional ceremonies such as the sacred Shaking Tent Ceremony.

The **ABI Community Support Program** and the **Aboriginal ABI Community Support Program** are designed around the clients' goals and strive to integrate clients into their communities. Survivors of ABI are able to access support services at any time after their brain injury, with no time limit whatsoever. Clients are self referred by family members or caregivers or are referred by the **ABI Outreach Team** at **City Hospital** who are usually in contact with a client while he or she is hospitalized. The ABI Community Support Supervisor goes out to meet the client, learning more about his or her needs and beginning an individual goal attainment. The client can begin the program immediately if there is a community support worker who matches what the client is looking for in a community support worker (e.g., age, gender, common interests) The frequency with which clients meet their community support worker is up to the client. Some clients and community support workers meet once a week and others meet daily. Program activities are either recreational or life skills based, depending on each clients' goals and interests. Examples include the following, with an emphasis on cultural learnings for Aboriginal clients.

➤ golfing

➤ swimming

➤ working out

➤ sweat lodges

➤ movies

➤ community events

➤ healing circles

➤ meal planning and shopping

➤ setting up a weekly schedule on a whiteboard, etc

After each outing, a time for the next outing is made, and the community support worker calls the client the day before and the day of the outing with a reminder.

Outreach Program

The **Outreach Teams** play a significant role in the **ABI Partnership Project**. There are three teams (Regina, Saskatoon and Prince Albert), and staffing varies for each team, with the team in Regina having the most staff and varied professionals, as their service area is the most populous and has the most registered clients compared to the other two. The teams match clients with services, one of which is the Aboriginal ABI Community Support Program, that meet their needs and help them achieve their goals for community integration, independent living, and increased quality of life. The goals for the team are the goals for the client, and Outreach Teams work with clients for as long as assistance is desired.

Each team works a bit differently to meet the needs of their clients; however, a closer look at the inner workings of the **Sask South Outreach Team** provides an overview of the processes of outreach teams within the Partnership. The Sask South Program has an open referral policy and receives referrals from inpatient programs, insurance companies, and family members, with about 75% of referrals coming from neuro units in acute care. Therefore, the first contact members of the Sask South Team have with clients is often in the hospital, but the relationship continues when the client is discharged from acute care. The number of self-referring clients is increasing, as more people are learning about the **ABI Partnership Project** through regional websites and the partnership website. The Outreach Team is available to survivors of ABI and their families any time after the brain injury, working with clients for an average length of 12–18 months but sometimes continuing for ten or more years. The Sask South Outreach Team tends to follow children longer as they progress through school.

Each client is matched with a primary worker who is responsible for coordinating services and maintaining goal achievement sheets, tracking goals as achieved, partially achieved, or withdrawn (when goals are deemed by the client no longer appropriate). The client and his or her primary worker also work in collaboration with between one and four associates in the process of setting goals and finding appropriate services. Associate members of a client's team are usually professionals within the Partnership but also include those from outside the Partnership as well. Associates may include, but are not limited to, regional coordinators, occupational therapists, speech and language therapists, social workers, or **SGI** insurance adjusters who must approve certain services if the client had insurance with **SGI**. Primary workers meet their clients whenever and wherever, by phone, in person, in their home or place of employment, or even at Tim Horton's Coffee Shop. Some visits also take place in the **Outreach Team** office if the client happens to be coming in for outpatient therapy. Members of the **Outreach Team** are aware of the long term nature of the process of community reintegration for survivors of ABI, and they are committed to establishing and maintaining relationships with each client.

Community reintegration and participation means different things for different clients. Depending on the individual, **Outreach Teams** help clients resume employment or get involved in a former recreation activity. They also help children and adolescents go back to school and find employment in whatever form that may take. For clients who are unable to pursue employment opportunities, outreach team workers connect them with recreation and other life enrichment activities that are of interest and already taking place in the community in which clients live. The team tries to capitalize on existing community programs and activities and make them work for their clients. For example, recently various art groups have formed as a result of clients' interests, and an artist in residence was able to work with clients for two months. As a result, the Sask South team is further incorporating what is available locally by collaborating with Regina's local art centre. The **Outreach Team** tries new programs for a set period of time, and depending on clients' interests, expand from there.

The members of the Sask South Outreach Team find that refraining from creating dependency is of great importance. In order to prevent dependency, the teams focus on empowering clients and creating opportunities for them to make their own choices, focusing on the clients' interests and what they are motivated to do. Sometimes clients set goals that are not achievable due to the severity of their brain injury; however, members of the team remain nonjudgmental and support the client in working toward his or her goal. The client's team works with the client through the process of becoming more and more aware of his or her abilities and limitations, presenting alternative possibilities. For example, one client survived an ABI when she was in Grade 12. She had her heart set on being a teacher and had already been accepted to university before the event; however, due to her brain injury, she was not capable of a four year B.Ed. program. Through working with her team, she came to accept this limitation and chose to take early childhood education courses at a community college that would not qualify her to teach in the same capacity that she once hoped for but would allow her to work with children in a child care setting. She was successful in completing her coursework and obtained a position at a daycare; however, she came to realize that she could not remember the children's names and that this was unacceptable for her position. With the help of her team, she has attained a government job where she still has memory struggles, but she functions very well in this setting and has been quite successful because of her people skills.

Sometimes **Outreach Teams** are more involved with family members of a client than they are with the clients themselves. There are some situations in which survivors of ABI do not believe they are in need of assistance and that everything is fine. In such cases, spouses of ABI survivors may be having trouble adjusting to the changes that follow their loved one's brain injury, and social workers are able to help them with coping strategies. In addition, once or twice a year, the Sask South and North Outreach Teams hold family panel nights where family members are able to tell their stories. The Central Outreach Team has started a family support group as well. The Sask South Team has tried family support groups in the past, but they found that many family members want to talk with other family members in similar situations. In response, the Sask South Outreach Team tries to connect families.

The **Outreach Teams** view helping survivors of ABI reintegrate into the community as more of an art than a science, recognizing that there is no cookie cutter approach and that getting to know each client is paramount.

Challenges

To better meet the needs of ABI survivors, better linkages with other disability groups and other human service providers (Housing, Income Security, Mental Health, Addictions, Justice) would be beneficial. However, it is sometimes difficult to achieve full collaboration from other human service providers to meet client needs when their direct mandate is not to serve individuals with brain injury even though these ABI survivors might have issues (addictions, mental health, and criminal justice system involvement) that these systems are to address.

Over the past several terms, the Provincial Advisory Group has included First Nations representation; however, it has been difficult to maintain because of competing pressures for past representative's time. There is currently not a First Nations representative for the 2010-2013 term.

While the services provided by the **Partnership** are quite comprehensive, there has been and continues to be a gap in residential services for individuals with ABI in Saskatchewan. The Partnership does not have a dedicated system of residential care for survivors of ABI (e.g., group homes, supported living environments, etc.) in Saskatchewan. In addition, within the Partnership, there is currently only one program that provides dedicated services for children and youth.

OUTCOME

Four evaluations of the **Partnership Project** have been completed, and the first three can be found on their website—www.abipartnership.sk.ca. The first examined the implementation of the pilot project (1998); the second explored client and program outcomes (2004), and the third explored four core areas of the Partnership: clients, families, service providers, and education and prevention (2006) (**Program Evaluation 2004 – 2006**). The most recent evaluation (2007 – 2010) has not been publicly released because its intended audience was internal. Its main purposes were to maintain accountability and program monitoring expectations and to record program improvement areas for ABI Provincial Office and funded agency follow-up. Some data from an excerpt of the report are provided below.

Program Evaluation 2004–2006

In the **Program Evaluation 2004–2006**, the ABI Partnership used a variety of both quantitative and qualitative measures to evaluate the effectiveness of services provided. For clients, the Community Integration Measure, Problem Checklist, Sense of Coherence Questionnaire, Mayo Portland Adaptability Inventory (MPAI), Quality of Life Questionnaire, Goal Attainment Template, Change in Functional Status Report (ABIIS), and Client Representative Case Studies were used. The case studies were used to gain the perspectives of clients, family members, and service providers on service appropriateness, referral effectiveness, and the responsiveness to client and family needs and how well services are helping clients meet their goals. The results showed that all the stakeholders in each region thought that the services provided "were appropriate, responsive, and demonstrated a high degree of referral effectiveness" (p. 24). When asked about responsiveness, one client responded,

> They really listened to me and that is what I like about it…I can call
> people at ABI and they will help me…they help me get information

> when I need it…I can talk to them. I stop by and they will talk to me when I need to talk. If I asked about a service they would find it out and get me into it. They were responsible and wanted to help me. (p. 24)

In addition, those interviewed also felt that the services offered through the ABI Partnership Project helped clients meet their goals and enhanced their quality of life. One parent of an ABI survivor commented,

> Without this program I don't think he would have half the quality of life that he now has. For the fact that they are more than willing to find any information or any answers to any questions that you could have. If they don't have the answers they would find them. Trust me, our son threw a lot of things their way. I don't think they have ever skipped a beat. I don't think they have ever said to our son it's not achievable. They have always encouraged him. Whether between them and us they have had to maybe guide him in a different direction, which you can do with our son if you do the right way, without him realizing that the direction has been changed. They're always eager to help him. They helped him in a way that encouraged his autonomy; they empowered him. Looked at pros and cons of the situation, always letting him make the decisions so that he has the feeling that 'I did this, it's my decision,' but he also knows where the help comes from to make those decisions. He has a lot of respect for everyone here so it makes it easier for him to ask for help. He feels very comfortable around the team. He will pop in and say hello, which tells me, because we know our boy, that he really likes and respects them. We definitely feel comfortable coming to ask them for help or ask questions. I can't think of service that we have seen or been through in the last five years that would have given him what he got there (p. 24 – 25)

The demographics of individuals with ABI reported in this evaluation speaks to the long term support possibilities the Partnership offers survivors of ABI, as the range in months since time of injury was quite wide, 5 months to 364 months (33.3 years) prior to survey completion.

Family Members, Services, and Prevention and Education programs were also reviewed. Family members were given the Family Needs Questionnaire (FNQ). Analyses showed that almost one-half of the family needs that family members themselves deemed important were unmet or only partially met. However, only 42 of 74 respondents said they had accessed available services, indicating that program staff members need to make themselves more available to family members beyond concerns of clients with ABI through individual open discussions and support groups, possibly dedicating a group of program staff to family needs. Family focus groups also revealed strengths and areas for improvement. Among the strengths were coordination of and access to services; meaningful life activity; and employment and residential support. Areas for improvement included more support and respite for families; specialized resources; access to resources; and social and recreational opportunities for meaningful life activity. Suggestions were made to make information more readily available through the website and kept up to date.

Program Evaluation 2007–2010

For the most recent evaluation (2007–2010), the Partnership divided rehabilitation outcomes into short-term, intermediate, and long-term in an effort to measure one of the Working Group's major objectives of improved rehabilitation outcomes and quality of life after program implementation.

ACTIVITY

Client-Centered Activities provided by Partnership

SHORT-TERM

Improved skills:
- physical skills
- cognitive skills
- social skills
- communication skills

INTERMEDIATE

Increased independence, productivity, and community involvement

LONG-TERM

Improved Quality of Life

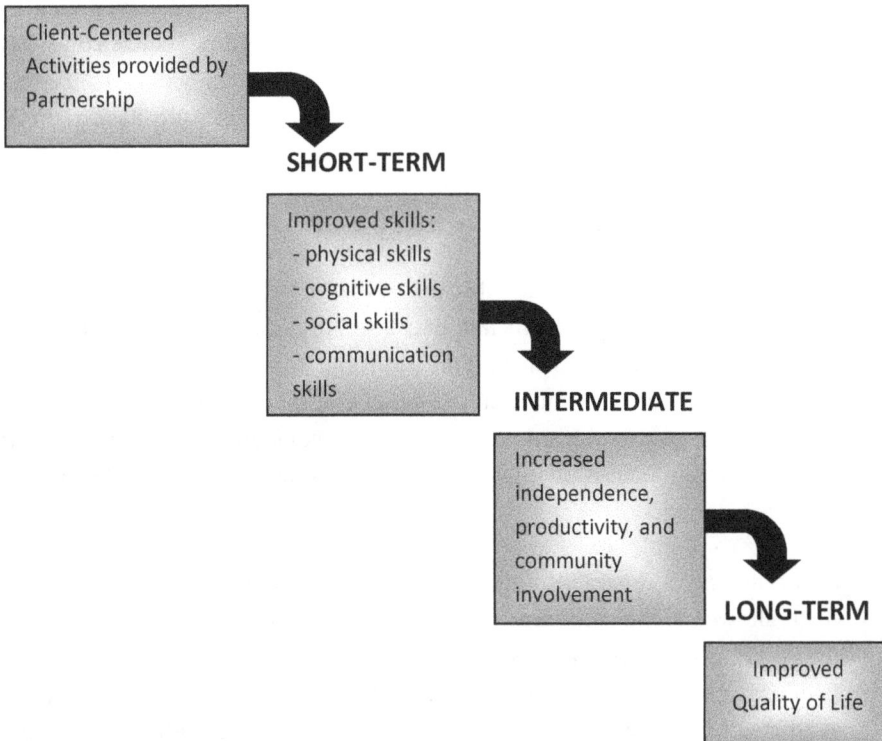

Flow Chart taken from ABI Partnership Project: 2007 – 2010 Program Review

To measure short term outcomes, the Partnership used the Mayo-Portland Adaptability Inventory – 4th edition (MPAI-4), which uses three subscales: ability (physical, cognitive, social, and communication skills), adjustment (e.g., controlling anger and managing fatigue), and participation (e.g., engaging in recreation or leisure activities). Intermediate outcomes were assessed with the Change in Functional Outcome data, which looks at how demographic data is related to employment, education, and living situation. Goal Attainment was used as a bridge between short-term and intermediate goals, as it is a way of capturing the diversity of client's needs and goals that is characteristic of brain injury.

To make the evaluation process more manageable for both clients and staff than the previous evaluation packet, only the MPAI-4 and Goal Attainment were used. In the 2004-2006 Evaluation, the MPAI-4 was administered at intake and at a client's one-year anniversary or when a client stopped using Partnership services. The protocol was changed to intake and a client's 18 month anniversary or when services ceased to be used in hopes of statistically significant improvements.

Of 28 outcome packages that were completed and returned for the 2010 analysis, 24 of them were used for demographic information. At time of injury, ages ranged from 16 – 86 years (average being 44.6 years; standard deviation of 19.6), and 75% identified as male. The most common cause of ABI was a stroke at 33% and motor vehicle collisions following at 21%. Forty-six percent of respondents had no auto insurance, and 21% had SGI No Fault insurance. Most respondents' home Health Regions were Saskatoon at 38% and Regina Qu'Apelle at 29%.

Mayo-Portland Adaptability Inventory – 4th Edition

A paired t-test was conducted on the three subscales of the MPAI-4-*ability, adjustment, and participation*-to identify statistically significant decrease in difficulties related to ABI. Significant improvements were found in participation and for total score ratings from survivors and staff. Reductions were found in the *adjustment subscale and the average scores,* but they were not statistically significant. The Partnership concluded that survivors and staff report relatively the same level of ability and adjustment at intake and at 18 months or program inactivation.

Fifteen of the 28 outcome packages also included ratings from clients' significant others, analysis of which showed significant improvements on all subscales and the total score. Analyses of the same 15 outcome packages for self and staff ratings revealed significant improvements in only participation and total scores. This indicates that significant others perceive a greater improvement in clients' functioning than did either the clients themselves or the staff. T-tests were used to examine improvement for each item of the MPAI-4. Survivors, their significant others, and Partnership staff reported significant improvement in many functional areas (physical abilities, cognitive abilities, mood, and symptoms) and some community participation areas (such as independence—residence, money management, and transportation).

The 2004 – 2006 evaluation report showed no significant improvements; whereas the 2007-2010 evaluation report shows significant improvements in several areas. Significant improvement was detected for 18 month pre-post measurement but not for the one year pre-post measurement, which suggests that improvements in skill attainment and community participation for survivors of ABI occurs over a **long period of time and that long term support is needed.**

Goal Attainment

The goals of the clients are the goals of the Partnership; thus, the goals of the clients drive the programs and services of the Partnership. All services of the Project are in place solely to support clients in achieving their goals. The Partnership recognizes that survivors of ABI have unique needs; thus, work with each client in the Partnership is client-centered. Goal setting involves the client, family, and staff. The 1999-2003 evaluation report recommended a standard tracking tool for individual goal attainment, and the Partnership has been using Goal Attainment since April of 2004. From 2005, each program has submitted annual Goal Attainment Templates. The goals are divided into five areas: Cognitive, Functional Independence, Psychosocial/Emotional, Community Activities, and Other. The following diagrams show the breakdown of client goal areas as well as percentages achieved, partially achieved, not achieved, and withdrawn.

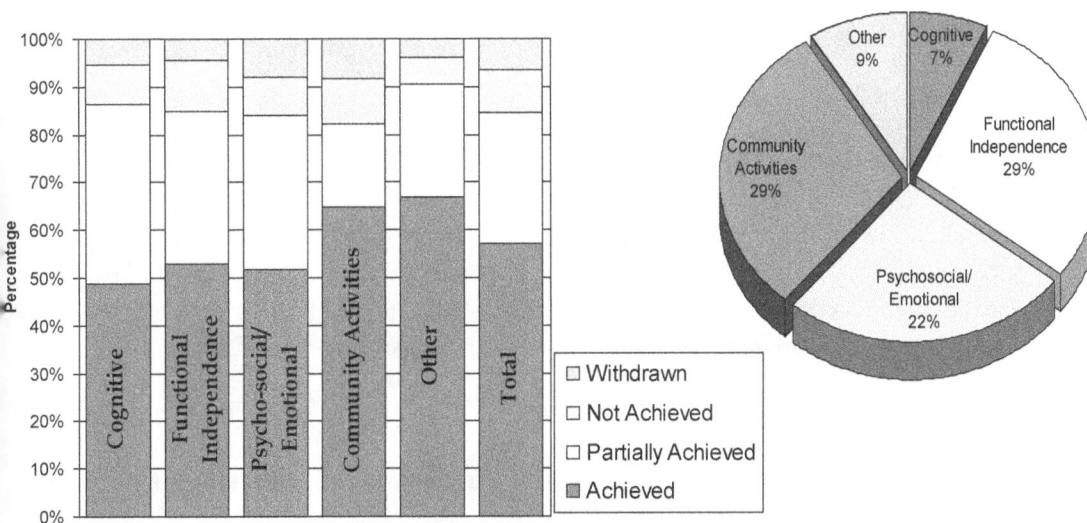

Breakdown of 2007-09 Client Goals by Area

(ABI Partnership Project – 2007–2010 Program Review)

The first evaluation of Goal Attainment in 2004-2006 showed positive results. Of the 5,342 goals submitted, 62% were achieved, 29% were partially achieved, and 10% were not achieved. The 2007-2010 evaluation reveals similar results. Of the 4,426 goals submitted, 60% were achieved, 28% were partially achieved, and 10% were not achieved. For both evaluations, the number of goals does not include those that were withdrawn.

The graphs below show that more goals were recorded as 'withdrawn' or 'achieved' for inactivated clients, and 'not achieved' by active clients. This can be attributed to the fact that clients achieve goals over time as well as develop the insight necessary to withdraw goals that are not appropriate.

Inactivated Clients   *Active Clients*

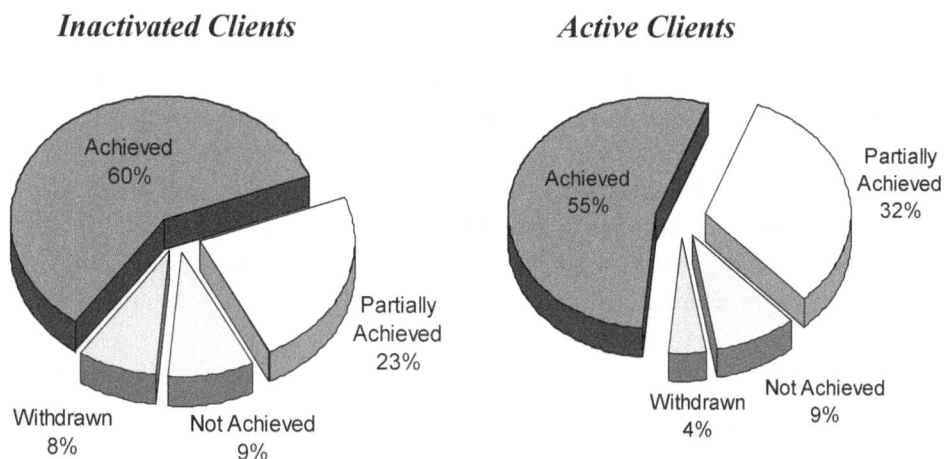

Client Goal Attainment 2007-2009 (ABI Partnership Project – 2007-2010 Program Review)

Overall, results from both the MPAI-4 and Goal Attainment show that the programs and services of the ABI Partnership Project help survivors of ABI maintain level of functioning and community participation in the short term, with improvements in skills and independence and increased quality of life occurring over the long term.

From the Clients

One client participating in the **Aboriginal ABI Community Support Program** had the following to offer: "[I] find it difficult to have no support left...even the Aboriginal agencies let me down...[I'm] glad I always have this program to count on" (personal communication, August 31, 2010). Another client from this same program commented, "It has been a big part of my healing being back involved with my cultural practices...never thought I would get the opportunity again to participate since I moved here [long term care facility]" (Personal Communication, August 31, 2010). One last client from the ABI Community Support Program is 46 years old and lives in a nursing home where the average age is in the mid 50's. She is grateful for the community activities in which she participates, such as going out to dinner, to movies, and hockey and football games. This client recognizes and appreciates that the program takes pressure off of her family. She also remarked, "Without this, I have nothing; I stay shut in. I wouldn't go out to the community, and it'd be pretty boring. I live in a place that has some programs, but the kind of person that I am, I think I need more" (Personal Communication, September 12, 2010).

Three clients of the **ABI Partnership Project** recently shared their experience with the Outreach Team in Regina. All of the clients spoke highly of the **Outreach Team** workers and the relationships they have built with them. In addition, they all recognized increased access to and awareness of opportunities with which the Outreach Team has connected them in order to fulfill their needs and desires.

One client is a 30-year-old woman who experienced a brain injury through a car accident in 1998. She has been in the program for 10 years and said that without her support worker, "I'd be lost. [My support worker] is just awesome! Basically, when I call and ask [him] for help with something, he has found ways to help me" (Personal Communication, August 25, 2010). Over the past ten years, her support worker has connected her with services and programs that have helped her rebuild her motor skills, meet new people, build confidence, and find employment. At the time of her car accident, she was pregnant. Once she was able to leave the hospital, the Outreach Team helped her regain the skills she needed to live independently and care for her newborn child. After she had her baby, she was struggling with balance due to the change in how her weight was distributed. She contacted her support worker who connected her with a physiotherapist who helped her regain her balance. This client also lost many friends after her accident and has made new friends through various social gatherings the Outreach Team facilitates, such as going fishing and bowling. In addition, this client feels encouraged by her support worker and feels more outgoing and confident. She often volunteers at her child's school and is willing to help out whenever she can.

Another client is the sister of a survivor of ABI. She lives two and a half hours away from her brother, which makes it difficult to provide the assistance he needs. However, her brother has been in the program for about 10 years, and she finds that her brother's support worker keeps her updated and helps her brother fulfill his needs. The family just recently lost their parents, which was exceptionally difficult for her brother with an ABI. His support worker went to the funeral with her brother, stood by his side while he spoke in front of his whole family, and walked with him to the gravesite. Her brother perceives his support worker as a friend and is able to talk with him about personal issues about which he does not feel comfortable talking to his family members. This client "could not say enough" about her brother's support worker and associate workers (Personal communication, August 25, 2010). Before her brother was in the program, interacting with the public and his coworkers in a socially acceptable manner was a challenge and sometimes and at times resulted in him being arrested. His sister feels that the members of the Outreach Team have helped her brother cope with his challenges and live a more meaningful life by providing relational support as well as opportunities to socialize and contribute to the community.

She admits that she wishes there would have been more support for the family at the beginning, when her brother first acquired his brain injury. Some family members do not understand that their brother's behaviour is due to his brain injury. She feels that if characteristics of brain injury would have been explained early on, the family would be more understanding now, several years later. She also wishes that her brother could be compensated for the work he does as opposed to just volunteering. Her brother often becomes frustrated that he is working so hard, building chairs and other furniture, but not receiving anything in return. His sister feels that, for her brother who is 50 years old, receiving compensation for his work would add even more meaning than having lunch and talking with his support worker and attending meetings give to his life. Even with these suggestions, this client is deeply grateful for the Outreach Team and does not know what she or her brother would do without them (Personal communication, August, 26, 2010).

The third client of the Partnership is 29 years old and experienced his brain injury when he was 15 years old. The Outreach Team was extremely helpful when he was transitioning back into high school by assisting him, his teachers, and principal to devise a plan that allowed him to be successful. The team also helped this client transition into university. He has earned a degree in Kinesiology and is beginning a Bachelor of Education program this fall. He speaks very highly of the Outreach Team. This client recognizes the importance of having a strong support system, which may or may not include a person's family. For him, he considers the Outreach team, his teachers, and his principal to be part of his family, as they have all supported him in his most difficult times. He says that he has talked with one of the support workers so much that he has become like a second father to him. He also greatly values one of the psychologists on his Outreach Team with whom he has discussed relationships and spirituality. He says that the members of the Outreach Team are extremely approachable and always willing to get together for a chat. In addition, SGI has been "very understanding and accommodating," and has helped him financially from the time of his accident through his graduation from university (Personal communication, August 25, 2010). This client finds that the best way to cope with the difficulties associated with his brain injury is by sharing his story. He enjoys writing poems as well as public speaking. He is one of the main speakers for a program that goes to high schools to educate students about the realities and dangers of motor vehicle collisions. Sharing his struggles and successes is a deep passion of his, and he would like to do so whenever and wherever the opportunity arises. He believes that one of the best therapies for survivors of ABI is to share their stories.

This small snapshot of clients' experiences with the **ABI Partnership Project** speaks to the program's success in helping clients achieve their goals and live fulfilling lives. The Partnership's coordination of services, **Outreach Teams**, and **Aboriginal Community Support Program** are particularly unique amongst programs for people with ABI and significantly contribute to helping people with ABI optimally participate in their communities.. Because Ontario and Saskatchewan have similar provincial health care delivery structures, such a program is viable in Ontario. Much can be learned from the Partnership's collaboration and coordination of services, relationship building between staff and clients, attention to clients' needs and desires, and a focus on clients' goal attainment. Implementing a program with these key features has the potential to better serve any ABI community.

REFERENCES

ABI Partnership Project. (2006). Acquired Brain Injury Prevention Project: Program Evaluation 2004– 2006. Retrieved from **http://www.abipartnership.sk.ca/images/file/8%29%20ABI_Evaluation_Report.pdf**

ABI Partnership Project. (n.d). Retrieved from **http://www.abipartnership.sk.ca//index.cfm**

Ontario Neurotrama Foundation. (2010). An outcomes framework for the ABI community of practice. Kitchener, ON: Author. [Draft].

Saskatchewan Health & SGI. (1995). Acquired Brain Injury—A Strategy for Services. Retrieved from **http://www.abipartnership.sk.ca/images/file/9%29%20Strategy%20Apr%202007-1.pdf**

Saskatchewan Health & SGI. (2010). ABI Partnership Project: 2007–2010 Program Review [Unpublished], p. 29–34; 66-70.

CHAPTER 9

ACQUIRED BRAIN INJURY IRELAND

By Georgios Fthenos & Danielle Hryniewicz

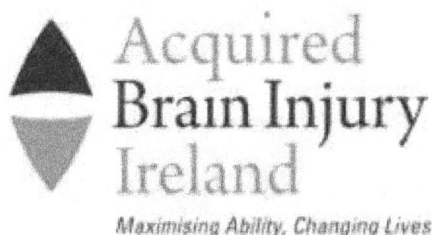

Acquired
Brain Injury
Ireland

Maximising Ability, Changing Lives

"We are committed to being there, to make a difference, to maximize ability and change lives for the better for those with and affected by ABI..."

- ABI Ireland

Population Served: Life Span
Contributing Author Contact Information
Christine Flynn, Project Manager Acquired Brain Injury Ireland 43 Northumberland Ave Dun Laoghaire Co Dublin 01 280 41 64 ext 201 230 4630 (fax) **CFlynn@abiireland.ie**

BACKGROUND

In recent years, various studies have pointed out a need to provide appropriate services to survivors of acquired brain injury and their families throughout the rehabilitation process (**Bissett, 2008**). In Ireland, professionals, ABI clients and family members have recognized a regional inequality in the provision of services and thus have been advocating for greater national coordination—to avoid people getting lost in the system or "falling through the gaps" (**Bissett, 2008**). The absence of suitable services has resulted in many ABI clients being inappropriately placed in nursing homes and psychiatric wards, while others have remained at home, creating a strain on their families and resulting in social isolation. A lack of knowledge and information exists among professionals and carers regarding ABI (**Bissett, 2008**).

The identification of a gap in services and the consideration of experiences elsewhere led to the establishment of a community-based reintegration program. Established in 2000, **Acquired Brain Injury (ABI) Ireland** has grown to serve people with ABI across the country, providing essential brain injury specialist therapy in the community. ABI Ireland's services are person-centred: every brain injury is unique and therefore each service must respond to individual needs. Services are supported by qualified clinicians and staff members, with an emphasis placed on extended activities of daily living, community integration, education, training and employment. ABI Ireland's interventions focus on enhanced community participation, improved quality of life, psychological adjustment, and carer stress. The organization is committed to filling a vital gap in services available in collaboration with statutory bodies (**ABI Ireland, 2009**).

Formerly the **Peter Bradley Foundation** (see Box 1), the organization changed its name to ABI Ireland in 2009. In the words of Maurice O'Connell, Chairman of ABI Ireland, "...the reason for our change of name was very simple—we believe that our name should reflect the people we serve, the work we do and the regions in which we operate" (ABI Ireland, 2009).

Box 1: The Origins of ABI Ireland: The Peter Bradley Story

Peter Bradley attended primary school in Strabane and Clongowes Secondary School in Co. Kildare, where he achieved an excellent Leaving Cert in 1975. From a very young age Peter demonstrated his love of words through his constant chat and love of English and debating. He had an extensive vocabulary, which often exceeded that of his contemporaries. Peter went on to UCD to study law where he graduated with his BCL in 1978. His college years in Dublin were spent in the usual student fashion—socialising and having fun. He learned to play the clarinet, saxophone and bass guitar. He also enjoyed going to concerts and gigs and adding to his extensive music and comics collection. In March 1980, a week before his final solicitor's exams, Peter was knocked off his motorbike by a car and sustained a severe head injury. Too ill to go to London for an operation, he underwent pioneering neurosurgery in St Vincent's Hospital, Dublin, which was given a 20% success rate. He survived but suffered short-term and long-term memory problems.

Peter didn't recognise his parents and much of his college learning was gone. He had also forgotten his relationship with his long-term girlfriend who continued to offer much support during the early days of his recovery. His accident left him blind in his left eye and deaf in his left ear. Following a short period of recovery in hospital, he went home to his family in Donegal to try to piece his life back together. The family remembers the terror of not being given any information regarding his condition or his prognosis. There was no guidebook to deal with the multitude of problems resulting from his accident.

Life continued...

Peter was never able to go back to college and there were no support services available. He attended Headway, then a new organization, which proved to be invaluable to both Peter and his family. Headway offered information, counselling and training for Peter. He went to live in Metro Manila in the Philippines with Sister Teresa, a family friend, where he worked as a volunteer in a prison. At this stage, Peter had made sufficient recovery from his motorbike accident to live independently and manage his own financial affairs. However, he did suffer residual problems including short-term memory loss, changes in communication style and fatigue.

All change again...

Devastatingly in February 1992, Peter was involved in a second road traffic accident, this time in the Philippines as a passenger in a car. He was left in a coma. Following neurosurgery, facial reconstruction and with a smashed pelvis, he was flown home on a stretcher in a critical condition, minded only by his parents. He went for rehabilitation in the National Rehabilitation Hospital, Dublin. Following a successful programme there, he was discharged to his own home, Anvers, in Glenageary, Co. Dublin. Despite two further emergency admissions to hospital with loss of consciousness, Peter lived independently in his home from 1993 until June 1998, when he fell and hit his head. This fall resulted in a slight stroke and further neurosurgery.

As a result of this, Peter could no longer live independently as his memory was not good enough to ensure he took his medication and ate regular meals. Peter almost died six times. He contracted meningitis in November 2001 and was again at death's door. Each time his family prepared for the worst. His stubbornness and will to live was extraordinary.

Still a young man, and with a total lack of community services for people with ABI, the only place for Peter to live was a nursing home for older people, even though all he needed was supervision. With their clinical background, Peter's sister Barbara O'Connell (CEO, ABI

Ireland) and her husband Maurice O'Connell (Chairman, ABI Ireland) knew that a nursing home was not appropriate for Peter. They also knew that he was not alone in his need for supports and services. They identified a much broader need for community rehabilitation services, which would provide a supportive living environment and help people with ABI to live in the community.

With financial assistance from the Health Service Executive and help from Peter's family they set up the Peter Bradley Foundation in 2000 which is now known as Acquired Brain Injury Ireland. The Foundation acquired Peter's family home at Anvers, Glenageary, Co. Dublin and so set up the first ABI Ireland Assisted Living Residence where Peter lives. Within eight months Peter progressed from being able to walk a maximum of 10 metres, sleeping most of the day in a chair in the nursing home and having little interest in his hobbies or surroundings, to going out on his own, shopping and visiting friends.

Life Today...

With continued support from ABI rehabilitation staff, Peter and two other men with similar needs live together in their community in Glenageary, taking an active part in everyday life. In 2008, Peter celebrated his 50th birthday with his family and friends, an important milestone for both Peter and the organization which was set up in his name.

(Source: ABI Ireland Annual Report 2008)

ABI Ireland's Current Range of Services

ABI Ireland has developed a range of ABI-specific community services in direct response to local identified needs across Ireland. As the needs of the individual client change over time, ABI Ireland provides a flexible approach, focusing strongly on individual development and incorporating person-centred planning (PCP) (ABI Ireland, n.d.).

Person-Centred Planning ensures that the client served is fully involved in all decisions that affect his/her life. A personal profile is compiled for each person, identifying their current abilities and their support needs. In partnership with the client, a personal therapy programme is drawn up, tailored to their needs and which enables them to realize personal goals which are meaningful to their lives. This approach ensures that the services provided are never generic or based on assumptions of what is best for the individual (ABI Ireland, n.d.).

Values

ABI Ireland strongly supports and promotes the following values:

➢ **Dignity & Respect**: The dignity of each person is upheld at all times and personal information is kept strictly confidential. Persons served are consulted regarding their personal therapy programme. At all times their privacy and individuality is respected in every way.

➢ **Choices**: Wherever practical and appropriate, choices are offered in all areas of a person's life; we respect the right of all to manage and control their own lives.

➢ **Relationships**: Everyone is encouraged to relate in an adult way using dialogue and negotiation. Good relationships make any therapeutic programme successful.

➢ **Sharing Everyday Places**: At ABI Ireland the focus is on the everyday experience of the person served, their abilities and their needs. The use of regular community facilities and meaningful everyday routines is encouraged, and normal community interactions are promoted.

➢ **Contribution**: ABI Ireland encourages everyone to make a personal and appropriate contribution within their physical and cognitive capabilities. Each person's involvement is to be respected and valued.

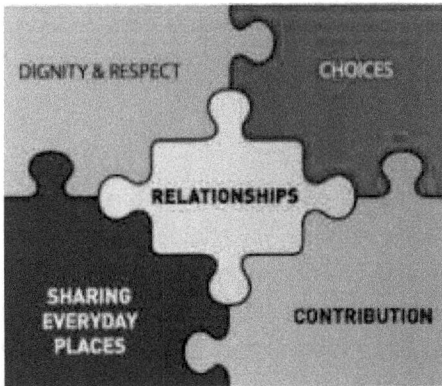

Figure 1: ABI Ireland Values

(Source: ABI Ireland Annual Report 2008)

Best Practice Guidelines

According to **ABI Ireland**, **Best Practice Guidelines** for Acquired Brain Injury recommend that: people with ABI have access to specialist services; there is a clear pathway regarding continuum of care; people with ABI may require different services at different times; people with ABI may require multiple services; specialist support for the family is an essential component of reintegration; services should be co-ordinated and integrated; people should have access to lifelong support, if needed (**ABI Ireland, 2009**). Effective community-based programs (addressing ABI) incorporate best practice guidelines in their service delivery and operations (**ABI Ireland, 2009**).

CARF Accreditation

In 2002, **Acquired Brain Injury Ireland** became the first service provider in the Republic of Ireland to achieve international recognition from the **Commission on Accreditation of Rehabilitation Facilities** (CARF), an independent, non-profit accreditor of organizations that provide services in a range of areas, including rehabilitation facilities.

In 2006, **ABI Ireland** achieved the highest level of **CARF** accreditation in ABI Residential Rehabilitation Services, ABI Long Term Residential Services and ABI Home and Community Rehabilitation Services. **ABI Ireland** is the first, and to date only, Irish service provider to achieve **CARF** accreditation. Recently, ABI Ireland has been successful in achieving re-accreditation by **CARF** for a further period of three years, up to November 2012. The accreditation survey was carried out in September 2009 and highlighted a number of areas where ABI Ireland either demonstrated exemplary performance or a particular strength.

The achievement of international accreditation from **CARF** is extremely important to **ABI Ireland** and its clients. It reassures stakeholders that the organization has been reviewed by an independent and internationally recognized agency.

Quality Measurements and Operating Standards

Everyone working in the organization is committed to providing a personal, quality driven service to its clients on a daily basis. **ABI Ireland** is stakeholder centred and outcome focused. Quality measurements are integral to the organization and include: (1) personal development plans and written service agreements for persons served; (2) regular consultation with families; (3) annual key performance goals and annual accessibility plan; (4) regular consultation with funders at national and local level; (5) annual independent auditing of finances; (6) Commission on Accreditation of Rehabilitation Facilities; and (7) annual survey of people using ABI Ireland's services (**uSPEQ survey**).

ABI Ireland carries out an annual uSPEQ survey of client satisfaction to seek the opinions and input of persons being served. The uSPEQ survey measures ABI Ireland's performance in the context of its core values. In 2008, every effort was made to ensure a very high response rate to the survey.

RESOURCES

Human Resources

Community Rehabilitation Support Team

An experienced **ABI Ireland Community Rehabilitation Support Team** assesses the individual needs of a person with ABI. The team is also responsible for developing a person-centred programme of services and support, which helps the client to maximize his/her abilities. The Rehabilitation Team consists of Clinical Staff, Local Services Managers, ABI Case Managers, and Rehabilitation Assistants, who work together with the client and family members.

ABI Ireland's Pathway of **Community Rehabilitation** has one point of contact for the client and his/her family. Under the direction of the Regional Manager, the point of contact may be either an ABI Case Manager (where one is in place) or the Local Services Manager. Following assessment by the Community Brain Injury Rehabilitation Team (CBIRT), individuals are referred to services, as to their needs and wishes.

The community support team consists of ABI Case Managers, ABI Local Services Managers, Rehabilitation Assistants, ABI Social Work-Family Liaisons, Occupational Therapists, and Clinical Psychologists.

Many board members and stakeholders have personal experience with ABI. Board members include healthcare professionals and business people.

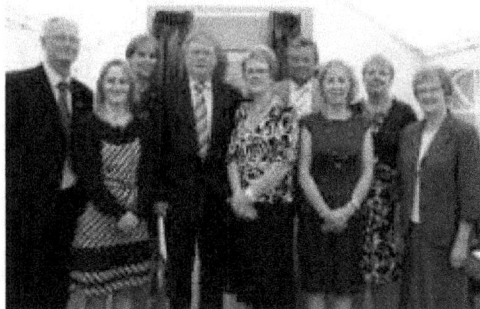

Financial Resources

Core funding from the **Health Service Executive** (HSE) is provided to **ABI Ireland**. In recent years, the HSE granted additional funds to the Side by Side Day Service. Service-users and family members alike have confirmed the effectiveness and appropriateness of the model in use (**Bissett, 2008**).

In 2009, **ABI Ireland** was privileged to have been allocated a number of grants throughout the year, including **Family Carer Training—Brain Aware** (National Programme, 2009–2011) supported by **Dormant Account Funding**, from the Departments of Social Protection & Community, Equality & Gaeltacht Affairs; Certificate in Brain Injury Specialist (CBIS) (National Programme, Pilot Programme 2009), supported by Monkstown Hospital Foundation; Purchase of an Accessible Vehicle—**Side By Side Day Resource**, Dun Laoghaire, supported by the people in need trust (PIN)—telethon; A variety of ABI initiatives including the development of an ABI Quick Guide, supported by the HSE & National Lottery / Respite Grant (**ABI Ireland, 2009**).

Like all organizations in the not-for-profit sector, funding of services continues to be a major issue for **ABI Ireland**. Since 2004, core funding has only marginally increased despite significant organizational growth and expansion. HSE funding for 2009 and 2010 has not been agreed upon, placing an enormous pressure on ABI Ireland. The organization resolves to press for delivery of its core funding commitments from the HSE (ABI Ireland, 2009).

Reporting System

In the past year, **ABI Ireland** worked with the HSE as a pilot organization to produce and sign off fifteen Service level Agreements, which formed part of a national Service Arrangement for the organization. At this time, the Finance Department worked to have a reporting system in place that would produce income and expenditure reports for all services on a monthly basis. These reports were ultimately created, along with a regional report and overall national report.

In 2010, **ABI Ireland** intends to build on this information system, improving the data input system so as to make it more user friendly (ABI, 2008).

IMPLEMENTATION

ABI Ireland provides a range of services throughout Ireland. Among the services provided are **Assisted Living Service**, **Day Resource Service**, and **Rehabilitation Support Team**.

Assisted Living

Assisted Living provides individualized, community-based support service designed to maximize the quality of life of each person living with ABI, while fostering autonomy, personal growth, and development. The emphasis of the assisted living model is based on individual need: over time, clients learn to maximize their abilities, reducing their dependence on support from **Acquired Brain Injury Ireland** staff. The assisted living model supports and promotes independence for the individual (ABI Ireland, n.d.).

ABI Ireland Assisted Living residences are conveniently located with access to local shops, transport, and amenities (ABI Ireland, n.d.). The physical environment in which the residences are located provides stimulation, support, and security.

Day Resource Service

Side by Side Day Resource Service provides resources, support, and advocacy to assist members in achieving their personal goals for community living. It is designed to help individuals move away from an environment where treatment is administered to an environment where they can once again participate, reciprocate and contribute to the community, empowering them with responsibility in their own lives (ABI Ireland, n.d.).

Side by Side is a service run by members for members, a life-long anchor support to assist people with ABI to set and achieve realistic short, medium, and long-term goals. The program model is flexible, variable, person- and client-driven (**Bissett, 2008**). The primary focus of the day resource service is on maximizing sources of intrapersonal support and independence in the functionality of its members. Each member has a key worker to help them develop an Individual Rehabilitation Plan (IRP), which is reviewed every two months. A weekly meeting of clients provides a forum for communication, and for reviewing and planning the on-going life of the centre. There are a variety of meaningful activities, such as drama, arts and crafts, photography, computers, environmental awareness, cooking, and music, which help members develop skills and interests. Cognitive exercise, such as crosswords and brain gym exercises, are organized on a daily basis.

An important aspect in **Side by Side** has been its flexibility in meeting the needs of a wide range of members. Some enjoy having a place to come Monday to Friday, while others prefer to pick and choose their hours of attendance, depending on their particular needs (Personal Communication, T. Bissett, September 27, 2010).

Side by Side is "inserted in the community" (Personal Communication, T. Bissett, September 27, 2010), where many facilities are located nearby. Program coordinators have further developed the aspect of a work-ordered day, whereby the members take a more active part in practically running the Centre and participating within the larger community. Efforts are made to connect clients with community facilities for educational, vocational and/or recreational purposes (Personal Communication, T. Bissett, September 27, 2010).

Rehabilitation Support Team

The **Rehabilitation Support Team** is responsible for assessing the individual needs of a client and for developing a person-centred programme of community services and support. The team consists of clinical staff, Local Services Managers, ABI Case Managers, and Rehabilitation Assistants together with the person with ABI and family members/carers affected by acquired brain injury. Various sources of interpersonal support are accessible to the individual client, by way of the team approach.

➤ Local Services Managers

Local Services Managers coordinate assisted living residences and/or Home & Community services in their area. They work as part of the Rehabilitation Team, managing a team of Rehabilitation Assistants, taking the lead in the provision of person-centred services, and linking in with families and the wider community (ABI Ireland, n.d.). The role of the Local Services Managers is to facilitate and assist optimal independence and participation in activities within a client's own home or work environment, and in the community. The investments of effort that a client makes on his/her own behalf facilitates independence, personal growth, and change.

➤ ABI Case Managers

Case Managers seek out and coordinate appropriate resources, monitor progress, and communicate with the person with ABI, the family/carer, and other professionals, including all statutory and non-statutory agencies. Case Managers identify local sources of help or support, educate and support carers, explore activities that may be available, and help the client structure time and live as independently as possible within her or his local community.

➤ Rehabilitation Assistants

Rehabilitation Assistants are key members of the team; they work in partnership with clients, directing and adapting their input in response to individual needs. They assist their clients in realizing the goals identified in the person-centred plan, and promote independence in the home and community. Rehabilitation Assistants are supervised and supported by clinicians and other qualified staff (ABI Ireland, n.d.).

A Promising Practice: Brain Aware, ABI Family Carer Training

In response to an identified national need, ABI Ireland introduced into its services the **Brain Aware Family Carer training programme** for those caring for and supporting a family member with ABI (ABI Ireland, 2009). In May 2009, a pilot programme ran in Kilkenny. The training, funded by the Department of Social & Family Affairs and the Department of Rural, Community and Gaeltacht Affairs, is supported by Pobal through the Dormant Account Fund (DAF) management team. Following an evaluation of the pilot, two more studies and evaluations were completed in Blanchardstown and Castlebar, with a further thirteen programmes scheduled between 2010 and 2011. Each programme is comprised of six sessions for groups not exceeding fifteen family carers. Topics in the training modules include: how families cope with acquired brain injury; living with ABI—a practical everyday approach; health promotion and wellbeing of carers; emotional and behavioural changes following brain injury; communication and the challenges after brain injury; attention and memory difficulties following brain injury; and children with an acquired brain injury. **Brain Aware** will run until June 2011, at which stage over 240 family members will have received training. The programme will be delivered in eight geographical locations across the country (ABI Ireland).

OUTCOME

Evaluation

Both external and internal service evaluations have been conducted on ABI Ireland's services (**ABI Annual Report, 2009**; **uSPEQ, 2009**; **Annual Report, 2008**; **Bissett, 2008**). These include an evaluation of the service as an appropriate model, assessing how the service meets the needs of clients, family members and carers, and how well it addresses the gap between service provision and need. Questionnaires have been administered to the clients and interviews conducted among the carers.

External evaluations are conducted by uSPEQ, a consumer survey questionnaire designed to capture common concerns and domains across varied setting and diverse populations. The primary purpose of uSPEQ is to gather feedback from persons served regarding their perceptions of the quality of service they are currently receiving or have received in the past.

The 2009 survey—conducted externally—indicates a very high positive response from the clients. There were particularly strong responses under the headings of Respect by Staff and Informed Choice, while the responses under the heading of Participation showed a marked increase on the 2008 results. With respect to the latter, Participation is operationalized as ten terms: "Able to deal with everyday activities", "Able to make important choices", "Know where/how to get help in the community", "Able to do needed things without barriers", "Able to do things I want now", "Participate in activities I want", "Opportunities to make friends", "Have friends I like to be with", "Do better in social situations" and "Got help to do things in community".

In the 2009 survey, each of these terms were measured and compared to responses obtained in 2008. The results indicate that the percent positive (agree and strongly agree) has increased for each term, with "Able to deal with everyday activities" scoring 90.1% compared with 80.6% (2008), "Able to make important choices" scoring 96.4% compared with 82.8% (2008), "Know where/how to get help in the community" scoring 84.9% compared with 77.8% (2008), "Able to do needed things without barriers" scoring 86.1% compared with 75.3% (2008) and "Able to do things I want now" scoring 75.7% compared with 68.8% (2008).

"Participate in activities I want" scored at 82.9% (79.1% - 2008), "Opportunities to make friends" scored at 80.7% (74.7% - 2008), "Have friends I like to be with" scored at 88.2% (80.0% - 2008), "Do better in social situations" scored at 84.4% (81.3% - 2008) and "Got help to do things in community" scored at 87.0% (76.1% - 2008).

An internal service evaluation of the Side by Side Day Service was released in 2008. The evaluation considered the appropriateness of the service model and assessed how well the service met the needs of clients, family members and carers, and how well it addressed the gap in service provision. In response to the specific needs of ABI survivors (Bissett, 2008), the results demonstrate that service-users and family members alike have confirmed the effectiveness and appropriateness of the model in use. To the question "Does Side by Side day service meet my needs?" 87% responded "yes", while 13% were unsure or did not reply. Ninety three per cent felt they were offered sufficient opportunity to voice their opinion, and thus meet their need to participate in the service. An issue of poor internal wheelchair access was identified in the study. This indicated the need for a change of premises, which is currently being sought (Bissett, 2008).

In the unstructured interviews with parents, several issues emerged: the existing lack of community services for persons with ABI, the drawbacks of rehabilitative training programs as distinct from day services and the need for programs, such as the Side by Side Day Service, to meet the needs of persons with ABI and the wider community.

Brain Aware

In the Internal Interim Report of **Brain Aware**'s Carers Training Project (2010), Carol Rogan, the report's author, indicates that the training programmes have been well attended. In the first year, 135 participants had signed up for the programme, exceeding the target of 120 participants. Feedback from participants has been extremely positive: participants completed pre- and post-course evaluation sheets and informal feedback was obtained at each session through informal chats during tea/coffee and lunch breaks. Pre- and post-course questionnaires were completed by 118 participants with the majority (82%) being female and 18% being male. The most represented age range was 46-55 years for both males (40%) and females (35%). Notable findings reported in the Interim Report include the following:

➢ When asked if the training programme met their needs, the majority of participants reported that it did. Some carers reported that they developed a deeper understanding of ABI in general and in particular to their own personal circumstances. Carers also reported that they learned a lot from each other as well as from the trainers.

➢ Further training needs were identified such as sexuality and brain injury, training in epilepsy, relaxation skills, cognitive stimulation and training for children/siblings of person with an ABI.

➢ There were a number of positive developments from the training programmes including strong peer support, friendships formed and participants feeling comfortable enough to share their very personal stories with the group. Participants gave examples of how their knowledge and confidence had increased as a result of attending the training programme.

➢ Some challenges that impacted on the training were an unsuitable training venue that had to be changed, fluctuations in attendee numbers, the need to change the content of one of the modules and the need for more exercises/interaction on some of the modules.

➢ In relation to future action, participants reported that they would access more services following the training. There was a general desire from groups to meet again on conclusion of the training programme, and this has been facilitated as much as possible.

Participants rated their knowledge on Acquired Brain Injury (ABI) and confidence in dealing with ABI both before and after the training programme. There was a significant increase in knowledge and confidence levels reported by participants after the training programme (Rogan, 2010).

Client Testimonials

In addition to external and internal evaluations, ABI Ireland solicits **client testimonials** from its members. Publicly accessible testimonials include *"A Different Light – But a New Light by Risteard Lloyd:* Re-establishing one's identity after Brain Injury (a story of survival)" (**http://www.abiireland.ie/docs/TheRisteardLloydstory2009.pdf**), "Paul Hughes—ABI Survivor Tells His Story" (**http://www.abiireland.ie/case_study2.html**), and "After My Stroke" (**http://www.abiireland.ie/case_study3.html**). Each case demonstrates ABI Ireland's operating model, as clients discuss the ways in which the program helps them to achieve personal goals. Paul Hughes' story is featured here:

Paul Hughes

My aneurysm troubles began when I flew to California in 2004 to meet up with old friends in Los Angeles and San Diego with my sons Jamie and Aaron.

On the flight over I sustained a slight headache but thought no more of it. We stayed for 10 days in LA before driving down to San Diego where I met up with my sister and booked into the Bahia Resort Hotel. Overnight my headache worsened and my sister sent for a doctor, who in turn sent me to Mercy Scripps hospital where I was diagnosed with having a brain aneurysm.

I had not seen my friend in San Diego for the best part of thirty years (we come from the same town in the North of England), so the first time we met again was in the hospital in the intensive care ward, and remarkably I recognized him immediately. My wife informs me that my treatment in Mercy Scripps was excellent—I was insured for once.

As my brain began to recover from the surgery I began confabulating wildly and was apparently a great source of amusement to the nursing staff as I regaled them with tales of my adventures up the Amazon, kidnapping the queen of England and accusing an eminent brain surgeon of being a member of the Israeli Secret Service. But I finally relaxed and knew I was in good hands when while being examined I looked down and saw my doctor was wearing cowboy boots. The cavalry had arrived!

The operation would appear to have been successful and I am extremely grateful to all at Mercy Scripps for the good care they took of me. My wife flew over the day after the aneurysm to be with me and apart from taking a shine to my cowboy doctor was a wonderful support.

On leaving the hospital we were taken by chauffeur-driven stretch limo to the airport in LA (insurance again) and flown back to Ireland and on to Beaumont Hospital where I stayed for another 2 and a half months recuperating, while my wife struggled long and hard to get some after care for me.

Eventually we were blessed to find Acquired Brain Injury Ireland (formerly the Peter Bradley Foundation) through her efforts at an opportune time when they were expanding their services into the community. Their advice and help has proved invaluable—both to myself and the rest of the family. Not only have they given me tremendous support but they have also come to the aid of my wife on several occasions when the going got tough for her. Unfortunately she could not be here today, but she wants me to sing the organization's praises on her behalf. They have been a life-line for her on numerous occasions.

When they first began their support programme with me, I was visited four or five times a week and over the years as I have improved this was reduced and we are now down to once a month and they continue to keep check on my progress.

I would like to thank the Rehabilitation Assistants and all the others from Acquired Brain Injury Ireland who have helped me move on and restart my life after what it quite a life-changing and traumatic experience.

It goes without saying that I can never repay my family for the love and patience they have shown me in what has been a trying and testing time. I love them more than I will ever be able to express. All of this love, effort and patience has allowed me to reintegrate myself into a working environment and this is proceeding apace with my son Jamie now talking about joining me in the carpentry/joinery business.

My work so far has consisted of general carpentry work—fitting kitchens, repairing furniture etc. But we have longer-term projects in mind such as producing rocking horses, and we have six of these on the go at present. The challenges I have faced since resuming work have been varied. Memory is still a problem. If I am on my own I have to make sure I make a note of everything –down to the last screw, or the job will slow down.

Confidence is on the up. Initially I was wary of taking too much on and worried about my own ability to complete tasks. This is improving however. Friends' reactions have been much better than I feared—not at all negative or wary, but caring—giving me small jobs, taking me to concerts and the like.

As far as getting back to work again, planning and making notes is imperative and Acquired Brain Injury Ireland has been instrumental in instilling this into my daily routine. Where I would once have been able to rely on my memory as to what I needed for a job the following day, this is no longer the case, so again, note-taking is important to ensure flow and continuity, particularly if I am working alone.

This was particularly difficult initially after my youngest son Aaron stopped working with me, as he would act as the company memory for the both of us. Again, strategies such as work sheets, diary and phone reminders have come into their own.

I am also determined in myself to move on. My skills are still extant and if I use my memory aids that they have drummed into me, I see no reason why I—we—shouldn't be able to move onwards and upwards—and if our rocking horse business takes off, that will be a positive to have come out of all the negatives. The Children's Hospital in Crumlin will certainly benefit, as they will receive a horse in return for treating both of my sons when they were small. A further positive was that I passed a driving test again—I had to go through this to prove to the insurance company that I was capable of driving safely.

Just one last thought again about my wonderful family—Chris, my partner for the last 30 something years (I know I probably don't look old enough for that to be the case!) has taken over as head honcho like a duck to water—doing her job, looking after the house and me in her wonderful, cheerful fashion (most of the time anyway) and I love her to bits—my sister and my sons have also been wonderful and supportive and I am so proud of them.

So that's it. I would like once again to thank everybody in the various hospitals and Acquired Brain Injury Ireland who have got me to where I am at this time.

Thank you.

Paul Hughes, ABI Survivor

(Source: ABI Ireland n.d.)

Program Replication

This year, six representatives of three Slovenian private, not-for-profit centres and one public institution (providing long-term rehabilitation support and residential care to adults with ABI), accompanied by a representative of the **Ministry of Labour, Family and Social Affairs of Slovenia**, visited **ABI Ireland**. The visit was funded under a Leonardo da Vinci Mobility project, which is part of the European Commission's Lifelong Learning Programme. The project is designed to improve the vocational skills of the workforce through European partnerships. The objective of the visit to ABI Ireland was to learn about the organizations' aims and objectives, to exchange knowledge and experience, and to compare services and programmes between partners. ABI Ireland decided to get involved in the project because of the growing need for new, innovative services and programmes for people with ABI in Slovenia.

ABI Ireland is currently being replicated in Slovenia; ongoing collaborations exist between ABI Ireland and the the **Ministry of Labour, Family and Social Affairs**. Strategies to transfer ABI Ireland best practice strategies are now being implemented.

Conclusion

Acquired Brain Injury Ireland was founded on the belief that "…with the correct environment and appropriate supports, people with ABI can live a meaningful life in the community. If you maximize ability you can change lives" (ABI, n.d.). ABI Ireland continues to expand its services to meet the individual needs of those with ABI. In addition, the organization strives to meet the individual needs of those who are struggling to cope within their family home settings.

As a **CARF** accredited organization, ABI Ireland offers on-going consultations with clients, their families, and carers. With a range of pioneering, flexible and tailor-made services that include assisted living and home and community services, day resource services, case management, education programs and individual person-centred planning—all with a critical emphasis on client-centredness, quality, and effectiveness—**ABI Ireland** serves as a national strategy to provide support and services that advance community participation for survivors of acquired brain injury across the country. The **2008** and **2009 Annual Reports** reflect significant achievements in ABI Community Rehabilitation and Participation. The **Side By Side Day Service** has shown that it leads to personal growth, community integration and improved independence (**Bissett, 2008**).

ABI Ireland has been involved in significant partnerships with the **Health Service Executive** across the country, delivering services locally in response to local need. Community support greatly enhances the work of the organization, enabling stakeholders and collaborators to positively impact on the lives of people affected, either directly or indirectly, by acquired brain injury. The growing number of people living with long-term consequences is a severe and complex circumstance. The implications for the provision of appropriate health services in the coming years are enormous (**Bissett, 2008**).

References

Acquired Brain Injury Ireland. (2008). **Annual Report: 2008**.

Acquired Brain Injury Ireland. (2009). **Annual Report: 2009**.

Bissett, T. (2008) Needs assessment for the provision of appropriate day services for people with an Acquired Brain Injury. Institute of Public Administration.

Rogan, C. (2010). BRAIN AWARE Carers Training Project Internal Interim Report: 2010.

uSPEQ (2009) **Consumer Survey Annual Report: Abridged Version: 2009**.

CHAPTER 10

SCHOOL TRANSITION AND RE-ENTRY PROGRAM (STEP)

A Promising Practice

By Sherry L. Ally

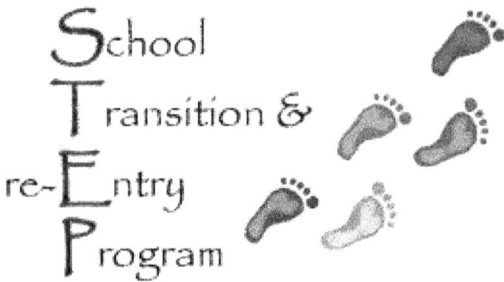

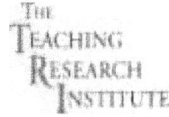

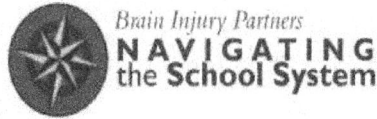

Population Served : Children aged 5 -18 with moderate to severe TBI/ABI	
Contributing Author Contact Information	
Kevin Prier PMP Project Manager Teaching Research Institute 99 W. 10th Avenue, Suite 370 Eugene, OR, 97401 Phone: 541-346-0592	Ann Glang, PhD Senior Fellow, Research Professor Teaching Research Institute 99 W. 10th Avenue, Suite 370 Eugene, OR, 97401 Phone: 541-346-0594

BACKGROUND

For children in the United States, brain injury has been cited as one of the most frequent causes of death and disability (**Center for Neuroskills, 2010**). The **Centers for Disease Control and Prevention (CDC, 2010)** indicate that infants (aged 0 – 4 years), adolescents (aged 15 – 19 years), and adults over the age of 65 are most likely to suffer a TBI. In the United States, in each year between 2002 and 2006, an average of approximately 380,000 school aged children visited the emergency room and over 35,000 were hospitalized as a result of TBI (**US Department of Health and Human Services, 2010**).

Provisions do exist in North American schools to assist students with TBI under the rubric of special education services. However, as is the case with referral to rehabilitation services for injury, a number of interrelated factors influence whether a child will be referred for special education services upon return to school (**Agency for Health Care Policy and Research, 1999**).

Researchers at the **Teaching Research Institute of Western Oregon University** note that among the over 2 million children with TBI currently residing in the United States, in 2004 only 24,000 school aged children were being provided formal services in public schools. Since school is characterized as a setting within which to practice skills gained or refined in rehabilitation (**Agency for Health Care Policy and Research, 1999**), this lack of service provision in public schools may limit a child's opportunities to participate fully in the classroom, with their peers and in their community, with obvious implications for their educational experience and quality of life (K. Prier, personal communication, July 27, 2010).

A Lack of Referral

A group of researchers reviewing the provision of special education for children with TBI argue that there exists a perceived "low incidence" of TBI within the North American public school context leading to a lack of service provision. Based on empirical research, these researchers propose that an interrelationship exists between under-identification of children with TBI within the school system and a number of associated factors, as illustrated in Figure 1.

Under-identification Cycle

Apparent Low Incidence

Lack of Awareness

Under-identification

Lack of Training

Lack of Research Money

Lack of Appropriate Services for Kids who *are* ID

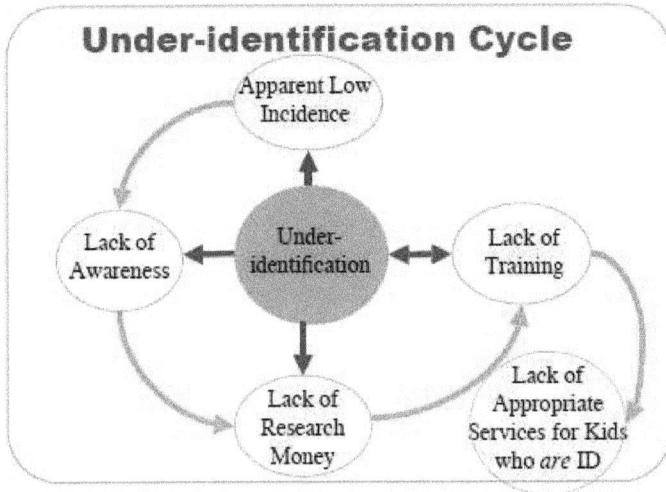

Figure 1: The under-identification cycle for children with TBI.

Under-identification is highly interrelated with perceived low incidence of childhood TBI; a lack of awareness of TBI and its manifestations in the school setting; a lack of funding for research; and finally, a lack of training for staff that may interact with children in the school setting. These factors all contribute to the lack of identification of children with TBI in the school setting and ultimately, a lack of service provision, whether formal or informal, in the classroom. This relationship is supported by empirical research and has prompted the development of research into effective initiatives designed to improve and therefore increase identification of children with TBI in school.

One such initiative is the **School Transition and re-Entry Program** (STEP) which supports facilitated transitions from the hospital to the school for children with TBI. **Glang, Todis, Hooda, Bedell & Cockrell (2008)** note that the provision of hospital-to-school transition services has been shown to increase a child's chances of receiving formal special education services. Therefore **STEP** may contribute to breaking the cycle of under-identification of children with TBI in the North American public school context, thereby allowing children with TBI to more fully participate in their schools and communities.

STEP is a five year research project being executed in three phases: planning, piloting and testing of strategies to improve identification. This case study will review the three research phases of **STEP** with particular reference to its current manifestation as a randomized control trial (RCT) of hospital-to-school transition services in three US states: Ohio, Oregon and Colorado. This portion of the research program—referred to as **STEP**—will be reviewed as a promising practice in the present work. That is, a program that seeks to improve community participation for individuals with TBI, but one which has not yet been evaluated.

Childhood TBI and the Changing Profile of Need

As with adults, TBI may affect a wide range of function, including "cognition, learning, behaviour, personality and social interaction" in school-aged children (**Glang, Todis, Hooda, Bedell & Cockrell, 2008**). Of particular importance in childhood TBI is that this injury occurs during a period of rapid change and development in the brain. Therefore, manifestations of TBI impact both learned skills and future learning and development. As children age, they are expected to develop new and fundamentally different skills, such as those associated with executive function and advanced reasoning (**Glang, Todis, Hooda, Bedell & Cockrell, 2008**).

These authors cite evidence to suggest that the effects of pediatric TBI may persist or even increase over time as expectations for learning and development change during childhood. Therefore, the needs of children change as they learn and develop post-injury. Social, psychological, and special education needs persist for varying amounts of time depending on the severity of the child's injury, from several months (as profiled in Figure 2) to the rest of the child's life.

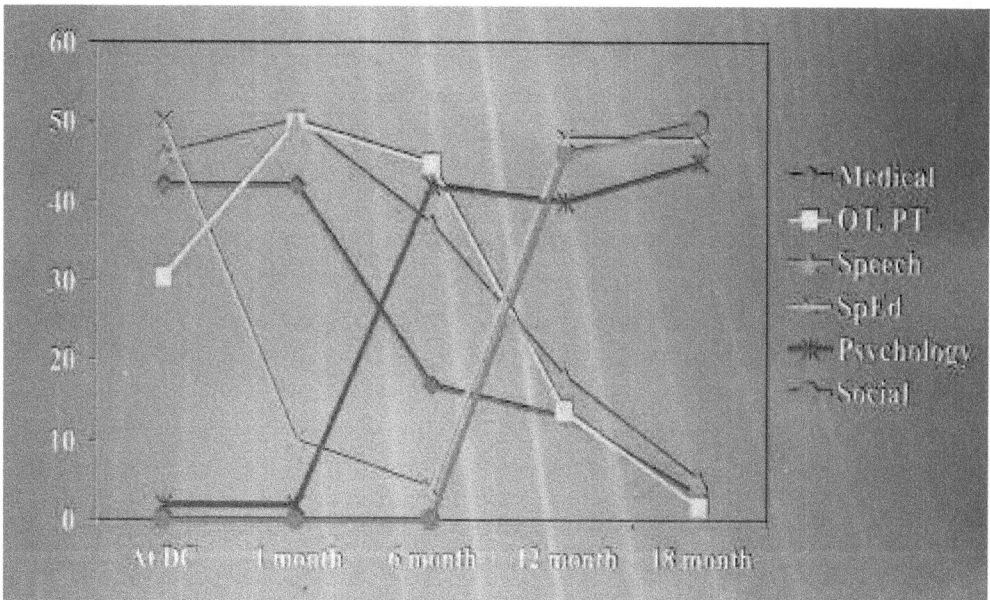

Figure 2: The changing profile of need for children with TBI (Dise-Lewis, 2006 as cited by Glang, Todis, Hooda, Bedell & Cockrell, 2008)

Legislation for Special Education

The provision of special education services for children with TBI was legislated in 1990 and revised in 2007 under the federal **Individuals with Disabilities Education Act** (IDEA), also referred to as the Special Education Law, and defined as "an acquired injury to the brain caused by an external physical force, resulting in total or partial functional disability or psychosocial impairment, or both, that adversely affects a child's educational performance" (Public Law, 101-475, as cited by **Glang & Todis, 2007**).

This provision covers open or closed head injuries that create impairments in any of the following areas: cognition; language; memory; attention; reasoning; abstract thinking; problem solving; psychosocial behaviour; physical functioning; information processing; speech; judgment; or sensory, perceptual, and motor abilities (Public Law 101-476, as cited by **Glang & Todis, 2007**). To qualify for special education services under this legislation, the majority of U.S. states require the following: medical documentation of TBI; documented change in performance in school related activities post-injury as compared to pre-injury; and a demonstrated capacity to benefit from particular modes of instruction offered within special education services.

In cases where a child qualifies for special education services under the **IDEA**, an individualized education plan (IEP) may be designed for the child. The IEP is typically designed collaboratively by the child's parent(s) or guardian, their teacher, a special education teacher, and a district school board representative. In some cases a child has suffered a TBI but does not meet the above criteria; that is, they suffer negative consequences of TBI but continue to perform at or near grade level in school. These children may not be eligible for an IEP, but schools and teachers may provide supports within the classroom for this population through a 504 plan (Rehabilitation Act of 1973). 504 plans allow for the provision of accommodations in the classroom for children with disabilities such as the allowance of extra time to complete tests or assignments or assistance with note taking. These types of informal services may be provided in the classroom even without a 504 (**Glang, Todis, Hooda, Bedell & Cockrell, 2008**; K. Prier, personal communication, July 27, 2010).

Lack of Formal Service Provision under the IDEA

Despite the evident high incidence of TBI as discussed above, research as early as 2001 highlighted a growing concern: children were not receiving the formal educational assistance services they evidently needed. Although not all children who suffer from mild to moderate TBI need special education services such as those provided under an IEP, even conservative estimates of the prevalence of severe TBI in school-aged children in

2003 revealed that only a comparatively small number of children were receiving formal special education services under the **IDEA**.

Glang and associates (2008) are in consensus with scholars in the field who argue that this population is underserved due to a particular constellation of factors (Figure 1). They argue that increased identification of children with TBI in the school system is critical to breaking this cycle (see Figure 3). Given this context, a line of research was taken up by Ann Glang Ph.D., Bonnie Todis, Ph.D. and researcher Kevin Prier, B.S., PMP, all of the Teaching Research Institute of Western Oregon University, to explore effective strategies to increase the identification of school-aged children with TBI.

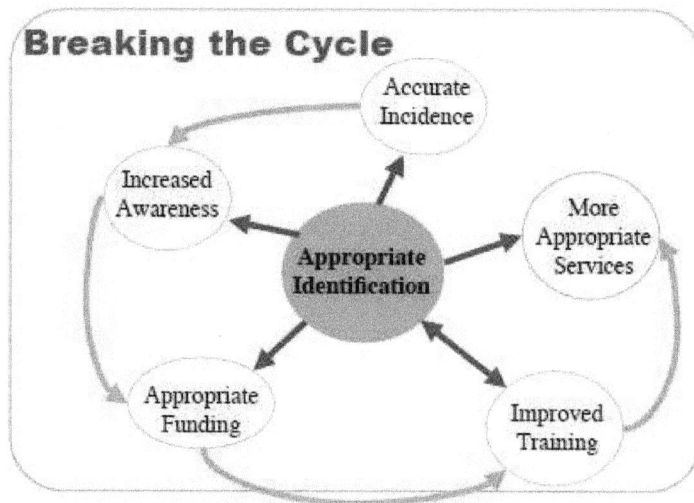

Figure 3: Breaking the cycle of under-identification of children with TBI.

The Back to School Study

The purpose of the Back to School study (**Glang, Todis, Hooda, Bedell & Cockrell, 2008**) was to explore factors that increased the likelihood that children with TBI would be identified for special education services in school.

Using primarily qualitative interviews with parents, this study revealed that both severity of injury and the provision of hospital-to-school transition services increased the likelihood that a child would receive special education services in the form of an IEP or 504 upon returning to school. Children with severe injuries were 8 times more likely to receive special education services. Conversely, children who received transition services were 16 times more likely to be recommended for special education services in school. These findings suggest that even though severity of injury might prompt the implementation of an IEP or 504, hospital-to-school transition services are a more effective strategy in promoting the provision of special education services for children with TBI.

Glang, Todis, Hooda, Bedell & Cockrell (2008) suggest that teachers may not understand the needs of students with TBI, even if they have had a severe injury. However, communication with hospital personnel or those with an increased understanding of TBI—provided by hospital-to-school transition services—may help to bridge this gap in information or understanding.

The results of this 2008 study prompted the development and validation of **STEP**. In follow up to the Back to School study and its results, Ann Glang, Bonnie Todis and Kevin Prier designed and piloted a hospital-to-school transition service for children with TBI and their families. Focus groups and interviews in Phase One of the research program (planning and development) led to a program design (Phase 2) that was piloted in Portland, Oregon (STEP booklet; Prier, personal communication, July 27, 2010).

Phases One and Two

The objective of this research initiative was to develop, validate, and disseminate information regarding effective measures or intervention practices for assisting children with TBI as they transition back to school. The intended outcome of this research was to increase identification of school aged children with TBI, thereby increasing the chances that they would be referred for special education services. Ultimately, the researchers hoped that this would allow children with TBI to more fully benefit from their educational experience and more fully participate in their schools and communities.

Within Phase One of the research project, focus groups were conducted in Colorado, Hawaii, Kansas, Ohio, and Oregon with TBI survivors, parents and any hospital and school staff that would potentially have been in contact with or providing information to children with TBI and their families. Consultation with other research groups in the area of childhood TBI also proved beneficial in designing an appropriate and effective transition service. Data collected in Phase One, from focus groups and consultation, showed that the following conditions were characteristic of an effective transition service:

➤ Met the needs of all groups involved: families, staff in schools and hospital personnel;

➤ Was accessible to parents across the spectrum of injury severity;

➤ Made use of features of successful hospital-to-school transition services already in operation; and

> ➢ Was flexible enough to be adopted by various American hospitals and departments of education.

In Phase Two of the research project, data collected from focus groups was compiled and transformed into a hospital-to-school transition service that was piloted in Portland, Oregon. Two outcomes of the pilot project were of particular importance.

First, pilot testing revealed that the intervention needed to demand as little as possible from hospital staff. Second, the process by which families were recruited in the pilot project—having information packages mailed to their home upon return from the hospital—was less effective than anticipated with regard to enrollment. The researchers decided that the point of information exchange had to be the hospital. That is, Boards of Education and therefore schools and teachers, had to be informed directly by the hospital. This provided the impetus for **STEP** to be incorporated into a standard hospital discharge protocol for children with TBI. That is, when a child is discharged from a hospital, hospital staff will provide an alert, in the form of a paper document, to a single point of contact at the state's Board of Education.

Upon completion of the pilot, a randomized control trial of a comprehensive hospital-to-school transition intervention was begun. This is the current phase of **STEP** and the portion of the project under review as a promising practice in the present work.

RESOURCES

The entire 5-year research project supporting **STEP** is being funded by a **National Institute on Disability and Rehabilitation Research** (NIDDR) grant administered by the U.S. **Department of Education's Office of Special Education and Rehabilitative Services**. This grant provides primarily salary support to the three primary researchers, Drs. Ann Glang and Bonnie Todis and project manager, Kevin Prier for research, development and dissemination of research findings.

STEP also operates with the assistance of local hospitals, school boards and staff. Local hospitals allow access to the population and provide a space within which data is collected and participants recruited for the RCT. State level departments of education involved in **STEP** allocate a portion of time for their salaried staff to work as facilitators within STEP. School boards allow teachers to contribute salaried time to participating in STEP (completing surveys; collaborating with facilitators, families, and students on 504 plans and IEPs).

This type of support from state departments of education and local school boards increases the sustainability of **STEP**. Although this is a short term project—primarily designed to be an evaluation of a program model and is therefore not intended to be sustainable in itself—**STEP** has been designed in such a way as to be sustainable should it be taken up by departments of education in the future. Explicit in the design of **STEP** was that facilitators were volunteers. They offered to participate in the study and their funding bodies allocate a portion of their time to the project. The project was designed in this way to decrease the chance that implementation of the project could lapse when the research grant expired.

IMPLEMENTATION

STEP Protocol

STEP has three components that revolve around the child with TBI: parents/families, the facilitator and hospital staff, seen here in Figure 4:

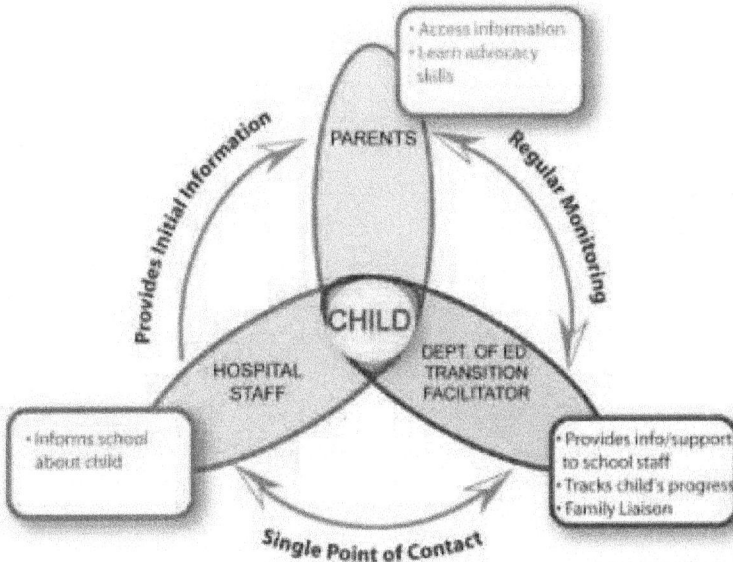

Figure 4: The three components of STEP: Family, Facilitator and Hospital

As outlined in Figure 5, the **STEP** protocol is as follows: a recruiter, who is an existing hospital employee, works within a participating hospital. The recruiter's status as an employee provides them access to hospital records that they search each day to find children who meet the criteria to participate in **STEP**. That is, children between the ages of 5-18 years who have visited the hospital and been diagnosed with a moderate to severe brain injury. **STEP** recruiters began enrollment for the RCT in late 2008 and ended recruitment in March 2011.

The recruiter approached the families and children within the hospital setting and provided them with information about **STEP**. This differs from the pilot protocol in that within the pilot, families were contacted by mail after they left the hospital. Contacting families at the hospital resulted in a much higher participation rate at the point of recruitment. When families consent to participate, medical information is recorded by the recruiter and sent to the Project Manager. In addition, parents complete a demographic information form, a teacher nomination form and two other questionnaires. This provides the research team with a point of contact within the school system and preliminary data for comparing children between control and experimental groups in the RCT.

The project manager documents the information and randomly places the child into one of two streams: half of the children are placed in the control group and half in the facilitator or **STEP** group. Children enrolled in the control group do not receive the hospital-to-school transition intervention. Implicit in this protocol is that once a family decides to participate in the program, decision making related to that child's participation in the **STEP** program is handled by one person, the Project Manager.

Currently, there are approximately 70 children in each condition. Fifty children have completed the **STEP** program (they have been enrolled for 12 months post-injury). Parents with children enrolled in the control group complete the surveys but do not receive an Information Booklet or access to the advocacy training program, and are not contacted by a facilitator (as discussed below). However, they may receive standard rehabilitation (based on the hospital's assessment) and special education services from their school based on need. Although it is impossible to prevent parents from inferring their assignment to the intervention or control group, this should have little effect on the outcomes of the intervention. There has been no differential attrition between the control and intervention groups from the first 50 families to finish the study period.

For children enrolled in the **STEP** group, information about the child is passed onto the facilitator, one per educational region. The Project Manager provides a Letter of Information and an Information Booklet to the families in the **STEP** group. At this point, the facilitator makes initial contact with the family and the child's teacher.

STEP Protocol

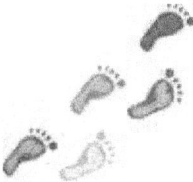

Items in BLUE are in the Service line and fall to the department of Education. Items in GREEN are in the Data line and only pertain to data collection for the life of the project. Once project is complete, hospital will notify DOE SPOC directly.

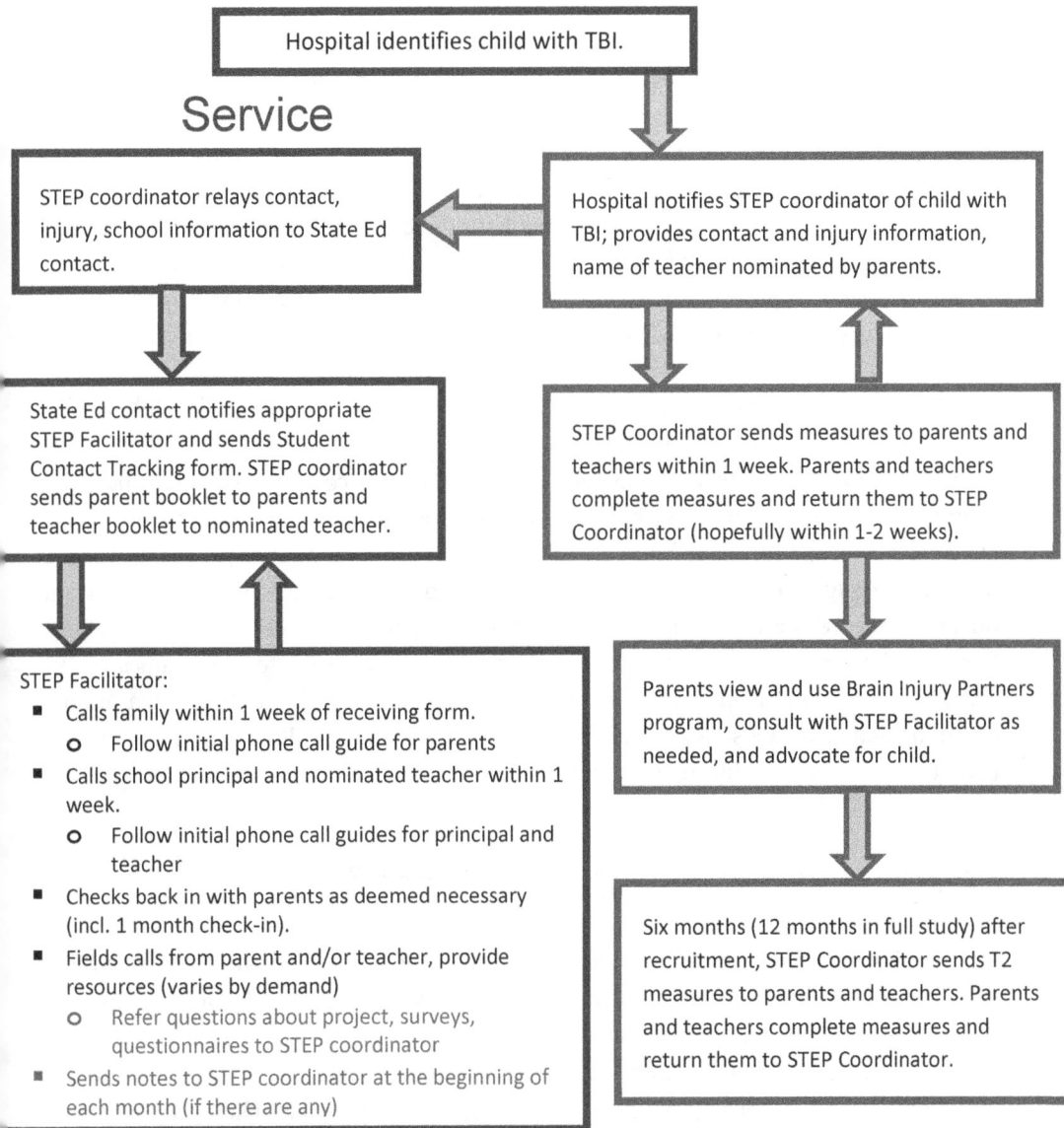

Hospital identifies child with TBI.

Service

STEP coordinator relays contact, injury, school information to State Ed contact.

Hospital notifies STEP coordinator of child with TBI; provides contact and injury information, name of teacher nominated by parents.

State Ed contact notifies appropriate STEP Facilitator and sends Student Contact Tracking form. STEP coordinator sends parent booklet to parents and teacher booklet to nominated teacher.

STEP Coordinator sends measures to parents and teachers within 1 week. Parents and teachers complete measures and return them to STEP Coordinator (hopefully within 1-2 weeks).

STEP Facilitator:
- Calls family within 1 week of receiving form.
  o Follow initial phone call guide for parents
- Calls school principal and nominated teacher within 1 week.
  o Follow initial phone call guides for principal and teacher
- Checks back in with parents as deemed necessary (incl. 1 month check-in).
- Fields calls from parent and/or teacher, provide resources (varies by demand)
  o Refer questions about project, surveys, questionnaires to STEP coordinator
- Sends notes to STEP coordinator at the beginning of each month (if there are any)

Parents view and use Brain Injury Partners program, consult with STEP Facilitator as needed, and advocate for child.

Six months (12 months in full study) after recruitment, STEP Coordinator sends T2 measures to parents and teachers. Parents and teachers complete measures and return them to STEP Coordinator.

The facilitator contacts the family to provide preliminary information as outlined in a phone call guide—for instance, to remind parents about the information packet they will receive, identifying needs and concerns, linking with resources, etc. These facilitators are trained in TBI/ABI and its effects on education and learning. Therefore, facilitators are encouraged to probe for specific issues the child may have and offer pertinent advice for handling these issues during initial contact with families. The facilitator then contacts the child's teacher to inform them that one of their students has had an injury and convey any parent concerns regarding the child's return to school. The facilitator provides the teacher with an information package and her or his contact information.

At this stage, both parents and teachers complete a "pre-injury assessment" on the child by way of a set of surveys. These surveys assess and provide baseline information on the child's behaviour and academic performance before the injury. At the close of the school year, the teacher completes the same assessment of the child's behaviour and academic performance. At the beginning of the following school year, the facilitator checks in with the family again and the new teacher to see how the child is progressing. At 12 months post-injury (whether the child has moved into a new school year or progressed to another grade), parents complete a survey on the child's behaviour and academic performance since the injury was sustained. Children are not asked to complete their own assessments.

Another resource or another program intervention offered to parents through **STEP** is access to the **Brain Injury Partners Website** (2010). Funded by the National Institute of Child Health and Human Development and developed in collaboration with the Brain Injury Association of America, this website offers tools to parents to help them become effective advocates for their child as he or she recovers from injury. The website is designed to augment the role of the facilitator in the hospital-to-school transition and offers various web based training and information for parents of a child with brain injury. Some of these resources include: information on effective ways to communicate with school staff; recommendations for self care and learning about your own unique parenting and advocate style; and practical information on special education and what to expect when a child graduates from high school.

Program Implementation After STEP: Scale Up

The recruitment process as outlined above will likely be adjusted in the case that **STEP** is taken up as a policy or program by state departments of education. In order to increase the efficiency of information exchange from the hospital to the school and the likelihood that children with ABI/TBI will be identified within the school system, **STEP** researchers argue that the recruitment process must be as simple as possible. They propose that if **STEP** is implemented or scaled up outside of the RCT the recruitment process should be altered such that one hospital employee would fax a paper form to a single point of contact at each state/regional department of education. In the proposed model for scale up, it would become standard hospital policy to inform the school board if a school-aged child suffered a moderate to severe TBI. Trained facilitators would be available in each region to continue the **STEP** process. Finally, since facilitators are state employees, the program eliminates some of the problems faced by schools in districts that may lack the funds to implement such a program independently.

The Facilitator as Advocate

As discussed with key informants, the role of the facilitator in STE**STEP** P is quite fluid. Facilitators are existing Board of Education employees (speech language pathologists, school psychologists, school nurses) and a portion of their salaried time with the Board is given over to working with **STEP** as a facilitator. They are expected to contact families and assist in data collection through the provision and collection of survey data, however, the ways in which they interact with families differs from this point in each case.

Each facilitator is trained by the **STEP** program, but as professionals they also have a unique skill set that they bring to their cases as facilitators and an insider view with regard to working with teachers and school boards. The Project Manager noted that their role in **STEP** is usually much greater than that of a medium of information exchange. For example, they may attend and participate in meetings with teachers and families and may also assist in the development of implementation of special education programming for a child. In this way, **STEP** researchers view facilitators also as advocates for children and families.

OUTCOME

Outcome Evaluation: STEP as a Promising Practice

Since **STEP** is currently in the RCT phase, a complete analysis of outcome measures of whether the program has been successful in meeting program goals is unavailable. However, preliminary data analysis on the first 50 families to complete the study period indicates the following. First, students in the intervention group were more likely to be identified for special educational services and received more services than those in the control group. Second, families who received the intervention protocol showed slightly less familial stress after one year. Third, parents were more satisfied with the services the students received, and parents felt more involved in the special educational process. Data analysis will continue as the investigators receive more follow-up data. Final follow-up surveys will be collected from families in March 2012 and a detailed multivariate analysis will be performed at that time.

The objective of **STEP** is to validate and disseminate information on effective hospital-to-school transition programs in order to increase identification of school-aged children with TBI. Increased identification may lead to a having a greater proportion of children who need special education services actually receiving them, allowing these children to more fully participate in, and benefit from, their educational experience. The RCT is ongoing and therefore, **STEP** may be considered a promising practice, as opposed to a best practice, in the promotion of community participation for children and adolescents with moderate to severe TBI or ABI.

When the RCT is complete, 12 months past the close of enrollment, ending in March 2011, the outcomes measures employed within the RCT to chart the child's progress through the program will be compiled in order to evaluate the efficacy of **STEP** as a hospital-to-school transition service. These measures include the following: the Child and Adolescent Scale of Participation; the Child and Adolescent Scale of Environment; the Child Behavior Checklist; the Behavior Rating Inventory of Executive Function; State/Trait Anxiety Index; and measures of service provision and satisfaction developed within **STEP** by program researchers.

Conclusion

Since its implementation, approximately 140 children have been enrolled in **STEP** and 50 children have completed the one-year study period, but the efficacy of this hospital-to-school transition model has not been examined through standardized outcome measure of the RCT results. However, based on preliminary data and anecdotal evidence from the student, school and experience of families, **STEP** is a promising practice. Indeed, even without statistical outcomes the **STEP** model has been taken up by school districts and local hospitals in Tennessee and Ohio.

This hospital-to-school transition model was developed to increase the provision of educational services for school-aged children with TBI. **STEP** makes efficient use of limited time and resources by working within a legal framework and in cooperation with school boards, teachers and local hospitals. In doing so, **STEP** is a promising practice that can meet the needs of a vast, underserved population—school-aged children with mild to moderate TBI who are not currently receiving or being referred for special education services.

REFERENCES

Agency for Health Care Policy and Research. (1999). *Rehabilitation for Traumatic Brain Injury in Children and Adolescents.* (Evidence Reports/Technology Assessments, No. 2S.) Rockville, MD: Carney, N., du Coudray, H., Davis-O'Reilly, C., Zimmer-Gembeck, M., Mann, N. C., Krages, K. P. & Helfand, M. [Online]. Retrieved September 4, 2010, from **http://www.ncbi.nlm.nih.gov/bookshelf/br.fcgi?book=erta2s&part=A2665.**

Brain Injury Partners. (2010). [Online]. Retrieved July 27, 2010, from **http://free.braininjurypartners.com**/

Center for Neuroskills. (2010). *Children and traumatic brain injury.* Retrieved August 25, 2010, from **http://neuroskills.com/children.shtml**.

Centers for Disease Control and Prevention. (2010). *Injury prevention & control: Traumatic brain injury*. Retrieved August 25, 2010 from **http://www.cdc.gov/TraumaticBrainInjury/causes.html**

Glang, A. & Todis, B. (2007, September). *Transition Tool Chest.* Presented at the Colorado TBI Educator's Conference, Denver, Colorado.

Glang, A., Todis, B., Thomas, C. W., Hooda, D., Bedell, G. & Cockrell, J. (2008). Return to school following childhood TBI: Who gets services? *NeuroRehabilitation*, 23(6) 477-486.

Ontario Brain Injury Association. (2010). *What is acquired brain injury?* Retrieved August 25, 2010, from **http://www.obia.ca/index.php?option=com_content&view =category&layout=blog&id=31&Itemid=41**

Public Health Agency of Canada. (2009). Introduction. In *Child and Youth Injury in Review: 2009 Edition: Spotlight on Consumer Product Safety*. Retrieved August 25, 2010 from **http://www.phac-aspc.gc.ca/inj-bles/index-eng.php**

Rehabilitation Act (1973). [Online]. Retrieved September 4, 2010 from http://www.dotcr.ost.dot.gov/documents/ycr/REHABACT.HTM

US Department of Health and Human Services (March, 2010). *Traumatic brain injury in the United States: Emergency department visits, hospitalizations and deaths 2002–2006.* Retrieved August 25, 2010 from **http://www.cdc.gov/traumaticbraininjury/pdf/blue_book.pdf**

CHAPTER 11

PEDIATRIC ACQUIRED BRAIN INJURY COMMUNITY OUTREACH PROGRAM (PABICOP)

By Georgios Fthenos & Danielle Hryniewicz

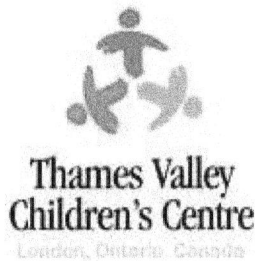

Thames Valley Children's Centre
London, Ontario, Canada

Population Served : Children and youth to 18 years of age
Contributing Author Contact Information
Sara Somers, MSW, RSW Community Outreach Coordinator PABICOP Thames Valley Children's Centre 779 Baseline Road East London, Ontario N6C 5Y6 519-685-8500 ext 53483 / 519-685-8152 (fax) **Sara.Somers@tvcc.on.ca**

BACKGROUND

The **Pediatric Acquired Brain Injury Community Outreach Program** (PABICOP) is an outreach program in Southwestern Ontario for children and adolescents with an acquired brain injury and their families. **PABICOP** is designed to complement services that are already available within each child/adolescent's own community. Community participation is key to program functioning. **PABICOP** regards the child/family and their community as the real "experts", encouraging and supporting as much community partnership as possible. "We want children and youth to be reintegrated into their home, school and community with relevant supports that are local and not based in a tertiary health care setting" (Sara Somers, Community Outreach Coordinator for PABICOP, Personal communication, September 21, 2010).

History and Development

The idea of a comprehensive program for children and youth with an acquired brain injury began to develop as a concept in the early 1990s. During this time, pediatric neurologist Dr. Jane Gillett observed that children and youth with an ABI continue to have ongoing problems after being discharged from traditional rehabilitation programs. Furthermore, these brain injury survivors and their families have a great need for support interacting with schools as well as in other settings and aspects of community life (**Gillett, 2004**).

Prior to the development of the **Pediatric Acquired Brain Injury Community Outreach Program** (PABICOP), families in Southwestern Ontario had access to some services through children's treatment and the **Community Care Access Centre** (CCAC). **Children's Treatment Centres**, funded by the Ontario Government, provide services and support to families with physical needs, such as cerebral palsy, spina bifida, neuromuscular disease, gross or fine motor delay, or speech language delay (**Gillett, 2004**). Most treatment centres have Physiotherapists, Occupational Therapists, Speech Language Pathologists, and Physician support through a family doctor or pediatrician. Other centres have access to medical specialists, such as Neurologists, Respirologists, Orthopedic Surgeons, Neurosurgeons, Maxillofacial Surgeons, and Otolaryngology (ENT) surgeons (**Gillett, 2004**).

Community Care Access Centres (CCAC) are found in every region of Ontario and provide a wide range of services for the entire population. A child or youth with an ABI can access physiotherapy, and/or school-based occupational therapy, as well as speech language pathology. A medical doctor's referral and school principal's acceptance of help are necessary for access to a CCAC (**Gillett, 2004**).

In 1992, Dr. Gillett formally began to arrange clinics in various counties in Southwestern Ontario. These clinics tended to be at **Children's Treatment Centres**or, in the case of Grey Bruce county, at a large community hospital equipped with a pediatric rehabilitation team. At these clinics, children with neurologic disabilities, and in particular those with an ABI, were frequently seen. As a result of this fact, patients and their families did not have to travel as far to receive treatment, and caregivers, individual therapists, and representatives of the educational system were able to attend appointments with the child and parent to discuss a range of issues and concerns. This "inclusive outreach" clinic format (**Gillett, 2004**, p. 2) improved care somewhat. There remained, however, a need for advocacy issues to be addressed within the school (on behalf of the family and child with an ABI), and educational outreach to be provided to families and community members. Identifying these issues, and recognizing that cutbacks, rather than program development or expansion, were the current norm within the health care system, provided an impetus for creative problem solving (**Gillett, 2004**). To this end, alternative methods by which to provide comprehensive, community based care—in a manner that was both inexpensive and effective—were explored and presented to the local district health council. Following several presentations, the local **Children's Treatment Centre**, tertiary Children's Hospital and Dr. Gillett consulted with community stakeholders to further refine the concept of an inclusive outreach clinic format (**Gillett, 2004**). Ultimately, the **Pediatric Acquired Brain Injury Community Outreach Program** (PABICOP) was established in 1999.

Guiding philosophy

PABICOP's philosophy is holistic, parent and family centered, and inclusive of the community at large in the ongoing care of the client with an ABI. For pediatric and youth populations, community participation and involvement largely centres in and around the school. Within the school environment, psychosocial, mental, cultural, and emotional factors interact with physical factors, generating outcomes that vary from individual to individual.

In addressing this finding, **PABICOP** aims to provide comprehensive and individualized forms of service, addressing, for instance, the finding that many children with an ABI demonstrate difficulty creating and maintaining peer relationships. The backbone of the program is one of prevention, as **PABICOP**'s developers recognize that preventing a brain injury is the most successful way of treating brain injury (**Gillett, 2004**). The program is committed to influencing individuals, as well as the community at large, to play and live in as safe a manner as possible. **PABICOP** has made linkages with individual safety community programs, as well as provincial and national safety programs, such as **THINK FIRST** and **SMART RISK** (**Gillett, 2004**). Primary and secondary forms of prevention are employed through education and advocacy.

A second aspect of the program pertains to community partnerships and length of service: long-term care of the client with an ABI must occur within his or her own community (**Gillett, 2004**). The family and extended community are the most important 'agencies' (**Gillett, 2004**, p. 3) in assisting the client throughout his/her life. Targeted partners include the family, hospitals, physicians, nursing, allied health professionals, the courts, lawyers, and insurance agents, **CCAC**'s, schools, teachers, principals, educational assistants, children mental health centres, and community, recreational and religious centres.

Objectives

PABICOP's Outreach Program has three primary objectives: 1) to improve integration and acceptance of children with an ABI into their home communities; 2) to improve the quality of life of children and their families with an ABI; and, 3) to minimize problems and to maximize the quality of life of children with an ABI as they enter adolescence and adulthood. To meet its objectives, the Outreach Program strives to ensure that children with an ABI, and their families, receive all of the services they require to support their social and emotional development, and well-being. Efforts to support and enhance an individual's personal resources encourage and facilitate intrapersonal development.

PABICOP educates families of children with acquired brain injuries, placing an emphasis on understanding a child's needs, learning to advocate for a child, and learning to serve as a case manager for a child. Individuals in the community, including therapists, mental health workers, school staff, tutors, physicians, and other local groups, are also educated about pediatric brain injury.

PABICOP's operational framework

According to Sara Somers, Community Outreach Coordinator, several values are encouraged and respected within **PABICOP**'s everyday operations. These include: empowerment, self-determination, and personal choice; full and inclusive participation as citizens in accepting and welcoming communities; the development and nurturance of meaningful relationships; a respectful and collaborative process between individuals, families, organizations, and the system; the unique contributions, strengths, and capacities of ABI survivors, rather than a focus on deficits; quality of life and well-being; the celebration of diversity (S. Somers, personal communication, September 21, 2010).

Clientele Base

Any child or youth between 7 days of age and 18 years of age who has sustained *any* type of ABI (mild/concussions/moderate or severe) and lives in **PABICOP**'s catchment area (five counties of Southwestern Ontario) is eligible to receive **PABICOP**'s services. Clients are assessed on an individual basis and services are tailored in collaboration with the child or youth and family (S. Somers, personal communication, September 21, 2010).

Client Referrals

Children and youth with an acute ABI are typically seen by a pediatric neurologist, who refers them to **PABICOP**. A client may be referred to **PABICOP** for assistance with medical, psychological, and educational issues, resulting from an ABI (**Gillett, 2004**).

Over 50% of client referrals are from **Fowler Kennedy Sports Medicine**, involving children and youth with complex concussions (S. Somers, personal communication, July 21, 2010). Review of data from clients of the **PABICOP** program indicates that youths in the 13-18 year old age group are at the highest risk for sustaining concussions and having ongoing and complex sequelae (**Somers et al., n.d.**). Although more males than females sustain concussions in all age groups, ongoing and complex sequelae are more prominent among females than males (in the 13-18 year old age group) (Somers et al., n.d.).

Understanding trends in the data allows program developers, collaborators, and staff members to provide a more targeted and proactive approach to educating and supporting children and youth toward alleviating stress and other difficulties associated with recovery from ABI.

RESOURCES

Financial Resources

PABICOP was established with funding from the Ontario Ministry of Health and Long-Term Care. Initiated as a partnership between the **Thames Valley Children's Centre** and **London Health Sciences Centre**, **PABICOP** originally received $348,000 per annum; the ministry continues to fund **PABICOP** at $369,000 per annum to provide services in Huron, London/Middlesex, Oxford, Perth, and St. Thomas/Elgin counties (**Thames Valley Children's Centre, 2006**). The lack of specialized brain injury support for children, adolescents, and families experiencing ABI in Grey and Bruce counties is an issue that has been brought forward on numerous occasions (**Thames Valley Children's Centre, 2006**) with proposals that seek funding for expansion of services to this area. To date, however, the proposals submitted have not yielded any increases in program funding. This is particularly concerning given the evidence that suggests benefits of providing appropriate supports and education within the client/families' home community. With adequate funding, **PABICOP** would be able to extend services into the Grey Bruce region (**Thames Valley Children's Centre, 2006**).

A Partnership Project between the counties of Middlesex, Oxford, Elgin, Huron and Perth, the **Children's Hospital of Western Ontario**, and the **Thames Valley Children's Centre** facilitates community participation through the accessibility and availability of community-based services.

Human Resources

The **PABICOP** team consists of multidisciplinary "panel of experts". A pediatric neurologist, community outreach coordinator, school liaison personnel, psychometrist, neuropsychologist, occupational therapist, and speech language pathologist coordinate community-based services for an ever-growing population of children and youth clientele (**Gillett, 2004**).

PABICOP's key stakeholders include the children and their families. Program Collaborators include the organizations who provide services to the clients and their families (e.g., schools) (S. Somers, personal communication, September 21, 2010). Both primary and secondary relationships are formed between the key stakeholders, program collaborators, and **PABICOP** team.

IMPLEMENTATION

The service delivery model of **PABICOP** recognizes that children and adolescents with ABI and their families have complex needs that are often long-term.

In attempting to address these long term complex needs, **PABICOP** aims to:

➢ **Support** children and adolescents with ABI and their families through the difficult transitions from hospital to home, school and community.

➢ **Support** children and adolescents who have a past history of ABI with issues in social, academic, medical or emotional spheres.

➢ **Assist** families to gain knowledge and skills to access the services needed for their child's health, education, social and emotional development.

➢ **Offer** information to the family, local service providers and the community about ABI to facilitate each child's reintegration into home, school and community activities.

➢ **Provide** health promotion regarding management and prevention of ABI to the community at large (e.g., schools physicians, allied health, community agencies).

Thus, **PABICOP** combines a consultative clinic model of relevant medical, therapy and psychosocial supports with education and community outreach supports to make a comprehensive service delivery model. The direct outreach consultation component is a feature that makes the **PABICOP** approach unique for pediatric brain injury services in the Southwest Region of Ontario. Following a referral, community outreach consultation services are provided primarily by school liaison, occupational therapy, social work and psychometry professionals.

Referral Process (within hospital settings)

At the children's medical centre, a package is provided to the prospective client's family with concrete suggestions for dealing with the symptoms that the client may display. In the most severe forms of injury—in which the child is hospitalized in the intensive care unit and/or in the hospital for a long period of time following multiple trauma—the pediatric neurologist works with the child and arranges for family meetings and discharge planning meetings. Therapies are initiated within the hospital, and the child is seen by neuropsychology specialist prior to discharge. A referral to **PABICOP** is made just prior to discharge (**Gillett, 2004**).

Services provided by the Outreach Team

Following a referral, the **PABICOP** team engages in rounds discussions to become familiar with potential new clients. If possible, the community outreach coordinator and school liaison (if the child is school aged) visits the family prior to discharge from the hospital. Contact is then made within 1-2 weeks of discharge (or on acceptance of referral), and an appointment is arranged for the community outreach coordinator and school liaison to make a home visit (**Gillett, 2004**).

Home visit

The home visit occurs at a time that is mutually agreeable to both the family and the team. During the home visit, information is gathered and a report compiled as to how the family is coping and functioning, and whether discharge supports, if any, have been initiated. Other issues (i.e., regarding community-based supports) are identified and permission obtained for the school liaison to talk to the school and schoolteachers. If crisis counselling seems to be indicated by the client and/or family member(s), the community outreach coordinator offers counselling support. If longer-term counselling appears appropriate, arrangements are made at this time (**Gillett, 2004**).

 Long-term counselling is initiated through an Employees Assistance Program (if the family has one), auto insurance (if applicable to the cause of injury), or through referrals to government funded community counselling programs. Counselling might consist of play therapy, art therapy, or more traditional psychological counselling (**Gillett, 2004**).

School visit

The school liaison obtains further information about school functioning prior to the injury. Once contact is established between the school liaison and school, a meeting is arranged. Upon arriving at the school, the school liaison contacts the principal, resource, guidance, and homeroom teachers to obtain more information. A problem-solving meeting is held with the child's teachers, addressing the specific needs of the particular child. Observation of the client in the classroom may or may not occur, depending on the needs of the particular student. The school liaison also participates in family meetings with the school and acts as a mediator between families and schools (**Gillett, 2004**).

Many pediatric clients may already have a diagnosis of attention deficit disorder, learning disability or behavioural disturbance (**Gillett, 2004**). As a result, one of the major roles of the school liaison is to try to improve the relationship between child and teacher. This is often accomplished by having both sides reconsider their stances (**Gillett, 2004**).

At times, the impact of the injury is such that the client requires more than "simple" modifications at school. For example, the client may need to be formally identified as a "special needs" student to access government-funded school resources (**Gillett, 2004**). In such a circumstance, the school liaison acts as an advocate to facilitate this process, which is often referred to as the IPRC process—Identification, Placement and Review Committee.

In Ontario, the formal identification of special needs requires medical documentation and support. The school liaison writes the required letters, which are in turn signed by the school liaison and pediatric neurologist. The school liaison also provides information within the school board system, liaises with the psychology support staff and the speech language pathologist support staff, and arranges for board-wide teaching sessions for professional development days (**Gillett, 2004**). All **PABICOP** team members assist in the presentation of professional development day sessions, which are tailored and designed to meet the needs of each particular school board (i.e., the needs of Mennonite students and predominately Mennonite school boards may differ from those of Catholic school boards).

Follow-up

During the initial contact with the family, formal follow-up in the closest community clinic is arranged. Typically, formal follow-up occurs about three months following discharge from the hospital. It may be completed earlier if specific needs are identified that require physician intervention (**Gillett, 2004**). At any time during their involvement with **PABICOP**, participating families are encouraged to contact the Outreach Team with questions or concerns. Many types of issues can be discussed at the clinic. The most common concerns are headaches, fatigue, sleep, and irritability. School issues are also discussed, and screening for other medical problems that may affect the client's learning and behaviour capabilities are undertaken as indicated (**Gillett, 2004**).

Although the family is strongly encouraged to bring the important people in the client's life to the meetings (e.g., service providers, schoolteachers and/or guidance counsellor, insurance agent, lawyer), the client's team consists first and foremost of the client, his/her extended family, and members of the community who interact with the client (**Gillett, 2004**). The school liaison attends each clinical appointment, as medical issues often impact on the client's school functioning. The community outreach coordinator also attends each appointment and participates in identifying services that are available.

Clinics

PABICOP currently operates in five counties of Southwestern Ontario, covering a region of approximately 30,000 sq. km (**Gillett, 2004**). A location for the outreach clinics in each of the other counties in Southwestern Ontario has been negotiated within each community (Gillett, n.d.) Newly diagnosed children are typically seen twice during the first year post injury and annually thereafter.

After the initial follow-up at three months, appointments occur at varying times. Each family is informed that they can contact **PABICOP**, requesting the Outreach Team's involvement at any time (S. Somers, personal communication, July 21, 2010). Any client with an ABI more severe than a concussion is followed as needed until age eighteen when transition into the adult service program occurs (**Gillett, 2004**).

Prior to clinic appointments, families are mailed a questionnaire and encouraged to bring the most recent school records and report cards, neuropsychological reports, and any other information they feel would be of some assistance (**Gillett, 2004**).

The clinics are run with an open-ended approach. Most clinics start with the pediatric neurologist asking the client to describe some of the "good things" that have happened to them since they were last seen. This could include such things as family trips, outings, recent gifts, marks on tests, achievements in extracurricular activities, or any other activities or feelings that the client identifies as a "good thing". The client is asked to identify three good things, if at all possible. Following this exercise, the client is asked if they feel that their health is good, and whether they have any concerns regarding their health. The family's input is solicited with the permission of the client. This is usually phrased in a way that would permit the parents to disclose information that the client may not agree with (e.g., "Do you think your parents agree with everything you said; if not, why not?"). Once the parents have had an opportunity to discuss the issues, the rest of the team is given an opportunity to speak. At this point, the client, family, service providers, and the schools identify future goals. Solutions to anticipated challenges (in achieving identified goals) are then devised (**Gillett, 2004**).

The clinical process provides the client with an opportunity to disclose concerns that he/she does not wish to discuss in front of his/her family and the other team members. Information that is disclosed by the client is kept confidential and not included in the report, unless it is felt that the information indicates a potential life-threatening problem (e.g., suicide ideation) (**Gillett, 2004**).

Clinical Specialists

The occupational therapist and/or the speech language pathologist may attend clinics to provide feedback on assessments they have performed. To this end, "mini assessments" (**Gillett, 2004**, p. 7) are performed to help identify issues and provide immediate feedback that will assist in problem solving at the clinic. A more detailed assessment can be completed at either the school or the home.

Assessments are sensitive to the needs of the clients, families, communities and clinics. The occupational therapist and speech language pathologist, for example, have extensive experience in the area of acquired brain injury. Both prefer to do their assessments within the community and within the activities that the client would normally be doing (**Gillett, 2004**).

Another role that the occupational therapist and speech language pathologist perform is one of peer-to-peer consultation. Within the province of Ontario, the **Community Care Access Centre** (CCAC) provides therapy services to people of all ages, following an appropriate referral. Therapists often deal with school-aged children with regard to speech problems, fine motor and perceptual problems, and physical problems.

The therapists have a large and diverse caseload. They treat not only clients with an ABI but also pediatric clients with cerebral palsy, spina bifida, spinal muscular atrophy, muscle diseases, peripheral neuropathies, neurogenerative disorders, metabolic disorders, postoperative cases, and developmental disabilities, among others. They are also able to treat clients with dyscoordination syndromes, and articulation and dysfluency problems (**Gillett, 2004**).

The therapists are also trained to perform assessments and devise treatment programs that are ultimately taught to teachers, educational assistants, and the families (**Gillett, 2004**).

Case Study: Anthony

Anthony was injured at age 14 in 1998. He had a younger sister age 11, and was a straight "A" student. His father works as a long distance trucker; his mother as a secretary. Anthony was a pedestrian in a motor vehicle collision. He received a Glasgow Coma Score of 4 at the scene, and his injuries included severe brain injury with seizure en route to hospital, multiple fractures on left and right sides, liver laceration/pneumothorax. Hospital course included 5 days in an intensive care unit, 12 days of bed rest for the liver laceration, and a chest tube for 10 days. Anthony required PEG feeding for 18 weeks. He was discharged home after 7 weeks with a Ranchos Los Amigo Scale of 4–5, and services through the Community Care Access Centre and Private Therapists.

PABICOP's role for Anthony, 1998 to summer 2003

Pediatric neurologist

-Talked to family doctor regarding medication and future medication.
-Saw at clinics August, October 1998; January, March, September, December 1999; March, September 2000, February, September 2001, September 2002, and April 2003.
-Treated headaches, sleep disturbance, fatigue, attention, feeding, seizures, tics, foot orthosis.
-Attended 2 school meetings and provided in-service.

Neuropsychology

-Did a preliminary assessment at discharge, upon return to school and with transitions in school.

Outreach coordinator

-Home visit 3 weeks post discharge.
-Facilitated application for respite care and attendant care.
-Facilitated counselling for younger sister.
-Helped find community resources to deal with special needs.
-Helped parents deal with anniversary reaction.
-Helped to find summer camp to facilitate functional application for therapies.
-Arranged marital counselling.

School liaison

-Worked with Anthony's family and team to plan for gradual re-entry into school.
-Wrote letters of support to obtain educational assistance (every year).
-Provided educational sessions to teachers every year.
-Provided education to Anthony's peers regarding ABI.
-Responded to requests to help determine behaviour management strategies and recommended Occupational therapy and Speech Language Pathology consults.

Speech language pathologist

-Provided consultation with community speech language pathology regarding cognitive and communication management issues.
-Completed a home visit and school assessment.
-Provided a cognitive and communication assessment and developed strategies to be used in the classroom in conjunction with the teacher, Anthony and speech language Pathologist.

Occupational therapist

-Assessment in home/school looking at memory, organization, sequencing. Helped facilitate strategies to be used by Anthony, the school and team.
-Repeated as needed.

Source: (Gillett, 2004)

Obstacles to Service Delivery

In Southwestern Ontario, there are at least 10 counties, 9 home care programs, and numerous school boards that *could* be involved with children with an ABI. Due to resource allocation, however, each county responds to the needs of the client in a different manner. Some counties lack certain services completely or have limited services and thus long waiting lists. Other counties may have potentially useful services, but their personnel are either unfamiliar with brain injuries or are able to provide appropriate services *only* if accessible support and consultation is available (Gillett et al., n.d.).

Identified Best Practices

The **PABICOP** team and clientele base have identified education, empowerment, and advocacy as effective and best practice factors (S. Somers, personal communication, September 21, 2010). Through **PABICOP**'s model of care, all facets of the client's life are acknowledged and supported. For example, the client's school is supported through **PABICOP**'s advocacy and outreach efforts, community therapists are provided access to a team of experts, the client's family MD is given resources to assist in the child's care, the client's siblings are provided with emotional support and knowledge, the community provides education and is involved in the ongoing life of the child (Personal Communication, J. Gillett, Oct. 9, 2010).

OUTCOME

In recent years, it has been argued that service provision should most often occur in the local area (**Emanuelson et al., 2003**; **Braga et al., 2005**). In this way, the cost and burden to the family is lessened. Further, children are able to maintain social contact with their peers and thus are able to practise social skills in a familiar environment.

PABICOP's objectives specify the provision of support and service in the client's home community. To facilitate this, partnerships with **Community Care Access Centres** are sought to ensure appropriate levels of therapy directly in the community.

Evaluation

McDougall et al.'s 2006 evaluation of **PABICOP** centres on the utility of the PABICOP model, a coordinated, family/community-focused program, in enhancing outcomes for children and youth with acquired brain injuries. Study findings indicate that clients and their families receiving services from the **PABICOP** program fared significantly better than a comparison group receiving standard care. Moreover, these group differences were maintained one year following initial involvement with **PABICOP**. These findings are consistent with previous studies which showed coordinated family/community-focused interventions are more useful than standard, clinic-based interventions for improving outcomes for children and youth with an ABI (**Swaine et al., 2000**; **Wade et al., 2006**; **Braga et al., 2005**). Further, family/community-focused interventions are better able to facilitate the dissemination of knowledge of ABI to families (**Wade et al., 2006**).

In addition to the demand for service, **PABICOP** strives to meet targets and best practices established specifically for the service. There are key transition points in a person's life, such as childhood to adolescence and adolescence to adulthood—and for those who have been hospitalized, the transition from hospital to home is also significant. Feedback from focus groups indicates that these times are especially important for children and adolescents with ABI and their families. Thus, it is particularly advantageous to have access to services in a timely and coordinated manner during these transition points. In the case of **PABICOP**, the referral to discharge trend complicates the application of this best practice: where client review is recommended and/or targeted for critical periods of time, the caseload volume does not always accommodate these reviews occurring where they may be intended (**Thames Valley Children's Centre, 2006**).

Community supports

With respect to community supports, it is reasonable to expect a significant need for behavioural support for many of the clients and families on the **PABICOP** caseload. Where private insurance is not in place, however, waiting lists for these services are lengthy. Further, in many cases these services have been found to be cost prohibitive and unattainable where insurance funding is not in place (**Thames Valley Children's Centre, 2006**).

As described in **PABICOP**'s 2006 Report, specialized knowledge is required from **PABICOP** staff to support therapists in the community in service provision for clients and their families. Support is required by all professions involved in the care and education of children recovering from ABI. These supports include occupational therapy, speech language pathology, social work, school liaison, medical and psychology.

Cost of Service Delivery

As with all healthcare services, the cost of providing **PABICOP**'s services has increased. Changes to the cost of service delivery have resulted from increases in cost of living, travel, and increases in overhead. Utilization statistics demonstrate that the demands for service have (and will continue) to surpass **PABICOP**'s ability to meet them effectively and within best practices (**Thames Valley Children's Centre, 2006**). In addition, the complexity of the clients' circumstances requires more than just clinical appointments: in order to maximize the benefit of these services, it is imperative that appropriate levels of support are also available (**Thames Valley Children's Centre, 2006**).

To serve an additional 70-100 clients a year, an increase of $350,106 ($318,349 for salary and benefit costs) per annum is required. Additional staff time would greatly enhance the Outreach Team's ability to participate in a broader range of community-based educational activities (**Thames Valley Children's Centre, 2006**).

Unmet Service Needs

Given that the complexity of the clients' circumstances requires more than just clinic appointments (**Thames Valley Children's Centre, 2006**), an ideal model of service delivery would benefit from the development of higher level skills in a physiotherapist that could be called on to provide occasional consultation and support.

Conclusion

PABICOP demonstrates a commitment to cross-sectoral, cross-organizational, and community collaboration, sharing, and dissemination of knowledge. In supporting innovation and best practices, **PABICOP** demonstrates an openness and responsiveness to system change. Program personnel work with the client and family "where they are at" (S. Somers, personal communication, September 21, 2010)—both geographically and during the rehabilitation and reintegration process. Its practice is dynamic and culturally sensitive, as the client and his/her family help to guide **PABICOP**'s Outreach Team in understanding what is meaningful to them (S. Somers, personal communication, September 21, 2010). Thus, the client and his/her family is offered a means of coping and an opportunity to bolster his /her personal resources (e.g., intelligence, appearance, strength, health, and temperament).

PABICOP was formed by directly asking the community what they wanted (Personal Communication, J. Gillet, Oct. 9, 2010). Although an initial sketch of the program was presented, the actual components of the program were revised and finalized with the help of the community. The community and/or local providers of service then helped to shape the program as they are most aware of the socio-cultural opportunities available. Moreover, community members are better able to understand what can be accomplished with local resources, such as support, stimulation, and security, offered by the physical environment (Personal Communication, J. Gillet, Oct. 9, 2010).

In efforts to facilitate community participation, **PABICOP**'s clinics are strategically located in the community. Teachers, therapists, and other interested parties can come together to participate in a client's plan of rehabilitation and habituation.

PABICOP is involved in trying to *prevent* ABI. To this end, the team works in collaboration with local Brain Injury Associations, Children's Safety Associations, and provincial and national associations. Education and advocacy are provided on an individual basis per family, as well as on a larger scale throughout the schools and community. **PABICOP** is involved in educating and advocating in the community about acquired brain injuries. Informal in-services are performed within the hospital, as well as the Community Care Access Centres, other hospitals, at the schools, within the school boards, at local brain injury association meetings, at provincial and national brain injury meetings, and at international brain injury association meetings (**Gillett, 2004**).

Several areas of **PABICOP** need to be developed further. The Outreach Team is currently working on the development of a database using pick lists. In using this database, there will be a collection of demographic data in addition to a detailed description of the brain injury. This will include data from the MRI, if obtained, CTs, EEG, SPECT scan, as well as neuropsychologic data. Occupational therapy and speech language pathology assessments, if available, will be collected. An ongoing record of conversations and interactions on behalf of each client and their parents, school, and other community persons, will be kept and stored. The database will be run on a real time basis. The client will have an opportunity to describe his/her history, which will also be recorded. Any recommendations and their outcomes will be subsequently quantified and evaluated.

The database is to be a long-term, ongoing project, allowing for appropriate data collection of long-term outcome measures. It is hoped that by collecting data on all clients with an ABI, a means of identifying clients who are at risk for lifelong problems (e.g., children with concussions) will allow for early and effective intervention (**Gillett, 2004**).

Interactions with family physicians, community physicians, and caregivers is another aspect of service that should be examined. It has been observed that a concise, yet detailed description of the injury, as well as a description of the current and anticipated problems, might assist in the client's provision of care. Descriptions could be kept at the front of the family doctor's chart for easy reference, should any problems appear (**Gillett, 2004**).

Finally, it has been recognized that counselling services for siblings and parents is greatly needed (**DeMatteo, 2008**). The community outreach coordinator is not capable of providing the degree of counselling requested, given his/her workload. As a result, an increase in psychological support, provided by another social worker and/or a psychologist, would be beneficial to clients and their families (**Gillett, 2004**).

PABICOP has grown to be an internationally respected service and model. This is evidenced by invited presentations in Denmark, as well as site visits being sought out by international agencies that provide or are intending to provide brain injury services (**Thames Valley Children's Centre, 2006**). With respect to the latter, recent site visits from a representative of an Australian service (looking to establish a brain injury service), and a planned site visit from representatives of Sweden and the Netherlands, demonstrate the transferability and applicability of the **PABICOP** model to various contexts. **PABICOP** has been successfully replicated in various sites across Europe, including Denmark, Sweden, the Netherlands, and Australia, among others

REFERENCES

Braga, L. W., DaPaz, A. C., & Ylvisaker. M. (2005). Direct clinician-delivered versus indirect family-supported rehabilitation of children with traumatic brain injury: a randomized controlled trial. **Brain Injury**, 19 (10), 819-831.

DeMatteo, C. A., Cousins, M.A., Lin, C-Y. A., Law, M. C., Colantonio, A., & Macarthur, C. (2008). **Exploring postinjury living environments for children and youth with acquired brain injury**. *Archives of Physical Medicine and Rehabilitation,* 89 (9), 1803-1810.

Emanuelson, I., Wendt, L. V., Hagberg, I., Marchioni-Johansson, M., Ekberg, G., Olsson, U., Larsson, J., Egerlund, H., Lindgren, K., & Pestat, C. (2003). **Early community outreach intervention in children with acquired brain injury**. *International Journal of Rehabilitation Research,* 26 (4), 257-264.

Gillett, J., Vriezen, E., Pigott, S., Sommerfreund, J., & Rosen, E. (n.d.). Acquired Brain Injury Community Reintegration Outreach Proposal: Submitted by Children's Hospital of Western Ontario, London Health Sciences Centre and Thames Valley Children's Centre.

Gillett, J. (2004). The Pediatric Acquired Brain Injury Community Outreach Program (PABICOP) – **An innovative comprehensive model of care for children and youth with an acquired brain injury**. *Neurorehabilitation,* 19, 207-218.

McDougall, J., Servais, M., Sommerfreund, J., Rosen, E., Gillett, J., Gray, J., Somers, S., Frid, P., Dewit, D., Pearlman, L., & Hicock., F. (2006). An evaluation of the paediatric acquired brain injury community outreach programme (PABICOP). **Brain Injury**, 20 (11), 1189-1205.

Rone-Adams, S. A., Stern, D. F., & Walker, V. (2004). **Stress and compliance with a home exercise program among caregivers of children with disabilities**. *Pediatric Physical Therapy,* 16, 140-148.

Sherwin, E. D., & O'Shanick, G. J. (2000). The trauma of pediatric and adolescent brain injury: issues and implications for rehabilitation specialists. **Brain Injury,** 14 (3), 267-284.

Swaine, B., Pless, B., Friedman, D., & Montes, J. (2000). **Effectiveness of a head injury programme for children: A preliminary investigation.** *American Journal of Physical Medicine and Rehabilitation,* 79, 412-420.

Taylor, H., Yeates, K., Wade, S., Drotor, D., Stancin, T., & Burant, C. (2001). **Bidirectional child-family influences on outcomes of traumatic brain injury in children.** *Journal of the International Neuropsychological Society,* 7, 755–767.

Thames Valley Children's Centre. (2006). Paediatric Brain Injury Community Outreach Program Proposal for Increased Funding.

Wade, S., Michaud, L., & Brown, T. (2006). **Putting the pieces together: Preliminary efficacy of a family problem-solving intervention for children with traumatic brain injury.** *Journal of Head Trauma Rehabilitation,* 21, 57–67.

Ylvisaker, M., Adelson, P.D., Braga, L.W., Burnett, S.M., Glang, A., Feeney, T., Moore, W., Rumney, P., & Todis, B. (2005). **Rehabilitation and ongoing support after pediatric TBI: twenty years of progress**. *Journal of Head Trauma Rehabilitation,* 20 (1), 95- 109.

CHAPTER 12

THE CHALLENGE PROGRAM -THE INSTITUTE FOR REHABILITATION AND RESEARCH (TIRR) MEMORIAL HERMANN

By Natasha Jamal

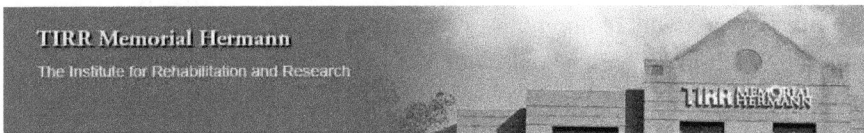

Population Served : Youth and Adults, 14 years and older	
Contributing Author Contact Information	
Joyce Leverenz Program Manager 2455 S. Braeswood, Houston, TX 77030 Phone: 1-713-383-5603 Email: **joyce.leverenz@memorialhermann.org**	Sandra Lloyd Director, Outpatient Services 2455 S. Braeswood, Houston, TX 77030 Phone: 1-713-383-5603 Email: **Sandra.Lloyd@memorialhermann.org**

BACKGROUND

The **Challenge Program** is a specialized outpatient day program for individuals with brain injuries, and is part of **The Institute for Rehabilitation and Research Memorial Hermann**'s rehabilitation continuum. The program is run from a hospital setting, with the benefits of connecting to leading research and resources in the field of Acquired and Traumatic Brain Injury (TBI), while simultaneously focusing on client rehabilitation or therapy for community re-entry. A key feature of the program is its comprehensive approach in helping clients achieve their rehabilitation goals. This includes encouraging the client to connect with a community in the program as a facet of the therapy as well as going beyond the traditional medical rehabilitation model by working with the client, their families and their community environments in order to meet mutually developed goals. The program has been structured and created for the purpose of successful community reintegration for clients with brain injury and will be explored as a case study.

The **Challenge Program** for community integration was developed in the early 1980s in response to a need for post-acute services for survivors of brain injury within the Houston, TX community. Prior to this, people with ABI/TBI had to travel several hours away to receive specialized outpatient services in Texas. In 1998, the program expanded with the hiring of dedicated staff and moved out of the hospital setting into a small community-based facility approximately four miles away. Due to a funding shortfall, however, the program is again operating as an outpatient service from **TIRR-Memorial Hermann**. The original objective was to help people with TBI to return to work, but currently the program uses a more holistic therapy approach in order to address its clients' needs beyond just functional rehabilitation. For instance program staff assess clients on their cognitive, behavioural, emotional, and social functioning in order to identify any impairments the client may be experiencing due to their brain injury. Furthermore, the therapy team ensures that the rights of the clients they serve are upheld by involving them in all of their therapy decisions and goal development.

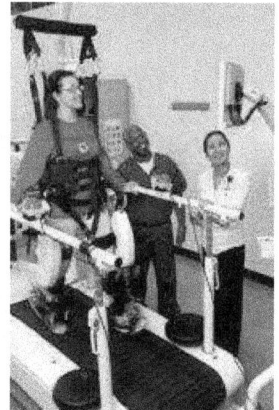

Community Participation

The therapy team at the **Challenge Program** has a dynamic understanding of the concept of community participation. Extending beyond a fixed notion of a therapy goal, the team believe the concept of community participation changes according to the client's progress and stage of therapy. For instance, clients may change their community participation goals during the course of their treatment, based on their capacity and progress. Furthermore, the program staff acknowledge that each client may have a different understanding of what successful community participation looks like, based on their contexts, interests, and involvement prior to injury. The program tried to help clients achieve community participation by recognizing that clients need to be able to take part in activities that are meaningful in personal ways and that connect them to their valued communities. One of the ways the program tries to support this is by connecting clients in specialized client groups as social support networks where individuals have similar goals, values, and injuries.

Three phases are noted within the continuum of helping clients connect with their communities:

1. Current community involvement.

At the time of admission, the client is assessed on the kinds of community participation and his/her level of involvement, such as:

    a) Whether they participate in home errands and meeting their living needs

    b) Whether they are part of a leisure activity in the community

    c) Whether they work or volunteer

The following questions are a sample of what is asked during admission in the Challenge Program: Do clients participate in grocery shopping? Do clients attend regular church or religious functions? Are they enrolled in a recreation class? Do they spend time with family and friends outside of their own home? Are clients currently employed or part of a volunteering organization? A base rate on the kinds of participation, as well as the number of hours per week of community involvement, are assessed, allowing therapists to have a reliable measure of the client's progress in therapy with the focus on community reintegration.

Upon admission, clients generally have few meaningful or sustained experiences of community participation—a primary challenge reported by people with ABI (**Willer, Allen, Durnan, & Ferry, 1990; Willer, Allen, Liss, & Zicht, 1991**). Staff at the **Challenge**

Program notice that many clients share the same sentiment; many seek therapy in order to re-connect with doing the things they love or are interested in. By assessing current levels of involvement, the program staff can then help clients move to the next phase.

2. Fostering meaningful community involvement.

The second phase of the program tries to foster meaningful activities and community connection as a means for community participation for the client. Specifically community participation within the rehabilitation setting is used as a therapy milieu— within the **Challenge Program**, the client is introduced and encouraged to become part of a specialized group of clients who have similar goals or shared experiences with their brain injuries and therapy plan. Some specialized groups of people in the **Challenge Program** also enter community areas outside the facility in order to practice the skills and strategies they have learned within the program. For example, if a client would like to re-enter the work force, he/she would be placed in a group of other clients who also share that goal. The group travels together, and, in this example, they enter a non-profit agency in order to meet others, interact together, and familiarize themselves with their capacities in a work setting. Another example is a specialized group travelling together outside the therapy setting for leisure purposes in order to enjoy each other's company and friendship.

The importance of connecting to a social support network that have similar goals, values and injuries is found to motivate clients and help them in their progress towards attaining their therapy goals (**Willer & Corrigan, 1994**; **Condeluci, 2002**).

3. Sustaining community involvement outside of the facility.

The third phase is based on progress and personal goals, where the client continues to be supported while being connected to the kind of community participation activity into which he/she would like to reintegrate outside of the formal clinic. Formal therapy is decreased, as the client is able to successfully implement the skills and techniques that they have learned in their external community setting. Program goals are achieved when the client is able to feel comfortable and adapt to their community settings outside the clinic.

The program staff acknowledges that each client may have a different understanding of what successful community participation looks like since this concept may differ according to the individual goals each client has during therapy.

RESOURCES

TIRR used to be a freestanding rehabilitation facility, however due to funding shortfalls it was acquired by Memorial Hermann in 2005. As a hospital TIRR has been nationally ranked in the top five within the United States for ten consecutive years. TIRR is also one of six hospitals to achieve a designation as a model system by the **National Institute on Disability and Rehabilitation Research** (NIDRR) which includes brain injury programs that considers the whole brain injury continuum including community integration. The program now falls under the rules and regulations of **Memorial Hermann**.

Funding for the **Challenge Program** is usually paid for by third party payers, including the **State Department of Assistive and Rehabilitation Services** (DARS). This is a state agency with two main programs, one for vocational and the other for independence. The client also has access to an interdisciplinary team since the program recognizes that community reintegration is a complex process. The program tries to merge different elements of the therapy and community integration process by setting up client team meetings. The client and the program team together set therapy goals and monitor progress. The program includes the people noted in Table 1, and each therapeutic team is tailored according to the needs of the client.

Table 1: *Team of Professional Staff and their roles within the Challenge Program*

Professional	Function
Physicians	Refers the client to the program, and act as consultants for the therapists. The therapy team works in collaboration with physician consultants.
Case Managers (or Primary Therapists who are licensed Clinical Social Workers within the Challenge Program)	Coordinates the client's overall program and communicates with insurance representatives. They also help the client and caregiver to understand and participate in the rehabilitation process, adjust to the changes in their lives, explore available options and services, and develop plans for return to home and the community.
Occupational Therapists	Assists the client with the development of daily living skills and provides training in the use of adaptive and mobility equipment to encourage independence.
Physical Therapists	Focuses on the client's mobility skills, and assess and treats impairments in strength, range of motion, balance, coordination and function.

Speech-Language Pathologists	Help clients to enhance their communication, cognitive skills and swallowing function.
Psychologists and Neuropsychologists	Assists clients with the emotional and mental adjustments to illness or injury and assesses cognitive function.
Cognitive Rehabilitation Specialists (includes Licensed Professional Counselors)	Assists clients with cognitive functioning, and implementation of learned strategies in community settings.
Vocational Rehabilitation Specialists	Assists clients in development and implementation of return to work plans. They also assist clients in preparing for work through practice work called job trials.

Additionally case managers or primary therapists also get to know the clients more intimately by knowing their individual goals, needs, barriers and facilitators towards their community integration. The primary therapists coordinate all areas of the program involving the client's care, including clinical needs, psychosocial factors, and financial constraints/issues. They also lead the team in team discussions and are responsible for progressing their clients through their program in order to meet their goals.

Challenges with the Program

The most significant issue the program faces is lack of funding for cognitive therapy services. Funding has become increasingly difficult for supporting community integration therapy programs. The **Challenge Program** manager and colleagues in TIRR Memorial Hermann's Managed Care Department continue to educate insurance providers regarding the need for cognitive therapy services for individuals with brain injuries. The Challenge Program manager and her colleagues have found that several insurance companies identify cognitive therapy services as a mental health issue and not caused by a medical condition. Furthermore, some funding agencies do not consider community integration services to be a medical necessity in the health care continuum. These issues continue to be the most significant barriers for clients' access to services.

Additionally, most third party payers do not cover vocational therapy services. Although **DARS** is a resource for funding, there is sometimes a delay in funds availability and a delay in access to services for clients. Furthermore due to funding restrictions, the program has found to be more sustainable while working out of a hospital setting. Most funding agencies have now adapted a medicalization model as a necessity for therapy services. Community reintegration goals for clients are required to be supported as a medical necessity in order for insurance providers and third party agencies to provide adequate funding for such essential services.

Other researchers and practitioners in the field of community reintegration have also acknowledged this unfortunate trend (**Sander, Clark & Pappadis; 2010**; **Willer & Corrigan; 1994**). Regrettably the impact of not gaining access to such services can become direct barriers to successful integration within their communities for people with brain injuries. Finding meaningful roles for participation in community life can actually prevent further injuries and greater dependency on social services and insurance funding.

IMPLEMENTATION

Program values

The program's approach is informed by the following mission statement: Empowering Individuals with Brain Injury to Realize their Maximum Potential and to Follow their Path of Purposeful Living.

Empowering Individuals

The program espouses that clients feel and perform their best when they are involved in some level of their community activities. These activities include participating in important decisions for their therapy services, as well as participating in the specialized groups where clients have the opportunity to meet with other clients with similar goals and injuries. The importance of involving the client stems from the program's adopted principle that all human beings need to feel as if they have worth and value in this world.

Purposeful Living

Community participation is addressed right at the admission of the program, where strategies, goals, and expectations are discussed and agreed upon before therapy. The **Challenge Program** tries to individualize its therapy approach by involving the client, his or her family, and the therapist within its plans and practices. This practice is in line with the recognition that community integrated therapy should extend beyond that of the institutional setting and into the homes and communities of the person with the brain injury (Rosenthal, 1990). The overarching therapy philosophy of the **Challenge Program** maintains that people will get better if they have something to do in society.

Steps in therapy

Program therapists first try to establish their clients' strengths and weaknesses in order to help clients figure out how they would like to participate in their communities. Next, the therapy approach tries to improve on the clients capacities by working on restoration, implementation of compensatory strategies and by identifying the kind of involvement clients see themselves working towards in their communities. Involvement in their communities can take the forms of going back to school, working, gardening, volunteering or living independently. Thus the program's main objective is to help clients identify what it is they would like to do in their communities; therapy is then focused on trying to help them meet these goals. Everything else within the program is tailored towards complementing this objective.

Program planning

The client and his or her family are integral parts of the program planning. The therapy team typically meets for 4 hours a week to talk about the client's progress and the planned approach towards a common purpose and goal for the team of professionals. Solutions and strategies to overcome program challenges are brought up as a group. Speech, Occupational and Physical therapists also have individual goals that take into consideration their distinct disciplines and the objectives that they are trying meet, all while leading to the common program goals as determined by the team, the client and family.

In situations where the program goals of the client and that of the staff may not be the same, the therapy staff supports the client by acknowledging their goals while negotiating with the client to work on achieving the smaller goals that may lead to the client's bigger goals. In such cases, it is common that clients may have reduced awareness of their own abilities and capacities after their brain injury, however other factors may also be involved. Nevertheless an element of trust between both the therapist and client is critical within the program's work. Thus the therapist is required to recognize and work with their clients' needs and service objectives, while clients are also required to trust the therapist to see whether certain strategies can work.

Clients with greater cognitive awareness and who can better identify what they are capable of doing are included to assist with outlining the steps towards the overall goal of the program, whereas clients with less awareness are still involved in developing the implementation of the program, yet do so by focusing on each step of the therapy as opposed to planning the greater extent of the therapy approach.

Components of the therapy approach

The therapy approach is comprised of the following four main components:

1. Cognitive Therapy

2. Physical/Occupational Therapy

3. Psychotherapy

4. Community Integration

Clients focus on these four integrated therapy components for a period ranging from 2 to 4 days a week, with the average being 3 days per week. Some clients may be part of 2 or 3 cognitive groups per day, working on developing their memory/cognition skills, awareness skills, community skills, and day time work skills. The therapy approach addresses various physical abilities, memory strategies, interpersonal community and problem solving skills in order to help clients establish sustainable strategies for long-term success. Most clients receive three to five hours of intensive therapy per day.

Community integration as a therapy feature

The **Challenge Program** also uses the community as a therapeutic milieu. The program provides group therapy, not only for cognitive issues but also for behavioural issues. Clients who have suffered from a brain injury may have challenges in their functional awareness and encounter challenges in their social skills. Group therapy enables clients to receive feedback from their peers and enables them to also feel part of a community. Clients also learn and share useful strategies by partaking in activities with their group and with other clients. Program staff have noticed that about 50% of the time, friendships are formed that continue beyond the program and facility. Furthermore clients' progress and motivation are also enhanced by sharing experiences with those who are also facing similar changes and seeing the success of those who are further along their therapy.

Application of program skills to clients' communities

Clients return to their own communities each evening to integrate the skills they have learned in therapy into their daily activities. Some immediately start the process of resuming their lives in their communities of school or work. The benefits of the program also enable clients to continue with the needed therapy, yet still be at home with their family, friends, and loved ones. The therapy strategies of the **Challenge Program** also take place within community settings, outside the clinic. The various community settings depend on the therapy goals of the client and can include places such as malls, grocery stores, parks, non-profit agencies, the client's own home, and job fairs. Therapists can assist with problem solving from the challenges and issues clients experience as they are practicing and applying the skills they have learned into their actual communities and real world settings. Thus frequent feedback and adjustments are made with the learned strategies in therapy as clients are able to recognize what works and what needs improvement while they apply these strategies into their lived experience and communities outside the therapy facility. For the best generalizability of learned behaviours, successful community integration therapy programs teach clients the skills and strategies they need for the environments appropriate to those skills and in which they will be used (**Willer & Corrigan ,1994**).

Service goals and program tracking

In addition to the client's personal goals, the therapy is also tailored according to the program track they are in (Table 2). Therapy tracks are chosen prior to admission and are based on clients' stated therapy goals. Therapy staff also recommend tracks from their experience, and observed capacity of the client on what can be accomplished during the admission. For instance clients can be placed in the employment track to assist them in returning to competitive or supported employment, develop preparation for being volunteer ready, focus on having greater involvement in their hobbies, or work towards having a greater sense of achieving personal independence in their daily lives.

Table 2: *Challenge Program Therapy Tracks*

Therapy track	Goal	Therapy
The employment track	Helps clients prepare for work re-entry based on their abilities and capabilities of fulfilling certain work based behaviours.	Focuses on compensatory strategies as well as pre-employment job trials, job coaching and consultation with employers. A vocational counselor is also able to help the client by assisting them in finding suitable work based on their interest and completion of capable work tasks.
The volunteer track	Helps clients prepare for volunteering in their communities based on their abilities, interests and	Prepares clients to interact with other people in their community, learn appropriate communication strategies and find volunteer opportunities

	capabilities of fulfilling certain tasks in volunteer agencies.	outside their homes. Supervisor education is also carried out in order to help the client feel more integrated within their structured volunteer activities.
The independent living readiness track	Allows clients to learn strategies and approaches to better their personal independence with a focus on safety and meeting daily independent living requirements and in their communities.	This includes working on strategies for medicine taking, accurately making change when purchasing or receiving money, shopping, going to a museum, preparing meals, communicating with others, taking the bus and more.
The educational track	Helps prepare high school and post-secondary students to re-enter their educational environments.	Therapists are able to consult with school staff to better accommodate the client's educational needs and foster a more inclusive learning environment.

The role of the family

One of the major requirements of admission to the **Challenge Program** is for the client to have a family or close loved member participate in the therapy program. Great importance is placed on educating and working with the family since many family members become primary caregivers to their loved ones who have experienced brain injury. The goals are to help family members acquire important information and skills and to better understand the capacity of the client, all in order to better care for the individual while providing the necessary independence. Caregivers and family are provided opportunities to practice new skills at the facility in collaboration with the staff. Family and caregivers' participation in daily care and decision making with the client and therapist is valued and encouraged as they are invited to all therapies and to collaborate with all the members of the rehab team.

Admission Criteria

Requirements for acceptance in the program include medical stability, basic self care skills, and the ability to benefit from the program. Additionally, the individual must have a friend or relative committed to serving as a partner in the therapy process. **Challenge Program** clients are also required to be 14 year or older.

Initially the **Challenge Program** only admitted individuals who were already "work-ready" in terms of their functional capacity. Recently the program has changed to have a more open door policy. Clients with more severe and potentially chronic conditions are regularly admitted. For instance in the case of a former client who was dependent on an oxygen machine, therapy staff accepted her enrollment into the program. After the program, the client successfully integrated within her community by actively volunteering and no longer relies on an oxygen machine.

Furthermore, the average length of stay has decreased through the year, however clients are open to have repeated admission to the program if they would like to work on another area of community integration in their lives. This may be noticed when a client has a three month visit to the program to work on individual independence in living, then returns at a later date to work on integrating into vocational employment.

OUTCOME

Continuous evaluation

The client's interdisciplinary team meets twice a month to review the client's progress towards the therapy plan goals. This also enables the staff to determine the length of time of the service required and to re-evaluate whether the therapy approaches are effective to the needs and goals of the client. If the therapy staff finds that the goals are not being met, the staff may need to change their approach and/or change the specialized group composition. This is done in order to help the client connect and meet with new groups of people who are relevant to his/her therapy needs. The team also takes part in a weekly clinical collaboration to speak about best practices of upcoming new models and/or social integration techniques to incorporate in their therapy practices. The approach follows a cyclical and ongoing process of assessment, goal development, intervention, evaluation and reassessment that is found to make the most successful impact for client progress and satisfaction outcomes for community integration therapy (**Sloan, Winkler & Callaway; 2004**).

Clients' subjective evaluations

Research has been able to demonstrate the importance of considering the client's beliefs and values in delivering therapy work. The client's subjective evaluation of services received can speak to whether he or she finds the program relevant, useful, and helpful towards therapy needs and goals. **Cicerone** suggests that a client's subjective feedback should be incorporated along with objective evaluation measures in order for the program to be considered as a best practice using evidence-based approaches in therapy (2005). The Challenge Program evaluates clients' overall satisfaction with the services they receive and whether they feel that they have been able to better connect and integrate within their communities in follow up measures after a one and five year post program progress. A satisfaction survey is administered to the client at discharge and the team uses the information to update and better inform their therapy approaches for future clients. The Challenge Program has administered three different outcome measures in order to gather useful information for their research and practice.

Past research has been able to share promising outcome measures for the effectiveness of the program using the Community Integration Questionnaire (CIQ). As indicated in Table 3 and seen in Figure 1, clients have shown a general improvement over time in terms of integrating into their communities in the domains of home competency, social integration, and productive activity.

Table 3. *Means (standard deviations) in CIQ survey scores over time (Sander, et al., 2001).*

	Admission	Discharge	Follow-up 1	Follow-up 2
Home competency	3.46 (1.98)*	3.92 (2.84)*	4.88 (3.35)	6.38 (3.29)
Social integration	7.13 (1.90)*	7.92 (2.12)*	7.92 (2.24)	8.67 (1.81)
Productive activity	0.83 (1.19)*	2.61 (1.67)*	2.91 (1.70)	3.26 (1.51)
Total CIQ Score	11.43 (3.31)**	14.43 (5.41)**	15.74 (5.34)	18.43 (4.22)
	*p < .05, ** p < .01			

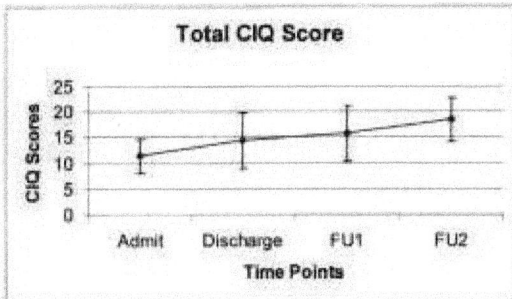

Figure 1. Total scores of CIQ over time (adjusted for time between injury and discharge) **(Sander, et al, 2001).**

The above results indicate that persons with TBI have made substantial gains in community integration after completing the Challenge Program. Specifically significant improvements from admission to discharge in measures of home competence, social integration and productivity were demonstrated within 8 months of the post-acute therapy program. These gains were generally maintained by a majority of the clients for as long as five years after discharge as seen in Table 3 and Figure 1.

Recently, it was felt that the measures being used no longer capture the client populations' progress as the program has continued to see individuals with more significant impairments. Thus in August 2010, the program changed to two main measurement tools. These measures are administered at admission, discharge, at a three-month follow up and at a one year follow up. The following measures are administered:

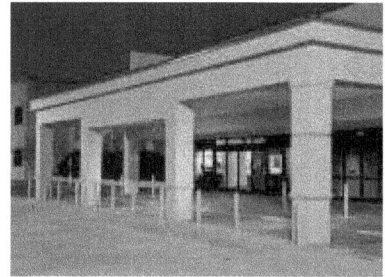

1) **Mayo Portland Adaptability Inventory 4:** is reported by clinicians and represents the range of physical, cognitive, emotional, behavioural, and social problems that people encounter after a brain injury. It also provides a clinical assessment of major obstacles to community integration. The Mayo Portland is well researched and is in its fourth edition.

2) **A Productivity measure**: asks clients to describe how many hours they keep busy whether in competitive employment, supported employment, or volunteering. Whether clients travel outside their homes more than once a week, whether they volunteer their services, if they partake in leisure activities outside of television more than twice a week, i.e., gardening outside or participating in a knitting group. If the client is in school, measures include whether they are taking and attending a class of any kind. The measure also takes into consideration non-productive behaviours. Most clients score high on non productive behaviours when they enter the program and score significantly lower on this measure after a three month follow up.

Recent measures find that 85% of clients have returned to community activities by the time of graduation from the program, and 90% of clients have significantly less need for supervision. Every quarter, a report is created from these measures and is shared with the **TIRR Memorial Hermann Quality Council**. The recent report from June 2008 to July 2009 had the following statistics reported (**TIRR Memorial Hermann, 2008**):

➢ 88% of clients who completed the program met their independence and personal safety goals, resulting in reduced assistance and supervision at home and in the community.

➤ 3 months after discharge, 96% of a sample of these clients reported that they had maintained these outcomes

➤ 90% of adult clients who completed the program met their volunteer or work goals

➤ 80% adolescent clients who completed the program returned to school by discharge

➤ clients rated the program as 4.5 for overall satisfaction (On a scale of 1 to 5, 1 being poor and 5 being excellent)

Conclusion

The **Challenge Program** is considered to be a best practice program for people with acquired brain injury since it has been able to integrate both the community integration as well as the cognitive rehabilitation aspects of therapy. Although situated in a medical hospital setting, the traditional medical model of client care is not endorsed since clients are empowered by being able to work with an integrated therapy team in creating and providing feedback for their own therapy goals and needs. Furthermore integration with a caring community is used as a therapy feature within this program. This is because family involvement and developing meaningful relationships within and outside the facility are found to further help the client with faster and better therapy outcomes and general well being. The successful outcomes of meaningfully integrating clients into their communities from this program is observed from the use of the community integration questionnaire, as well as the clients' own subjective evaluations which are monitored up to five years after discharge. Overall the program's practices are informed by the philosophy of trying to empower individuals with brain injury to realize their maximum potential and to follow their path of purposeful living.

REFERENCES

Cicerone, K. D. (2005). **Evidence-Based Practice and the Limits of Rational Rehabilitation**. *Archives of Physical Medicine and Rehabilitation,* 86(6), 1073-1074.

Condeluci, A. (2002). *Cultural Shifting: Community Leadership and Change*. Florida: Training Resource Network Press.

Fuhrer, M. J., Rossi, L. D., Gerken, L, Nosek M. A., Richards, L. (1990). Relationships between independent living centers and medical rehabilitation programs. *Archives of Psychical Medicine and Rehabilitation,* 71, 519-522.

Rosenthal, M., Forward. Kreutzer J. S. & Wehman, P. (eds.). (1990). Community Integration Following Traumatic Brain Injury. Baltimore, M.D.: Paul Brookes Publishing Company. In Sander, A. M., Clark, A., & Pappadis, M. R. (2010). **What Is Community integration anyway?: Defining meaning following traumatic brain injury.** *Journal of Head Trauma Rehabilitation, 25*(2), 121-127.

Sander, A. M., Clark, A., & Pappadis, M. R. (2010). **What Is Community integration anyway?: Defining meaning following traumatic brain injury.** *Journal of Head Trauma Rehabilitation, 25*(2), 121-127.

Sander, A. M., Roebuck,T. M., Struchen, M.A., Sherer, M., & High Jr., W. M. (2001). **Long-term maintenance of gains obtained in post acute rehabilitation by persons with Traumatic Brain Injury.** *Journal of Head Trauma Rehabilitation, 16(*4), 356-373.

Sloan, S., Winkler, D., & Callaway, L. (2004). **Community integration following severe traumatic brain injury: Outcomes and best practice.** *Brain Impairment, 5*(1), 12-29.

TIRR Memorial Hermann. (2008). Challenge Program patient outcomes. In *Day Rehabilitation at Kirby Glen.* Retrieved September 14 2010, from **http://www.memorialhermann.org/locations/tirr/forconsumers/content.aspx?id=388 8#challenge**.

Volpe, R. (2004). *The conceptualization of injury prevention as change in complex systems.* Unpublished manuscript, University of Toronto, Toronto: ON.

Volpe, R. (2010). *An outcomes framework for the ABI community of practice: Development and uses.* Centre for Community Based Research for the **Ontario Neurotrauma Foundation**.

Willer, B., Allen, K., Durnan, M. C., & Ferry, A. (1990). Problems and coping strategies of mothers, siblings and young adults with traumatic brain injury. *Canadian Journal of Rehabilitation, 3,* 167-173.

Willer, B., Allen, K., Liss, M., & Zicht, M. (1991). Problems and coping strategies of individuals with traumatic brain injury and their spouses. *Archive of Physical Medical Rehabilitation, 72,* 460-464.

Willer, B., & Corrigan, J. (1994). Whatever it takes: A model for community-based services. **Brain Injury**, *8*(7), 647-659.

CHAPTER 13

THE KREMPELS CENTER

A nonprofit organization dedicated to improving the lives of people
living with brain injury from trauma, tumor or stroke.

By Jami-Leigh Sawyer

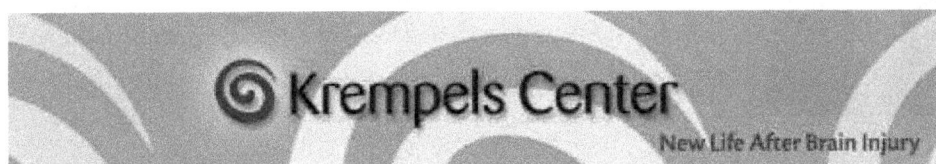

Krempels Center
New Life After Brain Injury

Population Served: Adults 18 and older	
Contributing Author Contact Information	
Dr. Michael Fraas Department of Communication Sciences and Disorders, USA 151 Hewitt Hall, 4 Library Way, Durham, NH 03824, USA Tel: 603-862-4591 Email: **Michael.Fraas@unh.edu**	Carol Davis Senior Program Coordinator Krempels Brain Injury Foundation – Steppingstones Program 100 Campus Drive Portsmouth, NH 03801 Email: **cdavis@krempelscenter.org** Tel: 603-430-7668
Website: **http://www.krempelscenter.org**	

Background

> "Cruising along the highway on a sunny June afternoon in 1992, feeling great. Just starting married life with my beautiful wife sitting right beside me. I was a successful building contractor; active in sports, my church, and the community; finally coming into my prime. And then, in a second, everything changed. Squealing tires, twisted metal, flying glass. A tractor trailer truck slammed into our car. My wife was killed. I was left fighting for my life, and facing the long, lonely journey through the no man's land of "recovery." Confused, angry, crippled, and heartbroken, I desperately tried to cling to the life I had known. But over the course of two agonizing years, I slowly realized that I was never going to be that person again." (David Krempels)

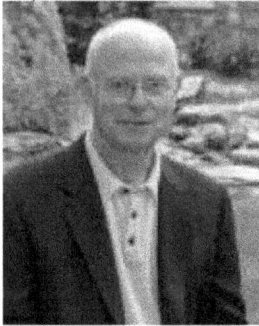

Founded by David Krempels in 1995, **The Krempels Center** is a nonprofit organization dedicated to improving the lives of those impacted by brain injuries as a result of trauma, tumor, or stroke. **David Krempels** was motivated to create this organization after being injured in a car crash. Following the crash, David attended support groups for people who survived a brain injury; however, he did not feel there was enough support for this population. This resulted in David using a large portion of his own jury award to fund the creation of the Krempels Brain Injury Foundation for People Living with Brain Injury. He did this with the help of four close friends—John L. Ahlgren, Jim Fisher, Lisa Hanson and Effie Malley.

The Krempels Center has undergone various transitions since its inception in 1995. Initially started as an emergency fund program, its original mission was to assist individuals and families who were experiencing financial strain as a result of a recent traumatic brain injury. With a budget of $30,000, the advisory committee met monthly to review applications from people with a brain injury. In 1998, this budget was increased to $120,000, and the first paid staff member, Lisa Hanson—social worker, was hired. The organization continued to focus primarily on grant applications, with Lisa assisting members with all phases of the application process and taking an active role in the lives of each member. The focus of this organization began to shift in 2000, when the foundation board became aware of the clubhouse model: a physical place where survivors could meet and spend time together. A consultant was hired to determine if the organization should move to such a model, and after demonstrating that this would be feasible, the Foundation expanded to a program called Steppingstones. In 2004 the name of this program was changed to The Krempels Brain Injury Foundation. This organization has grown in both size and quality over the years, and now offers a number of group activities tailored to members' needs. Members are encouraged to take active roles, choosing which groups they wish to attend, and how often. Overall, **The Krempels Center** organization is dedicated to engaging members in meaningful and productive experiences, while promoting community participation, inclusion, and education. **The Krempels Center** is a nonprofit organization dedicated to improving the lives of people living with brain injury from trauma, tumor or stroke.

The Krempels Center provides services to anyone who has survived a brain injury as a result of trauma, tumor, or stroke. Members must be 18 years of age or older. Survivors who are members of the Krempels Center are largely unemployed, and tend to use social security as their main source of income. **The Krempels Center** serves the Portsmouth, New Hampshire area, and works in partnership with Universities and community volunteers. Each year, the organization serves approximately 90 individuals and their families. Members are often referred to the organization by their families or by medical professionals.

RESOURCES

Funding/Cost

The **Krempels Center Community Program** is a client centered, comprehensive, member driven program, funded largely through grants, fundraisers, corporate sponsors, Medicaid and private insurance money, and gifts donated from community agencies. Members play a key role in expanding the program to meet the needs of those participating. There are approximately ninety active members involved in the Krempels Center Community Program, with an estimated thirty-five members attending groups on a daily basis. Member fees consist of a $65.00 daily fee, however this fee is assessed on a sliding scale basis, as no member will be turned away. According to social work employee Lisa Hanson, "we are very flexible. As a social worker, I love this about our program. We follow David Krempels' philosophy that no one is turned away due to inability to pay. Since we are not a medical model or rehab, we don't fall under any **Medicaid, Medicare** or insurance guidelines for funding. So, we look to grants, fund-raisers and donations to make up the difference in our budget" (**Feals, 2011**).

The majority of funding for the organization comes from community donations. Each year, the Krempels Center staff, members, and community volunteers organize a major fundraising event called the Runner's Alley/Redhook 5K Memorial Road Race and Health Walk. **The Krempels Center** is working towards a long-term plan to secure funding. They have developed a three-year strategic plan aiming towards financial stability and community awareness.

Staffing and Program Location

The Krempels Center consists of a multidisciplinary team to help meet the needs of members. The organization currently employs the equivalent of four full-time staff members specifically within the **Community Program**: two social workers and two occupational therapists. There is also a program assistant and an administrative assistant who help run the program. Other staff members within the organization include the executive director, and the development director who supports fundraising and training. Member groups take place in an afterschool program gymnasium, which is subleased by **The Krempels Center**. This building contains a gym, kitchen, cafeteria, and outdoor trails. Transportation to the Community Program is provided by **COAST** bus.

University Students and Faculty

A unique feature of **The Krempels Center** is its relationship with university students and Faculty from allied health disciplines (**Fraas, Balz, & Degrauw, 2007**). Approximately 100 students from undergraduate and graduate university programs assist with the implementation of group activities and provide individual support sessions to help members identify their goals and plans for the program.

Volunteers

Community volunteers are a crucial component of **The Krempels Center** program. Community volunteers assist by lending their skills in groups including arts, recreation, and leisure adventures. Volunteers are also central to assisting with the organization of fundraising events. **The Krempels Center** program maintains the philosophy that the mutual rapport developed by including volunteers in the program helps to eradicate misconceptions and negative stereotypes about people living with brain injury.

IMPLEMENTATION

Programs

The Krempels Center Community Program consists of two main member activities: Group Sessions and Community Education. Member autonomy is encouraged as members choose which groups they would like to participate in, and how often. Members are also encouraged to visit the organization prior to joining, in order to see first-hand the types of groups offered.

Group Sessions

The Krempels Center Community Program offers its members a number of Group Sessions that consider the individual from a holistic approach. Groups are based on seven main themes: creative, emotional, functional, physical, recreational, social and vocational activities. The overall goal of the groups is to improve member's quality of life. Groups are offered only three days a week: Monday, Wednesday, and Friday, in order to account for member fatigue. Members are able to choose which groups they would like to attend, in addition to how often they would like to attend. Early-bird groups are offered at 9:30 a.m., followed by Community Meetings at 10:15 a.m., Morning Groups at 11:00 a.m., Lunch at 12:00 noon, and Afternoon Group at 1:00 p.m. The Community Meeting occurs each morning to allow for introductions, announcements, program descriptions and learning objectives.

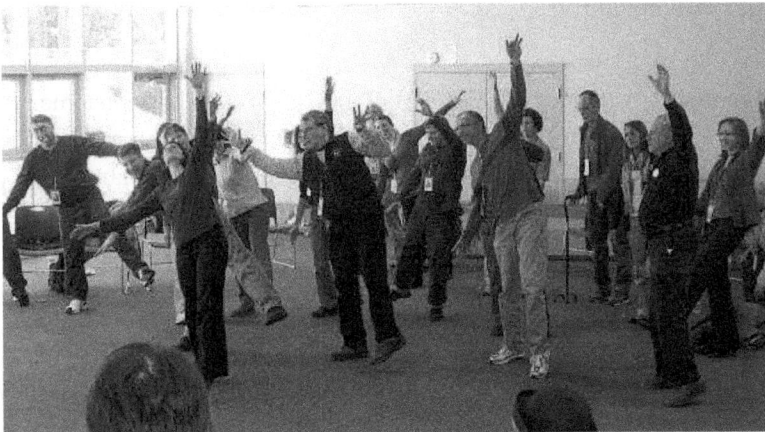

Figure 1: Krempels Center Community Program Group Photo

Members play an active role in determining the group schedule, in addition to the types of groups that are offered. Caregiver Support Groups are also incorporated into the program, and occur every Wednesday. The first hour of the Caregiver Support Group is led by a trained counsellor, followed by a one hour discussion session between the family members. One-on-one service for members and/or their families are also provided if needed. An example of the Community Program offerings is included in Table 1. A description of all of the groups offered within this program is included below.

Table 1. *Community Program Group Schedule*

Time	Monday	Wednesday	Friday
9:30-10:10	Computer Skills Saori Weaving Cards & Coffee 20-minute Tune-Up	Computer Skills Saori Weaving Cards & Coffee 20-minute Tune-Up	Computer Skills Saori Weaving Cards & Coffee 20-minute Tune-Up
10:15-10:50	Community Meeting	Community Meeting	Community Meeting
11:00-11:50	Open Minds Photo Safari Brain Power Wii Sports & Fitness Community Outing	Transitions What's Cooking? Travel Group Yummy Yoga Brain Power	Life Skills What's Cooking? Creative Expression Easy Reader
12:00-12:50	Lunch	Lunch	Lunch
1:00-1:50	Meditation Relationships Challenge Group Common Threads	Current Events Creative Expression Healthy Living Rain or Shine	Aphasia Support Spare Time Music Matters Sports & Fitness

Aphasia Support is facilitated by Dave Halloran, a Krempels Center member who is nationally recognized for his leadership in aphasia advocacy. The group is designed to provide emotional support to members and their families, while sharing and practicing compensatory strategies for aphasia.

Brain Injury 101 focuses on learning about brain functions, various types of injuries and the impact brain injury has on one's life.

Brain Power provides an opportunity to "exercise the brain" through a variety of activities that address common cognitive, speech, and memory challenges.

Cards & Coffee encourages members to gather informally to play cards and enjoy socializing with other members, staff, and interns.

The **Challenge Group** is designed to help members develop effective communication and problem-solving skills by engaging in fun, cooperative, challenging games. No "zip-lines" in this group includes mental challenges and team-building activities.

Community Connections is designed to help members set goals to engage in new or past leisure activities independently in the community. Individuals are able explore leisure interests and identify community resources, including friends and family they can access. Each group includes discussion of members' activities and helping each other resolve barriers such as transportation and limited finances.

Community Education is geared toward preparing for outreach opportunities that educate the public about living with and the prevention of brain injury. This group addresses presentation and public speaking skills and provides opportunities for advocacy and to practice these skills.

Community Outings explore the Seacoast via Coast bus and trolley while working on money management, transportation, and community integration skills. This group lasts the entire program day.

Computer Skills provides an opportunity for members to develop and practice computer skills under the guidance of staff and interns or utilize computers independently.

Creative Expression is designed to explore and express members' creative sides utilizing writing, drawing, collage, watercolor painting and craft activities. This group also provides time to weave using accessible Saori looms to create fiber art.

Current Events explores various media (radio, newsprint, Internet) to gain knowledge of current news, weather and sports as well as local, national, and world affairs.

Easy Reader is the Krempels book club. Krempels Center founder David Krempels reads and discusses books chosen by group participants.

Emotions provides a forum for sharing and discussion aimed at processing the emotions involved in living with a brain injury. This support group is facilitated by interns and social worker Lisa Hanson, the Krempels Center support and resources coordinator. Themes and topics vary depending on the needs of the members.

The **Happiness Project** is based on Gretchen Rubin's bestselling book of the same name. She spent one year looking at the wisdom of the ages, current scientific studies, and lessons from popular culture about how to be happy.

Life Skills, facilitated by interns and mental health therapist John Burbank, explores skills needed to balance and cope with issues encountered by people living with brain injury. Themes are developed and incorporated based on member need and include stress management, communication, and adjustment to change.

Meditation, led by interns and Gerry Duffy, a trained expert in eastern and western meditation, provides opportunities to practice meditative techniques to improve health and wellness.

Music Matters offers an opportunity to listen to and engage in a variety of music styles. Past themes included music through the ages, (60s, 70s, 80s), and types of music (rock, reggae, classical, etc). Musical instruments received through a grant from the Portsmouth Rotary are used.

The **Newsletter** group provides an opportunity to learn and practice writing, interviewing, and computer skills by publishing one or more newsletters during the semester. The Photo Safari group can also be a resource for photos to illustrate the articles.

Photo Safari, taught by master photographer Gene Paltrineri, teaches the fundamentals of camera operation, photography composition and utilization of computer software to enhance photographs. The group includes field trips around the Community Campus and Portsmouth, allowing opportunities for experiential learning.

Relationships is designed to help members build connections with others, establish appropriate boundaries, communicate effectively and enhance social skills through assertiveness techniques, active listening, role-playing, and discussion.

Sign Language teaches conversational sign language as an alternative form of communication. New skills are applied in a variety of activities including short stories, songs, and games.

Sports & Fitness provides opportunities to engage in sports and other physical activities, adapted for all abilities, including Wii Games, donated by one of the members and her family, and Wii Fit, donated by the Occupational Therapy Department at the University of New Hampshire.

Transitions provides an opportunity to discuss and process the many transitions encountered by people living with brain injury. This support group is facilitated by interns and certified grief and bereavement counselor Pamela Sollenberger.

Twenty-Minute Tune-Up is an exercise group geared toward improving strength, flexibility and endurance, utilizing hand weights and thera-band. The group takes advantage of the Community Campus walking trails.

What's Cooking brings together community members to prepare and enjoy lunch together. This group provides teaching and practice in the fundamentals of meal planning, budgeting, food preparation, kitchen safety, and healthy eating. There is a $3 fee to cover the cost of food.

Yummy Yoga, facilitated by interns and certified Kripalu yoga instructor Maddy Botari Eaton, is designed to teach and practice adaptive yoga in a comfortable, safe manner for health and wellness. Seeking balance and focus in all dimensions of life is a primary benefit of this activity.

Community Education Program

The Krempels Center is committed to community participation and prevention strategies. An example of this commitment is the creation of the **Community Education Program**, whereby members participate in a weekly group that teaches skills in public speaking. Members then participate in talks within the community to audiences such as elementary, secondary, and university students, health professionals, community agencies, and other individuals who have experienced a brain injury. Examples of speaking engagements include members telling their personal stories, in addition to providing education and offering prevention strategies. The goals of this program are to enhance members' public speaking skills, while increasing community involvement providing the community with important information. See Box 1 for an example of a speaking engagement.

Box. 1 The Boston Globe, Sunday Edition (01/11/09)

In his shoes : Sixth-graders get lessons on what it's like to go through life with a brain injury

How do you button a shirt or put on socks using only one hand? What's it like trying to get around in a wheelchair if you can't see? How isolating is it to not recognize or remember people's faces? These are just a few of the questions sixth-graders at the John C. Page School in West Newbury explored during a recent two-day program on brain injury. Presented by the Krempels Brain Injury Foundation of Portsmouth, N.H., the program was presented in conjunction with a schoolwide yearlong campaign titled We Can Make a Difference. "It's about how one small act can turn into something magnificent," said Susan Van Etten, counselor at Page. "And it's the idea of understanding people with differences and that we can reach out and not shy away." Van Etten said foundation founder David Krempels, who

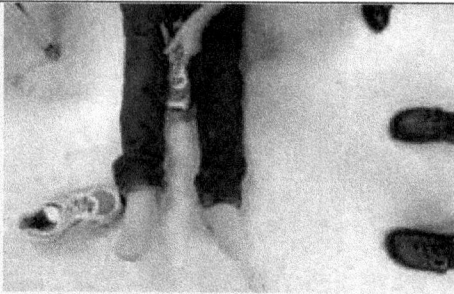

spoke to the students, epitomizes the far-reaching impact of one person's actions. On June 8, 1992, Krempels and his bride of two days were driving on the Maine Turnpike during their honeymoon. Traffic was stopped for a construction project, but the tractor-trailer behind the couple didn't brake and slammed into the car. Krempels's wife was killed. He was left in a coma and brain-injured. Krempels had a long, difficult recovery and was emotionally and financially drained for years. Eventually, with rehabilitation, he improved and remarried. Meanwhile, he won a monetary settlement relating to the accident. He used a portion of the money to start Krempels Brain Injury Foundation, which includes SteppingStones, a community-based day program for people with brain injuries, and a family support program. "Here's a man who could have taken the money and moved on with his life, but he decided one person could make a tremendous difference in the lives of so many others," said Van Etten. As part of the Page School program, organized by Barb Kresge of West Newbury, program coordinator for SteppingStones, students learned about the causes and physical, emotional, and social implications of brain injury; how to recognize and respond to someone who is brain-injured; and injury prevention, such as wearing a helmet while riding a bike and skateboarding. They also had a chance to interact with several people with brain injuries. But much of the impact of the program came from students participating in interactive activities that allowed them to experience what it's like living with a brain injury. Throughout several classrooms, stations were set up where they were asked to perform dressing and eating activities, with limitations and with adaptive equipment. They were asked to pick small matching objects from gift bags without looking and with mittens on, to simulate decreased sensation in the hands and fingers. And they completed memory and cognitive tests on computers. "Challenging," "impossible," and "frustrating," were students' reactions to chores such as cutting grapes with a butter knife or peeling a potato using their nondominant hands; trying to navigate a maze on paper by looking at it in a mirror, so up is down and left is right; and telling a joke to another person by tapping out letters on a communication board rather than speaking. "It was hard to understand what the other person was trying to say," Kelsie McNamara said of the joke-telling exercise. "It's harder than talking face to face. It shows how lucky we are that we can communicate." "I can't believe people have to live like this every day," said Caroline McDonough, after sitting in a wheelchair and steering it through an obstacle course using only her nondominant hand. "It must be hard." But there was also recognition of what can be done to improve the lives of the brain-injured. After meeting Jarrod Limbert, 29, of Newmarket, N.H., who was hit by a car when he was 7 and is in a wheelchair and unable to speak, Hannah Tew commented on the Dynavox that helps him communicate. "It's really amazing they have those tools," she said. "Even though he has a brain injury, we can communicate with him. It's nice we can treat him like a normal person."

Intakes are conducted with new members at the start of their involvement with the **Krempels Center**. These intakes assess areas of neuro-cognitive measures, language and cognition, community integration measures, and quality of life. This program uses a multidisciplinary approach, including social workers, occupational therapists, speech-language pathologists, and recreation staff. The main barrier identified in implementing this program is transportation. This is supported in the literature, as **Fraas and colleagues (2007)** found that transportation is one of the needs not addressed through this program. **The Krempels Center Community Program** typically relies on the bus system, thus, members are only able to travel where the bus takes them. This limits areas and activities within the community that members are able to access.

Theoretical Frameworks

The Krempels Center Community Program is grounded in frameworks that emphasize the person in their environment: **The Model of Human Occupation Theory**, and the Person, Occupation, Environment Theory. The Model of Human Occupation Theory was developed by Dr. Gary Kielhofner, and is one of the leading theories in Occupational Therapy. This theory is applicable across the life span (**MOHO Clearinghouse, 2010**) and addresses how human occupation is motivated within one's physical and emotional environment (**MOHO Clearinghouse, 2010**), and how illness and disability-related issues may arise (**Ramifiken & Van Niekerk, 2009**). Similarly, the Person Occupation Environment Theory describes the interaction between the person, the environment, and the occupation (**Ramifiken & Van Niekerk, 2009**), and was founded in 1996 by Law and colleagues. This framework is drawn upon within the Krempels Center Community Program, as they look at the member first, and then how that member occupies time (e.g., leisure, work, homecare), and lastly how the member lives in his/her environment.

Student Involvement

Krempels Center is considered to be a teaching center for local university students (**Fraas, Balz, & Degrauw, 2007**). Undergraduate and graduate students, largely from the University of New Hampshire, in allied health disciplines including Communication Sciences and Disorders, Occupational Therapy, and Therapeutic Recreation, assist with group activities and individual support sessions with members. Students are supervised by university Faculty, of which there are 8-10 from various Faculties associated with the Krempels Center. Each year, approximately 100 students provide a total of nearly 7500 hours of support to the Center. Each student is involved with the center for one academic semester, and receives academic credit for their participation in the program.

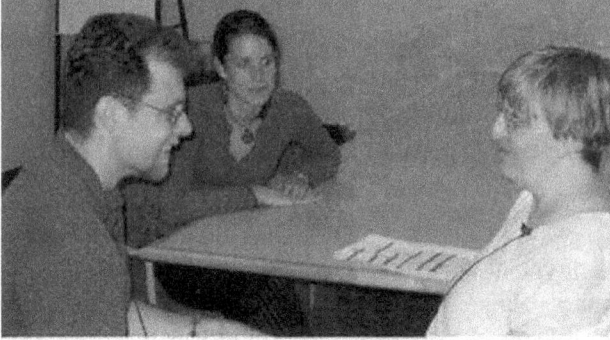

Figure 2: University Intern interviewing a Member of the Group Program

The Role of Culture and Diversity

The Krempels Center Community Program accounts for cultural and other diverse issues, particularly through their Enrichment Program. This program offers members the opportunity to partake in new cultural experiences, by exposing members to various activities within the community, or, by having those activities come into the Krempels Center Building. Examples of such activities within the Enrichment Program include African dancers, drumming, folk group, guest speakers such as TJ Wheller who lectures on the Civil Rights Movement, and lastly cooking groups that offer a variety of recipes from around the world.

OUTCOME

Evaluation Methods

1. Informal Evaluations with Members

Krempels Center strives to achieve outcomes that focus on the community members' experience. Staff members of the Krempels Center have attempted to complete formal evaluation of the program in the past; however, it was found that members often experienced memory difficulties. In light of this, staff and interns now facilitate conversations on a regular basis; sitting with members to have discussions after groups occur in order to gather their feedback. Members have been accommodated in order to provide feedback, using methods such as "give thumbs up, or thumbs down." The applicability of the Community Program within the actual community is measured by interns asking members questions such as "would you want to access this in your home life? How does what you did today impact you outside of here?"

2. Oral History Project—Evaluation with Practitioners and Students of Members Experience

Michael Fraas and colleagues have been instrumental in developing and supporting strategic research and evaluation of the **Krempels Center** programs. In 2007, **Fraas and Calvert (2007)** conducted a study investigating the influence of listening to oral histories told by members of the **Krempels Center** programs, on the attitudes and beliefs held by Speech-Language Pathologists, graduate students and undergraduate students studying communication sciences and disorders. Oral histories are defined as "a method of gathering and preserving historical information through recorded interviews with participants in past events and ways of life" (**Oral History Association, 2002**), and are considered to help facilitate better understanding of a population from within (**Fraas & Calvert, 2007**). Researchers have identified that in order for survivors of brain injury to succeed in society, individuals must be made aware of what it means to have an acquired brain injury (**Lefebvre, Pelchat, Swaine, Gelinas, & Levert, 2005**; **Swift, & Wilson, 2001**). Furthermore, misconceptions held by practising clinicians can have a negative impact on members' experiences (**Fraas & Calvert, 2007**). In order to examine the influence of such oral histories, a 10-item questionnaire was administered to all 87 participants (27 speech language pathologists (SLP); 21 graduate students; and 39 undergraduate students). Next, participants listened to oral history samples, and then completed the same 10-item questionnaire a second time. Results of this study indicated that listening to the oral histories of ABI survivors, particularly members of the Krempels Center programs, had an effect on all participants, as changes in response to the questionnaire indicated improved attitudes and beliefs toward ABI survivors. Undergraduate students demonstrated the most significant change in their responses on all questions related to ABI. Similarly, graduate students also showed a large change in their responses, particularly on questions related to items focusing on the role of speech therapy in rehabilitation, and on cognitive function. SLP's showed the greatest change in their responses to items focusing on social and vocational attainment for ABI survivors. **Fraas and Calvert (2007)** state that "by increasing public awareness of the impact of ABI, empowering survivors and their families through increased education, and improving the attitudes and beliefs of ABI held by allied health professionals, survivors of ABI will improve their rehabilitation process and experience a higher quality of life" (pp. 1453).

Box. 2 *Oral History Questions asked to Krempels Center Members*

Oral History Questions
1. Could you tell me about your life before your injury? <u>Additional Probes:</u> Employment, Family, Goals, Education, Friends, Social life, Religion
2. Describe your injury. <u>Additional Probes:</u> How long ago did it happen? Where did it happen? What happened to you?
3. What was your rehab experience life? <u>Additional Probes:</u> What types of therapy did you

have? Where did you have therapy? What was beneficial/nonbeneficial during therapy?

4. What changes have occurred since your injury? <u>Additional Probes:</u> Physical, Emotional, Communication
5. How has life been since your injury? <u>Additional Probes:</u> Social, Family, Vocation, Financially, Religion
6. How has your communication been affected since your injury?
7. What goals are you currently working toward? Or what would you like to achieve in your life now?
8. How has [the ABI program] played a part in your life?

3. Qualitative Investigations: The Use of Narratives to Identify Characteristics leading to a Productive Life following ABI

In order to better understand the characteristics that lead to a successful recovery and productive lifestyle, **Fraas and Calvert (2009)** conducted a study analyzing qualitative interviews with 31 survivors of ABI from the **Krempels Center** Organization. Using a phenomenological approach, four major themes were revealed from the interviews: development of social support networks, grief and coping strategies, acceptance of the injury and redefinition of self, and empowerment. From the original sample of 31 participants, four case studies were chosen in order to highlight quotes supporting the aforementioned themes. Empowerment was one of the key themes of this study, and it has a particular role in community participation. **Fraas and Calvert (2009)** state that "the participants in this investigation have achieved a number of accomplishments that have empowered them to become independent, resourceful, and eager to give back to their communities" (p.322). Much of the empowerment described in this study is said to come from members advocacy efforts in raising awareness in their communities, and a desire to help others facing similar issues. One member stated: "So far I have probably done 15 different speaking engagements through [the ABI] program and through the American Heart Association and through Train to End Stroke, kind of a little bit of everything" (p. 322). Empowerment through community participation is described as an important factor to quality of life and productivity for ABI survivors (**Fraas & Calvert, 2009**).

4. Qualitative and Quantitative Evaluation: Meeting the Long-term needs of Adults with Acquired Brain Injury through Community-based Programming.

The effectiveness of the Krempels Center Community Program was evaluated in a study conducted by **Fraas, Balz, and Degrauw (2007)**. In this study, both qualitative and quantitative measures were used to gauge how effective clinicians and program members felt this organization was at addressing the needs of clients. A focus group was also conducted with program members, student interns, and caregivers in order to supplement the findings. Results of the surveys and focus group identified three needs that varied considerably amongst groups of participants with respect to how "strongly" they reported each need being met. The three needs identified included: emotional, social, and transportation needs. Focus group findings identified emotional, social, and cognitive needs as the most important for ABI survivors, which program members, interns, and caregivers all felt were being met through the Krempels Center programs. Areas that participants identified as unmet included social support for caregivers, community education, and transportation issues.

5. Evaluation of Expressive Electronic Journal Writing of Members

Research indicates that survivors of ABI often experience deficits such as depression, impaired ability to communicate, and social isolation following their injury (**Fraas & Balz, 2008**). Such deficits have the ability to decrease ones quality of life (**Fraas & Balz, 2008**), which may in turn affect their community integration and participation. Because creative expression is a program offered to members of the **Krempels Center**, and given that expressive writing programs have demonstrated effectiveness in reducing impairments for other populations (**Fraas & Balz, 2008**), Fraas and Balz (2008) conducted a study examining the effects of online, expressive journal writing as a means to positively affect communication, emotional status, and social integration for ABI survivors. Conducted at the **Krempels Center**, this study used questionnaires including the Community Integration Questionnaire (**Willer et al., 1993**), the Brief Test of Head Injury (**Helm-Estabrooks and Hotz, 1991**), and the Beck Depression Inventory II (**Beck et al., 1996**) to gather information from six members (n=6). Demographic information of participants is included in Table 2.

Table 2: *Sample demographics of members who participate in the study.*

Cause of Brain Injury	Years Post-onset	Age
TBI/MVA	20	41
TBI/MVA	9	61
TBI/Gun shot	27	46
RCVA	1.5	56
RCVA	3	43
RCVA	2	59
MVA=motor vehicle accident; RCVA = right cerebral vascular accident.		

This study was conducted over a 10-week period, with Week 1 and Week 10 dedicated to pre- and post-testing respectively. Weekly writing sessions required participants to use their own computer to respond to a new writing prompt. If participants were unable to use the keyboard due to physical limitations, they dictated their responses to a research assistant. Quantitative analysis of the questionnaires revealed a significant difference between pre- and post-participation in the writing workshop for the Community Integration Questionnaire only. This finding was surprising, as it means that participants reported less community integration following participation in electronic journal writing. This is inconsistent with the qualitative findings, which highlighted the positive benefits that participants expressed. These researchers highlighted two possible reasons for such a surprising finding: 1) pre-testing occurred during a time when the Krempels Center was preparing for two very busy and popular fundraising activities (of which the clients are actively involved), and also during the active school term with high student involvement at the Center; 2) post-testing occurred after these fundraisers had occurred, and no active planning was taking place for any other activities. Additionally, post-testing was completed during the summer months when most students were away and not actively engaged in the program. Thus, the amount of community integration that participants were directly involved with at the time of survey completion may have played a role in the results.

Qualitative findings revealed four major themes: 1) improved communication, 2) personal fulfillment, 3) a newly revealed writing talent, and 4) empowerment (**Fraas & Balz, 2008**). For example, when asked to write about a gift participants could give to someone else, one client responded: "Right now I would say thank you to a lot of people. It makes people feel appreciated [...when I] realize what they have done for me. [This] would make me feel not quite so helpless because I could interact with people..." In conclusion, these researchers suggest further research be conducted to examine the potential benefits of electronic journal writing for those isolated by a brain injury.

Evaluation Summary

Findings from research conducted with members at the **Krempels Center** have been used to make changes within the organization. Specifically, two main initiatives surfaced as a result of research, both pertaining to a study conducted by **Fraas and colleagues (2007)**, which examined the effectiveness of the community program at meeting the long-term needs of members. As a result of the research findings, two needs were identified that were described as being unmet: 1) social support for members and caregivers, and 2) community education. In an attempt to address these need identified through the research process, changes were made within the **Community Program**. For instance, the facilitator of the Family Support Program used to focus on topics such as resources and grants, however, as a result of the research study mentioned above, the focus of this program was changed to address the emotional and psychosocial needs of families and caregivers. Additionally, survivors described a lack of brain injury information and awareness in the community. This finding stimulated the creation of the Community Education Program described above, whereby members develop presentations that they offer to the community through forums such as school, rehabilitation agencies, doctors, and university settings.

Dissemination

Information about the **Krempels Center Community Program** is disseminated in multiple ways. For example, members disseminate information about the program, in addition to information related to their personal journey, and brain injury prevention, directly to the community through **Community Education** sessions. Additionally, traditional ways of disseminating knowledge through academic forums are also used, as multiple research studies have been published in prominent journals such as *Brain Injury, American Journal of Speech-Language Pathology* and *Disability and Rehabilitation.*

Conclusion

The **Krempels Center Community Program** is a unique program that fosters community participation. The emphasis of this programs' dedication to community participation is evident by the recent name change. Previously referred to as SteppingStones—the newly named Community Program highlights the efforts being taken to facilitate community participation. When asked directly how this program fits with community participation, Carol Davis (Community Program Coordinator) explained that this program gives people an opportunity to increase their confidence to do more. It facilitates members being active within their community, and provides a safe environment for them to work towards their goals. Both individual members and their families work towards their own rehabilitation, and are responsible for their own growth.

References

Beck, A. T., Steer, R. A., & Brown, G. K. (1996). *Beck depression inventory.* San Antonio: The Psychological Corporation.

Centre for Community Based Research. (2010). An outcomes framework for the ABI community of practice.

Feals, J. (2011). *Krempels Center creates a sense of community for those with brain injury.* Retrieved July 2011, from **http://www.seacoastonline.com/articles/20110116-NEWS-101160333**.

Fraas, M., & Balz, M. A. (2008). **Expressive electronic journal writing: Freedom of communication for survivors of acquired brain injury.** *Journal Psycholinguist Res, 37,* 115-124.

Fraas, M. R., & Calvert, M. (2007). **Oral histories: Bridging misconceptions and reality in brain injury recovery.** *Disability and Rehabilitation, 29*(18), 1449-1455.

Fraas, M. R., & Calvert, M. (2009). **The use of narratives to identify characteristics leading to a productive life following acquired brain injury.** *American Journal of Speech-Language Pathology, 18,* 315-328.

Fraas, M. R., Balz, M., & Degrauw, W. (2007). Meeting the long-term needs of adults with acquired brain injury through community-based programming. **Brain Injury,** *21*(12), 1267-1281.

Helm-Estabrooks, N., & Hotz, G. (1991). *Brief test of head injury.* Chicago: ProEd.MOHO Clearinghouse. (2010). Introduction to MOHO. Retrieved September 10, 2010 from **http://www.moho.uic.edu/intro.html**.

Lefebvre, H., Pelchat, D., Swaine, B., Gelinas, I., & Levert, M. J. (2005). The experiences of individuals with a traumatic brain injury, families, physicians and health professionals regarding care provided throughout the continuum. **Brain Injury,** *19*(8), 585-597.

MOHO Clearinghouse (2010). Retrieved September 10, 2010 from **http://www.uic.edu/depts/moho/**

Oral History Association. (2002). Carlisle, PA: Dickinson College.

Ramifikeng, M., & Van Nieker, L. (2009). Occupation focus conceptual frameworks. Retrieved September 10, 2010 from **Http://www.oerafrica.org/FTPFolder/Occupation%20Focus%20Conceptual%20frame works/index.htm**.

Swift, T. L., & Wilson, S. L. (2001). Misconceptions about brain injury among the general public and non-expert health professionals: An exploratory study. **Brain Injury,** *15*(2), 149-165.

Willer, B., Rosenthal, M., Griffith, E. R., Bond, M. R., Miller, J. D., & Kreutzer, J. (1993). **Assessment of community integration following rehabilitation for traumatic brain injury.** *Journal of Head Trauma Rehabilitation, 8,* 75-87.

CHAPTER 14

BISCAYNE INSTITUTES OF HEALTH & LIVING INC.

By Gaayathiri Jegatheeswaran

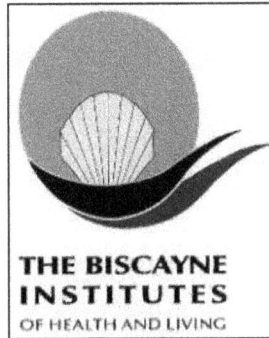

THE BISCAYNE INSTITUTES
OF HEALTH AND LIVING

Population Served : Children and Adults	
Contributing Author Contact Information	

Dr. Marie A. DiCowden

Executive Director and Founder

Biscayne Institutes of Health & Living, Inc.

2785 NE 183rd Street

Suite 100

Miami, Florida 33160

Tel: 305-932-8994

Email: **dr.d@biscayneinstitutes.org**

mdcatbihl@aol.com

BACKGROUND

Outcome studies reveal that many individuals affected by acquired brain injury (ABI) fail to integrate themselves back into the community (**Willer & Corrigan, 1994**). This occurs even though they have received standard rehabilitation. This very situation has paved the way for the development of community based programs—so much so that a 10-fold increase in such programs were noticed between 1981-1991 (**Willer & Corrigan, 1994**). However, the models that some of these programs used failed to differ from the standard rehabilitation model. As a result, **Willer & Corrigan (1994)** proposed Whatever It Takes (WIT). This model outlines a service approach that will successfully integrate ABI survivors back into the community. WIT proposes the need for an individualized, holistic therapy plan; skill development, and the development of supports (**Willer & Corrigan, 1994**). Coincidentally, the services at **Biscayne Institutes of Health and Living, Inc.** (BIHL), located in Miami, Florida, have been implementing this approach since 1988.

The idea behind **BIHL** came about when Dr. Marie DiCowden was working at the **University of Miami School of Medicine**. At the university, she noticed that individuals who had completed rehabilitation would often come back after being discharged. The very same problem was noticed by two local neurosurgeons in their practice with individuals with mild brain injury. The surgeons offered to find funding for the program's development and Dr. DiCowden established **BIHL** with this support. The success of **BIHL** as a community-based program is facilitated by the unique health care delivery model used by **BIHL**. This model, known as the **HealthCare Community™ (HCC) model** (see Figure 1), offers a novel way of delivering healthcare by integrating clinical practices, administration, and finances.

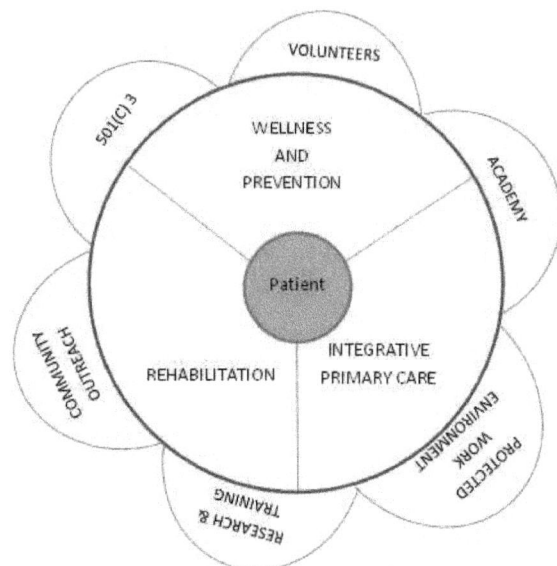

Figure 1: The HealthCare Community™ model encompassing the services at Biscayne Institutes of Health and Living, Inc. (DiCowden, 2007).

Biscayne's HCC Model

Clinically, the main focus is on treating the whole person through individualized therapy by a community team of professionals who address physical, cognitive, social, and behavioural aspects of the consumer. Further, traditional Western care, as well as alternative forms of medicine (e.g., acupuncture), is used to treat individuals. To integrate the administration of this institution, moreover, an office governing the program works with the team of clinicians and facilitates a seamless flow of communication between the concerned parties. Financially, patchwork funding composed of public and private funds is utilized to sustain the institution.

Quintessentially, **BIHL** specializes in providing community-based healthcare that serves as a cross between hospitals and practitioners. It is dedicated to following consumers through the span of the healthcare continuum ranging from wellness to rehabilitation, and the developmental stages of a lifetime. **BIHL**, furthermore, takes a concerted effort to follow individuals in both the family and community contexts. This feature allows **BIHL** to serve as a central hub for up-to-date information on the consumers. In essence, **BIHL**'s focus is on health and quality of daily living, and not on illness.

There are three core services that are offered by **BIHL** —integrative primary care, rehabilitation, and wellness and health promotion. Of interest to this particular casebook are the therapy services for Adult Traumatic Brain Injury (TBI) and Neurology, and Pediatric TBI. These services will be discussed in further detail in the subsequent sections.

"Community participation, as defined at Biscayne Institutes, includes the ability for an individual to participate in many aspects of emotional and physical interactions that enhance the quality of life for themselves and others. As with all aspects of health, participation is on a continuum. Community participation can include the ability to interact with spouse, children, grandchildren, friends both at home and at gatherings/activities (however minimal) outside the home. It may mean being able to again take up some of the responsibilities of living in the home, or in volunteer or work capacities—all aspects that contribute to an individual's sense of Self and meaning of their contribution to life. It can include the range of being able to go out in public or private transportation—or if the individual is truly able to make gains to go back to driving themselves; it may mean the ability to travel on vacation with others or find meaningful daily activities in their immediate surroundings. Biscayne's goal is to enhance each person's individual definition of quality of life and help them reach a full definition of living emotionally, cognitively, physically and spiritually."

- Dr. DiCowden (personal communication, November 26, 2010)

Adult and Pediatric TBI Services

There are three stages to these services: Assessment and Treatment Plan (Stage 1), Consolidation of Skills (Stage 2) and Life After Rehab (Stage 3). Information regarding the therapy plan in Stage 1 will be discussed in this section. More information about the stages will be presented in "Implementation". Notably, **BIHL**'s usage of terms such as "patient" and "treatment", which are often utilized by traditional rehabilitation facilities, do not negate **BIHL**'s dedication to offering services that foster community participation to individuals with TBI. The usage stems from the fact **BIHL** was developed in the midst of traditional rehabilitation programs nearly two decades ago using the observations from experience in such rehabilitation facilities.

Individuals admitted into the day TBI services are seen for post-acute care and are then monitored long-term in the community. The therapy for each consumer in the program is individualized and determined by administering a series of evaluations to assess cognition, behaviour, physical health, etc. Using the findings, an interdisciplinary care plan is developed with the consumer and his/her family in mind. Additionally for children, special care is taken to help them attain optimal functioning for their age. Failure to do so may delay or hinder the emergence of subsequent age-appropriate behaviour (**DiCowden, 2007**).

There are numerous interdisciplinary professionals and caregivers (e.g., psychologists, social workers, and speech, occupational and physical therapists) who work together to administer the plan. The service plan may consist of numerous services like cognitive retraining (to stimulate brain recovery), biofeedback (to create awareness of physiological functions), and other therapies and interventions (e.g., speech, behavioural and occupational). Additionally, alternate forms of medicine, like Chinese medicine, can also been used to aid healing. Furthermore, interventions may be applied alongside group/family therapy as well. In the Pediatric TBI Service, various therapies like physical, occupational and speech therapies are presented in conjunction with special education. **BIHL** is very flexible in when and how they offer these services to students—if the parent wishes, services can be offered after-school or, if the children are admitted into the Biscayne Academy, provided alongside educational programs. Biscayne Academy is a school at **BIHL** that works with the Pediatric TBI Service to offer special education to children/adolescents. Studies have shown that by offering such educational opportunities in parallel with therapy, a positive effect is seen physically, cognitively, emotionally, socially, and behaviourally (**DiCowden, 2007**). Consequently, by implementing such an extensive therapy plan, even clients who were deemed "difficult" were able to improve their level of functioning.

Case 1: Hope for Individuals with "Difficult" Brain Injuries

A psychotherapist by profession, "L" was left unable to walk or talk and lost her independence following a brain injury. After undergoing 7 years of holistic rehabilitation at BIHL, she is now able to live her life independently. Additionally, she has also taken the responsibilities of being a peer mentor helping to run psychotherapy programs for individuals with TBI and is the creator of family support groups with her husband who is a psychiatrist. She is also the president of a nonprofit organization that focuses on rehabilitation for seriously injured individuals. Furthermore, she is a strong advocate of long-term rehabilitation for individuals with TBI (even beyond the "24-month maximum recovery rule").

- DiCowden, 2004

Development of Strategies

The strategies used in the therapy services were mainly from Dr. DiCowden's work experience at the **University of Miami**. However, readings were done on the cognitive retraining program at the Rusk Rehabilitation Institute to further enhance therapy (personal communication, June 1, 2010). As mentioned, all the strategies used in the therapy plan exist to encourage and foster community integration. In addition to the ultimate goal of achieving community integration, the strategies used in the services have the following objectives: to increase emotional status and memory, decrease depression and anger, improve relationships and help consumers obtain work/volunteering positions. Additionally, for the pediatric population, the Biscayne Academy provides education, and facilitates mental/physical growth and development.

Notably, there are no cultural/diversity issues in implementing these strategies as Miami is very multicultural and this diversity is reflected in the staff as well as the populations served. These strategies, however, would be further enhanced by more funding.

Community Participation

BIHL offers a full continuum of services to the community ranging from integrative primary care to wellness and health promotion. It functions as a community based facility to everyone in the local community. This very environment facilitates the interaction between individuals with brain injuries and members of the community. This context also serves as a constant reminder to how community integration/participation is important to the lives of individuals affected by TBI. The reminder, furthermore, is woven into the interdisciplinary plan of therapy created for the consumers admitted to **BIHL**.

Every aspect of the therapy plan is geared towards helping consumers achieve their highest level of functioning in the community. The different types of therapies and modules help consumers develop skill sets necessary for them to participate in their life roles and integrate into the community. For example, occupational therapy provides the skills to function in the activities of everyday life. The importance of interacting with other individuals is further strengthened in group and family therapy. Moreover, when funding permits, field trips are also taken as a group by the consumers of the TBI services. Other important aspects of this program are the work and volunteering placements—whether it is in the community or within **BIHL**. These positions are supported and monitored by **BIHL**in Stage 3 of its therapy plan, "Life After Rehab". This plays a very important role in fostering community participation/re-integration. The stages of the therapy plan will be discussed in detail in "Implementation".

Consumers

In the Adult TBI Service, the ages of the consumers range from late-20s to mid-60s. In the Pediatric Service, consumers up to the age of 22 years are seen. Even though there are wealthy patrons who undergo therapy, the majority of the consumers are from the lower-middle class, many of whom are on either social security or disability. Furthermore, approximately one-third of the consumers who obtain the services are complex TBI cases (personal communication, June 1, 2010). The majority of these injuries are caused by motor vehicle accidents (MVAs). In addition to MVAs, injuries in children also occur as a result of recreational mishaps (e.g., near drowning accidents). Notably, cases of TBI due to gunshot wounds have also been reported among the client population.

Accreditations

The rehabilitation services at **BIHL** have numerous accreditations. At the federal level, **BIHL** is recognized as a Comprehensive Outpatient Rehabilitation Facility. It has also been designated as an Adult and Pediatric Brain Injury and Outpatient Medical Rehabilitation Program by the **Commission on Accreditation of Rehabilitation Facilities**. **BIHL** has also been given a **Medicaid** waiver by the state of Florida to provide services for low-income families. Florida's pride in **BIHL** is further reflected in **Florida's Brain and Spinal Cord Injury Council** designating it as a state-provider of services to both adults and children. These accreditations demonstrate that **BIHL** upholds the conditions needed for the recognition—**BIHL** is considered to have services that go beyond the traditional rehabilitation approach and gear their practices/stages to foster community participation.

RESOURCES

Collaborators and Stakeholders

The key players at the beginning of the **BIHL** initiative were Dr. DiCowden, the aforementioned two neurosurgeons and a number of investors in the community. They all joined forces to make Dr. DiCowden's dream of creating an integrated rehabilitation service for individuals with TBI a reality. All but one of the neurosurgeons (who has passed away), still serve as collaborators to **BIHL**, with Dr. DiCowden functioning as the executive director.

The stakeholders of **BIHL** are the consumers, the referral sources (e.g., hospitals, physicians and case managers) and the individuals/agencies that pay for the therapy (e.g., insurance and **Medicaid**). The reactions of the stakeholders, at the beginning and now, have been supportive. At the time of implementation, there were many rehabilitation clinics present within the community. These clinics, however, solely looked at the physical well-being of consumers (and hence, feared the competition posed by **BIHL**). The success of consumers who attended **BIHL** soon stood as a testament to the quality and validity of **BIHL**'s strategies. This further strengthened the community's support for **BIHL**.

Resources to Implement Strategies

At an annual operating cost of $1.4 million, **BIHL** is funded by a variety of sources and exists as a result of patchwork funding (DiCowden, 2007). These sources are as follows: **Medicare, Medicaid, Medicaid waiver, Florida State Brain and Spinal Cord Injury Program**, private insurance, self-pay**, Florida State Department of Education (McKay Scholarships)** and various grants. The contributions from these sources further allow **BIHL** to provide 25% of its services to consumers at no charge (**DiCowden, 2007**). However, more funding is needed as there are many individuals who are unable to afford the services offered at **BIHL**. This is the main reason why **BIHL**stands proudly behind the Healthcare Reform in the United States.

In terms of non-monetary resources, **BIHL** is a freestanding program that is dependent on its own services, contracts and the aforementioned grants. There are no collaborations that **BIHL** utilizes.

Inputs to the Participation Program

Since its initial implementation in 1988, when only the rehabilitation services and the student training program were present, **BIHL** established the integrative primary care, wellness, and health promotion services. These three core services were further supported by ancillary programs that came into existence in later years. The ancillary programs included a community outreach program, a professional training/research program, Biscayne Academy (established in 1995) and 501(c) 3 (a non-profit organization that raises funds for those who are unable to afford the services).

Case 2: Biscayne Academy and "C"

"C" was 9 years old when she was in an MVA and hit her head on the pavement during the accident. She suffered a moderate head injury and remained in public school for two years while attending the after-school pediatric program at BIHL. When she was 11, she entered Biscayne Academy and recently graduated from the school at the age of 19. BIHL was able to help her with her social skills though she was unable to reach the reading and math level for her age. At present, she is working in retail.

- DiCowden (personal communication, November 26, 2010)

IMPLEMENTATION

Effective Practices

BIHL's success in integrating consumers back into the community is greatly influenced by the fact that it is a community based, full service institute. As is their motto, **BIHL** considers "rehabilitation is for life" and gives importance to the community participation of its consumers. **BIHL** considers community participation as the participation in life roles in the community and family, establishing meaningful relationships, self-determination, and achieving well-being and quality of life.

BIHL: Healing Power of Place

The **BIHL** facility physically differs from traditional medical buildings and settings. Situated in an attractive location surrounded by lush gardens, **BIHL** places importance on the healing power of the environment. Inside the facility, **BIHL** is adorned with beautiful furniture and ample lighting. Additionally, there are many rooms (both community and group) in the facility that were designed to look like rooms found in a home. The most important room at **BIHL** is the meditation room, which not only serves as a place for meditation, but also as a place for community gatherings such as dances, transition or graduation ceremonies, as well as cultural events for consumers, staff and community outreach programs. Notably, consumers, staff and people from the community all join together (at no cost to the individuals) to engage in meditation in this room as it is offered in the schedule. Other wellness/prevention workshops and programs, including yoga and Tai Chi, also take place in this room.

Continuum of Care

BIHL offers a continuum of care that facilitates the interaction between individuals with brain injuries and members of the community (see the model, Figure 1).

➢ **Integrative Primary Care**: Consumers are treated in three contexts—as a supplementation to rehabilitation programs, as a primary care practice, and to provide health evaluations and follow-up.

➢ **Rehabilitation Services**: The three stages of TBI therapy are detailed throughout this chapter. In addition to these services, there are four other adult rehabilitation services and one other pediatric service. The adult services are as follows: Adult Outpatient Medical rehabilitation (treating consumers with health challenges like amputation, chronic pain and spinal cord injury), Elders program (addressing issues of consumers related to aging), Adult Developmental Disabilities program (helping individuals with developmental disabilities function) and Adult Dual Diagnosis rehabilitation (helping individuals suffering from alcohol/drug addictions along with injuries involving the brain, spinal cord, etc.). The Pediatric Outpatient Medical rehabilitation focuses on treating children with health challenges ranging from autism and cerebral palsy to learning disabilities and emotional disabilities.

Case 3: The Success of "N"

"N" was involved in a serious MVA in Greece when he was a late adolescent. He also sustained a prolonged coma. After receiving traditional rehabilitation from several facilities in Europe, he went to Miami at the age of 21. He was referred to BIHL by the University of Miami. He underwent therapy at BIHL for 3 years and entered a BIHL community program at an art college upon completing stage 3. At the college, he became well-acquainted with graphics and eventually went back to Greece to help his father with his international publishing business. Accommodations were made at the workplace to support "N". Through his family's support, he even published a few motivational books for individuals with ABI.

- DiCowden (personal communication, November 26, 2010)

➤ *Wellness, Prevention and Health Promotion:* This service area is made up of both clinical and education programs. The clinical programs serve as extensions to the integrative primary care and rehabilitation services. After discharge, consumers in the TBI services are able to participate in activities designed to maintain/promote health. These can be exercise programs and ongoing social support groups. In terms of educational programs, classes and workshops are offered on a weekly basis. These include yoga, Tai Chi, and meditation classes, as well as workshops on health education and promotion. Often, these workshops are sponsored and are presented in conjunction with university hospitals. Topics presented in these workshops have included weight loss, nutrition, stress management, etc. The goal of these classes and workshops is to help individuals develop an understanding of health and well-being.

➤ *Ancillary Programs:* These programs exist to provide added support to the core services provided by **BIHL**:

a) **The Biscayne Academy**: The Biscayne school serves as a support for the pediatric rehabilitation program and provides special education for the children in the program. Admission into the school is assessed case by case. Even though the rehabilitation services generally do not have an exclusion criteria, the Academy considers individuals with a history of violence or current gang relationships, dependency on ventilators or grandiose psychotic episodes inappropriate for this model (i.e., outpatient model). The curriculum follows the state's Sunshine Curriculum taught in other Florida schools. The main difference is that the curriculum is individualized to each child/ adolescent and includes academic, behavioural and social goals.

b) **Professional Training/Research**: Professional students from different medical schools and universities are supervised and trained by qualified practitioners at BIHL. Training also occurs in the TBI services. With regard to research, the primary focus is on the use of the Functional Assessment and Functional Impairment Measurements (FIM/FAM COMBI) as well as the implementation of the International Classification of Functioning, Disability and Health (ICF) in assessing clinical programs.

c) **Community Outreach**: BIHL sends different teams of clinicians into the Biscayne community to provide various services and information. For instance, teams from the Elders program are sent into nursing homes and assisted living facilities to establish holistic programs that address the interactions between the mind and the body. Also, wellness teams are sent to local businesses and schools to establish stress management initiatives. Further, BIHL allows local community groups to use their facility—for example, the local Kiwanis Club (an organization that serves children) has regularly met at BIHL to conduct fundraising activities.

d) **501(c) 3**: This service is also known as the Biscayne Foundation and functions as a nonprofit public sector program that raises money for community members who are unable to afford the services at BIHL. Additionally, it raises money for education and research. Some of the funded research projects include the assessment of the effect of art in healing and development of integrative summer camps for children.

e) **Volunteering/ Protected Work Environment**: Members from the community at large and consumers who are in stage 3 of their therapy are able to engage in volunteering at BIHL as well as other venues. Positions range from peer mentoring to the production of items to be sold. Stage 3 consumers can also work in protected job environments. More information regarding stage 3 and volunteering/work placements is presented below.

Case 4: Consumer "T" at the Biscayne Academy

"T" started attending the Biscayne Academy at the age of 15 after completing rehabilitation at BIHL. He encountered a traumatic brain injury from a go-cart accident at the age of 14. He did not demonstrate any developmental problems before the accident and was functioning averagely. After the accident, however, he had trouble with attention, memory and socialization. Additionally, he demonstrated aggression and other maladaptive behaviours. Following individualized care from the Academy for five years, his functional levels have increased substantially. He attended the Biscayne Academy full-time while preparing for business classes at the local community college. This is made possible by the joint effort by BIHL and the college for the students at the Academy. Further, "T" served as the treasurer of a local community club (Kiwanis Club) and owns a landscaping business part-time. He also went on to complete massage therapy school and is now a licensed massage therapist.

- DiCowden (personal communication, November 26, 2010)

Stages of Therapy

In addition to the previously outlined interdisciplinary therapy in the rehabilitation services, information regarding the stages and practices of the day program are detailed in this section. These stages/practices are very important in fostering community participation in the consumers.

Stage 1: Assessment and Treatment Plan

Individuals admitted into the program are first assessed and evaluated on an individual basis. The consumers are usually assigned to a unit consisting of cognitive retraining (for both the left and right hemispheres) and group therapy. All the other services (individualized therapy, occupational therapy, behavioural therapy, etc.) are tailored to the individual depending on the wishes and needs of the consumer and his/her family. All these services are provided at **BIHL**. Furthermore, project modules (developed by **BIHL** from research and experience) are used to help the consumers develop necessary skills.

Though the exact steps of the modules cannot be disclosed due to proprietary reasons, many modules are used by **BIHL** for memory strengthening, focus development, concentration, safety, activities of daily living, etc. Notably, there are 37 modules addressing skills associated with the left hemisphere of the brain and 22 modules to address the right side.

Even though it is a day program, modifications have been made to accommodate the few individuals who choose to continue their employment. For example, the modules were adapted for three working individuals—two postal workers and one office worker. They came to **BIHL** after work 3 days a week. **BIHL** was able to help them continue their jobs in spite of their TBI.

Case 5: Continued Employment

"A" was a doctoral-level instructor at a local college. He suffered a mild/moderate ABI from a MVA and attended therapy for 2-3 years at BIHL. At BIHL, he received a modified therapy plan that allowed him to continue teaching until his retirement. After he retired, he began to travel and went to South America. Presently, he and his son are running an internet company selling imported coffee from South America.

- DiCowden (personal communication, November 26, 2010)

Stage 2: Consolidation of Skills

This stage is characterized by the mastering of the skills developed in stage 1. For some this stage might take several years. The next stage is not reached until individuals are able to independently demonstrate the skills to their maximal ability. Ideally, **BIHL** hopes the consumers can reach level 5 (i.e., mild to no impairment) on the Functional Independence Measure or close to it before entering stage 3 (personal communication, June 1, 2010).

Field Trips/Special Olympics

Additionally, field trips, though becoming less available due to the decrease in funding, are also incorporated into the therapy plan. Field trips include visits to the grocery store, to restaurants, to local stores (e.g., book stores or a close-by outdoor shopping mall). These trips are geared to help individuals cope in public places, to make purchases, order food, keep a budget, plan meals and shop, etc. The trips are also supplemented with community events like Opera Day (where members of the **Florida Grand Opera** perform) held at the Institutes. Furthermore, long-term consumers who are moderately or seriously injured take part in the **Special Olympics**. They have done very well at the bowling event and have won many local competitions for several years.

> **Case 6: Maintaining Artistic Pursuits**
>
> A well-known entertainer in Miami, "P" suffered a combined head injury and stroke. She went to BIHL after undergoing traditional rehabilitation for 5 years. After 5 years at BIHL, she was able to talk and write—BIHL was even able to help with her aphasia. Even though she was unable to go back to performing (because she still suffers from dysarthria), she was able to write and direct for a local acting group.
>
> - DiCowden (personal communication, November 26, 2010

Stage 3: Life After Rehab

After successful completion of stages 1 and 2, consumers are able to decide their next course of action.

Work/Volunteer Placements

Individuals may decide to pursue employment, upon which several steps are taken by **BIHL** to ensure that they are able to manage the job. Work assessments are done and **BIHL** works closely with the employers to monitor the adjustment of the individual over a long period of time. Site visits are often done. Individuals may also decide to pursue volunteering opportunities, which are monitored the same way as work placements. **BIHL** volunteer positions have included peer mentoring, assistance with laundry in occupational and physical therapy, assistance in the children's programs, grounds care, etc. **BIHL** has also placed volunteers outside of its programs. These placements have usually been with local community hospitals where they have served as welcoming volunteers to the hospital, collecting dietary menus from patients, etc. The participation/re-integration of individuals in the community is further monitored by Community Participation logs on the individuals.

While the job or volunteer opportunities are being pursued, the individuals are required to check in to **BIHL** to undergo individual or group therapy as long as it's needed (even after program attainment). Ongoing support is given to individuals in stage 3, and they are able to return to **BIHL** as needed. According to Dr. DiCowden, over the years approximately 10% of individuals have returned to **BIHL** to continue their support (personal communication, June 1, 2010). Most notably, a Life Learning Lab is provided in this phase. In the Life Learning Lab, issues that are persistent after discharge when living independently are managed and addressed when the consumers come in several times a week. For instance, topics like proper nutrition and the importance of hygiene are discussed.

Case 7: Long-term Therapy Works

Thirty-four-year-old "R" suffered a brain injury in 1995 when he received a blow to the head resulting in his being comatose for 5 days. He attained close to 5 years of therapy at BIHL and now works as a heavy equipment operator following certification. Furthermore, he owns a company that subcontracts for larger construction companies. He also married and now has a child.

- DiCowden, 2004

Public Awareness

Information about brain injuries and **BIHL** is disseminated to the general public via peer-reviewed articles and other publications. Notably, in a book entitled "Humanizing Health Care", published in 2007 by Praeger Press, volume 1 is devoted to **BIHL** (**DiCowden, 2007**). Dr. DiCowden has contributed to the newsmagazine "ADVANCE for Directors in Rehabilitation". She has written an article titled "Shattering Myths" where she discusses the "24-month maximum recovery rule" for individuals with TBI (**DiCowden, 2004**). This rule, used by many insurance companies to deny further therapy beyond 24 months, states that recovery plateaus after this time for individuals affected by TBI (DiCowden, 2004). In the article, Dr. DiCowden provides evidence that demonstrates significant recovery even beyond 24 months (**DiCowden, 2004**). Moreover, she has offered expert opinion for an article by **Tisha Nickening (2004)**, "Finding the Way Back" in the same magazine. The article looked at how TBI survivors can successfully integrate back in the community and discussed the issues surrounding re-integration (**Nickening, 2004**). Dr. DiCowden briefly discussed the practices used in BIHL to achieve community re-entry (**Nickening, 2004**).

Actors in Decision Making and Planning

The senior leadership is comprised of the executive director (Dr. DiCowden), the administrator, the clinical coordinator and the heads of all the programs (brain injury, outpatient injury and pediatric brain injury), who meet to discuss options and to make decisions and plans. The need to make decisions usually occurs due to feedback from evaluations (e.g., target goal benchmarks and feedback from consumers) and is often concerned with individual programs within **BIHL**. Responsibilities for successfully running **BIHL**, furthermore, are shared among everyone involved with providing the services (i.e., the senior leadership, clinicians, etc.). These individuals are often cross-trained to gain experience in various positions so everyone is held accountable.

OUTCOME

Evaluation

All the consumers in the TBI services receive the FIM (functional independence measure)/FAM COMBI pre- and post-therapy. All consumers who have multiple years of therapy (not necessarily just the complex cases) receive the FIM/FAM COMBI every year. The categories measured by the FIM/FAM COMBI include self care, communication, psychosocial adjustment and cognitive function. Often, in almost all of the categories, there is an increase in functioning at time of discharge compared with time of admission into the program (BIHL Report, Biscayne Health and Living Institutes Inc. (2010)). Ratings are done yearly for long-term patients as well as each time they transition from stage 1 through 3. Discharge from rehab occurs in stage 3 (i.e., the "Life after Rehab" stage) of the therapy plan.

Further, **WHO's ICF** measure is additionally used to track complex cases and determine the individual's functional level (e.g., in terms of ability of lifelong relationships), activities and participation in life. The longest documented case study was for a 9-year period. The measures depicted a steady improvement for items such as higher cognitive functioning, physical health, memory and attention.

Additionally, to demonstrate the influence of the therapy on individuals with TBI both in the short term (progress at 1 year) and intermediate (progress at 3 years), data from two different individuals are presented below. The data depicts the short term progress of Consumer A and intermediate progress of Consumer B. The trends graph of specific functions for Consumer A (Figure 2) demonstrates a steady increase over time. The specific functions presented include learning, general tasks and demands, communication, mobility, interactions and relationships, self-care and domestic life. The overall trend showing recovery of these functions for Consumer A is shown in Figure 3.

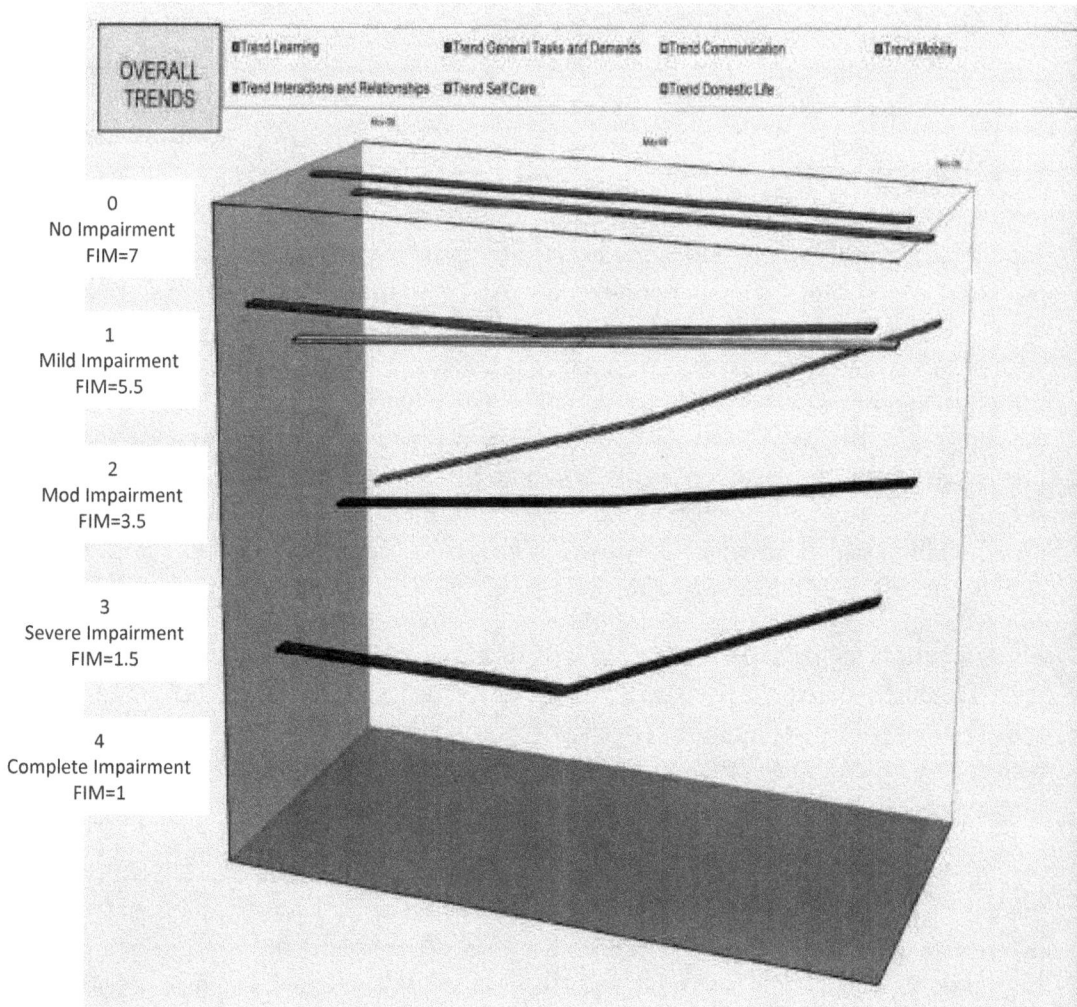

Figure 2: ICF trend analysis of specific functions of Consumer A tracked over a 1-year period (**DiCowden & DeGrand, 2010**).

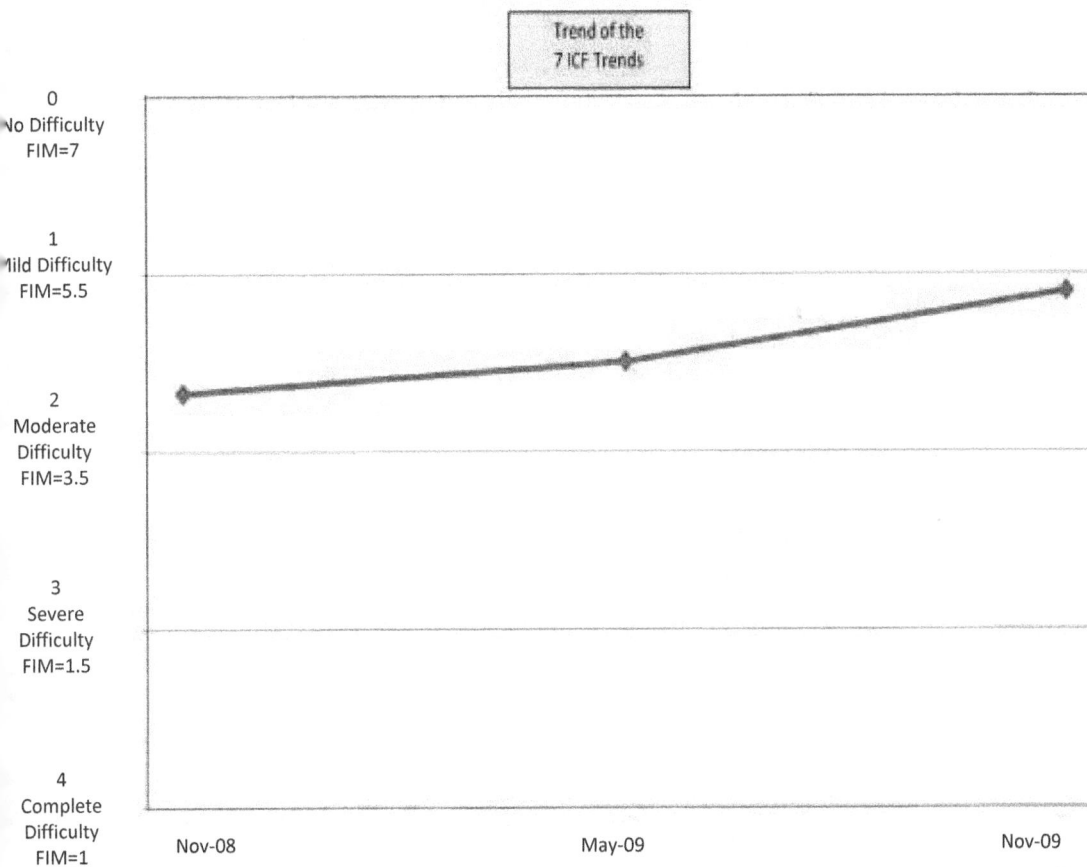

Figure 3: Overall trend of the functions of Consumer A over a 1-year period
(**DiCowden & DeGrand, 2010**).

Similarly, when tracked over a 3-year period, Consumer B also showed recovery in the
above-mentioned functions (Figure 4). The trend of these functions is summarized in
Figure 5.

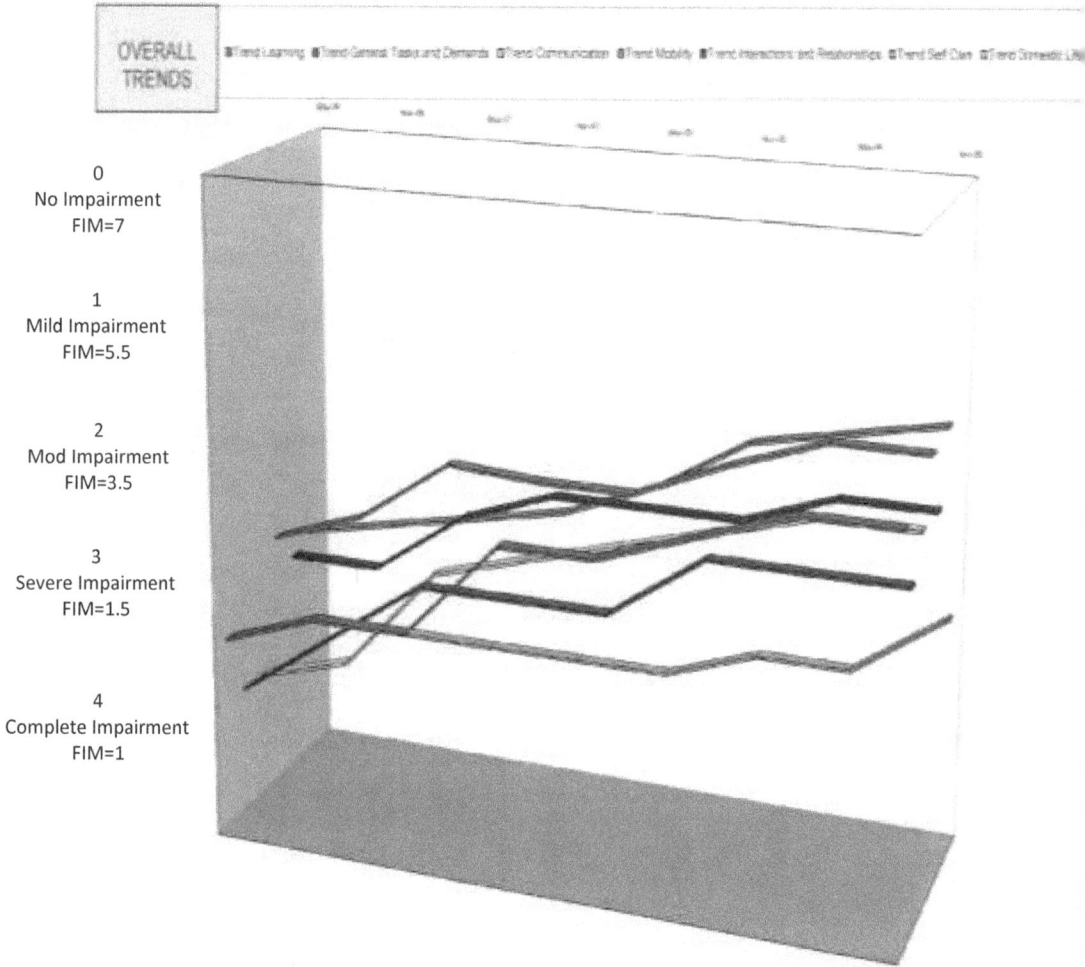

Figure 4: ICF trend analysis of specific functions of Consumer B tracked over a 3-year period (**DiCowden & DeGrand, 2010**).

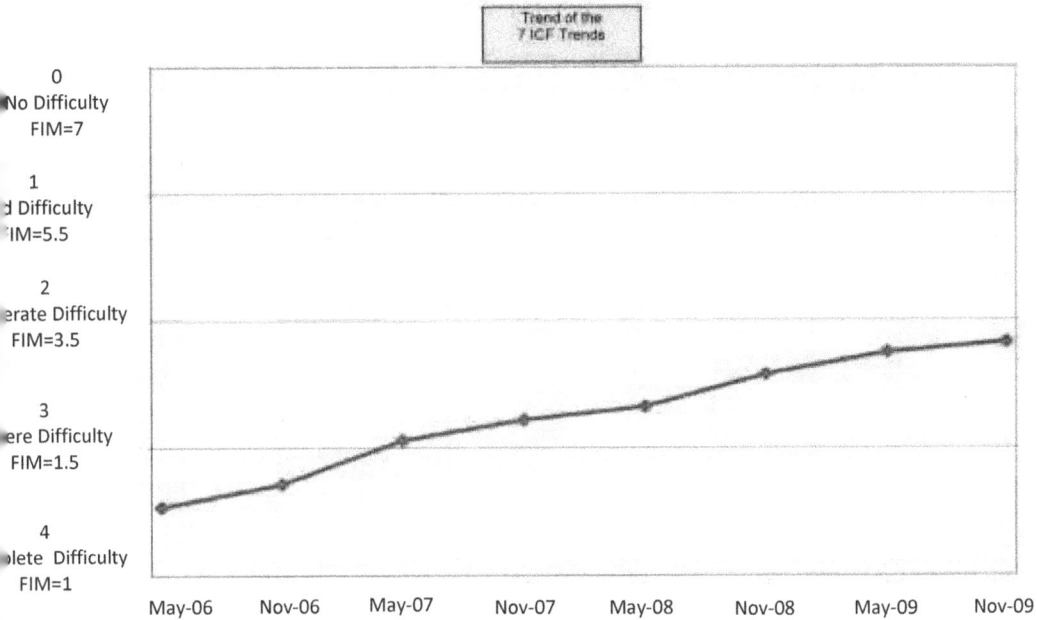

Figure 5: Overall trend of the functions of Consumer B over a 3-year period (**DiCowden & DeGrand, 2010**).

During stages 1 and 2 of the therapy plan, various short-term goals are also set each week by the team of interdisciplinary caregivers and evaluated the following week. The goal benchmarks need to meet 75% of the set goals to be deemed successful. These goals are physical, cognitive, emotional and behavioural in nature. The goals met in 2008 and 2009 are outlined in Table 1. TBI Services are shown in Figure 6 (**Biscayne Health and Living Institutes Inc., 2010**).

Table 1: *Percentage of goals met in 2008* (**Biscayne Health and Living Institutes Inc., 2009**)

	2008		2009
Goals	**Adult TBI Service**	**Pediatric Rehabilitation Service**	**Adult TBI Service**
Physical	73%	93%	50%
Cognitive	79%	97%	85%
Emotional	85%	96%	79%
Behavioural	74%	90%	65%

Additional goals, in consultation with the consumers, are set for 1-3 months as well. Long-term goals are set by the consumer and his/her family. An example of a very frequent long-term goal is the goal to one day live independently.

Moreover, a Community Participation log is also kept on all the consumers after being discharged to further monitor their successful integration and participation into the community. The case studies featured in this chapter are carefully summarized with the assistance of this log.

The findings from all these evaluations and measures are presented annually in the Information Outcomes Management (IOM) report. The cost-effectiveness of the **BIHL** services is also outlined in the report. Information from 2009 indicates that services were provided to individuals in the adult and pediatric programs at a rate of $112.21 per hour and $10.44 per hour, respectively (**Biscayne Health and Living Institutes Inc., 2010**).

Furthermore, evaluations, in terms of consumer satisfaction and stakeholder questionnaires, are also conducted at **BIHL**. These measures, along with the abovementioned measures and goal benchmarks, are analyzed to see if change is needed in any of the services. The questionnaires are done by mail, phone interviews, or on-site interviews. According to the IOM report released in 2010, in the adult programs, 67% and 33% of the consumers rated the quality of treatment at **BIHL** as excellent and good, respectively (**Biscayne Health and Living Institutes Inc., 2010**). Further, the effectiveness of the therapy was rated as excellent by 62% of the consumers and as good by 35% of the consumers (**Biscayne Health and Living Institutes Inc., 2010**). The data from the stakeholder questionnaires revealed that all responses from stakeholders were positive about BIHL—progress made by the consumers in terms of physical and emotional achievement, and maximum benefits, were positively noted by the stakeholders (**Biscayne Health and Living Institutes Inc., 2010**).

ADULT BRAIN INJURY TEAM
FACT SHEET

THE
BISCAYNE
INSTITUTES

2009

1. Biscayne Institutes has served the community for 21 years and treated hundreds of survivors of brain injury and their families.

2. Average of 5 to 8 patients with brain injury in full day treatment on ongoing basis.

3. Average patient age ranges from 43 to 70 years of age (mean age was 57 years old), although pediatric and geriatric specialty programs are also available.

4. Biscayne Institutes also specializes in reintegrating long-term "difficult to treat" individuals, who have sustained a brain injury, back into the community.

5. Patients report and data for the last year confirm:

    ➢ 79% Cognitive goals met
    ➢ 85% Emotional goals met
    ➢ 74% Behavioral goals met
    ➢ 73% Physical goals met

6. 17% of patients are minorities (Hispanic, African-American, Caribbean). Biscayne provides fluent, bi-lingual staff.

7. 58% are female, 42% are male.

8. Biscayne Institutes engages in significant advocacy with carriers and governmental sources for patients with brain injury.

9. All staff healthcare providers are licensed in their specialty and credentialed by Medicaid and/or Medicare.

10. Biscayne Institutes is acknowledged for its exceptional service and accountability by being accredited by both state and national agencies.

THE BISCAYNE
REHABILITATION
INSTITUTE

THE BISCAYNE
ACADEMY

THE BISCAYNE
HOLISTIC HEALTH
INSTITUTE

T: 305/932 8994

F: 305/932 9362

2785 NE 183rd Street
Miami, Florida 33160

Figure 6: A fact sheet on the Adult Brain Injury at BIHL distributed in 2009 (**Biscayne Health and Living Institutes Inc., 2009**). The statistics are based on data from 2008.

Dissemination of Information

Information is disseminated to the stakeholders primarily through IOM reports and fact sheets. Fact sheets, however, are often more favoured by the consumers due to their conciseness (for an example, see Figure 6 above). Informational brochures providing brief descriptions on **BIHL** and its services are also given to the public. In addition, as mentioned previously, information about **BIHL** is also disseminated to the general public via peer-reviewed articles and other publications. Specific case studies are also presented by Dr. DiCowden at conferences like the **WHO**'s North American Collaborating Centers meetings and at meetings at the **National Institutes of Health**.

Analysis: Community Participation and BIHL

The Whatever It Takes Model and BIHL

At the onset of this case study, it was stated that the WIT model outlined the approach necessary to successfully integrate consumers into the community. This section will briefly look at how **BIHL** fairs with the principles that govern WIT.

Principle #1: "No two individuals with acquired brain injury are alike" (Willer & Corrigan, p.650-651, 1994)

BIHL has individualized its program by administering individual assessments on all the consumers admitted into the program. Using this assessment, **BIHL** also tailors an interdisciplinary therapy plan for that individual. Goals are set for the individual and assessed on a weekly basis. A goal has been reached once it exceeds the benchmark set for it. Furthermore, a specific deadline is not placed for the completion of the treatment—an individual moves through the stages of the therapy plan at a pace all their own, determined by when they achieve the goals set for a particular stage.

Principle #2: "Skills are more likely to generalize when taught in the environment where they are to be used" (Willer & Corrigan, p.651, 1994)

Modules are administered at **BIHL** for the development of various skills. To account for the issue of generalizability of these skills to the real-life environment, field trips are taken and skills are further developed and taught in stage 3 (life after rehab) at their homes, and/or job/volunteer placements.

Principle #3: "Environments are easier to change than people"
(Willer & Corrigan, p.651-652, 1994)

The project modules are tailored for each individual and their needs so that they can develop new skills to integrate back into the community despite any handicap. Though environmental manipulations or assistive devices are not provided by **BIHL** directly, **BIHL** helps the individuals acquire these through other sources. Furthermore, **BIHL** participates in advocating and educating communities to provide an environment that is more accepting and welcoming of individuals with disabilities—an environment provided by **BIHL** itself. As well, **BIHL** participates in the Health Care Reform Hearings in the United States to advocate the need for access to quality care for individuals with disability.

Principle #4: "Community integration should be holistic" (Willer &
Corrigan, p.653, 1994)

Upon completing the assessment of an individual, information is provided to the individual on his/her impairment and a therapy plan is created with the consumer and his/her family. A series of goals are set to eventually reach the long-term goal of community integration. Various skills are developed and therapies are provided to address the person in his/her entirety so that they can integrate into the community to their full potential.

Principle #5: "Life is a place-and-train venture" (Willer &
Corrigan, p.653-654, 1994)

Supported employment and supported volunteer placement is provided by **BIHL**. A monitor from **BIHL** works closely with the individual and their employer (volunteer coordinator) to ensure that the individual is accommodated. Work assessments and adjustment reports are often done to ensure that the individual has adjusted to their position. These individuals are monitored for a long period. Additionally, **BIHL** personal will also monitor the adjustment of the individuals at home if need be. This too is followed for the long-term.

Principle #6: "Natural supports last longer than professionals"
(Willer & Corrigan, p.654-655, 1994)

A social support network is developed with fellow consumers in a group setting (i.e., group therapy). Many individuals regularly meet at**BIHL**even after leaving the services at the institutes. This network is further developed in the wellness programs when they interact with individuals from the community during mind and body exercises.

*Principle #7: "Interventions must not do more harm than good"
(Willer & Corrigan, p. 655-656, 1994)*

Even though exact details of the modules have not been published at this point, it has been stated that the regimens have been carefully created after perusing various studies (thus, it can be assumed that the harm and benefits of each module/therapy were carefully analyzed). **BIHL** is currently in the process of preparing the modules for publication and sale.

*Principle #8: "The service system presents many of the barriers to
community integration" (Willer & Corrigan, p.656, 1994)*

In the United States, funding for ABI/TBI services come from different sources in a fragmented format— individuals and their families are forced to jump from one funding source to another (**Willer & Corrigan, 1994**). A very disheartening situation exists where insurance companies (worker's compensation) and Medicare will decrease or remove funding of an individual's therapy past 24 months of therapy (**DiCowden, 2004**). BIHL itself tries to provide 25% of its services to consumers at no charge; however, it faces financial problems at times as it too runs as a result of patchwork funding (**DiCowden, 2007**).

*Principle #9: "Respect for the individual is paramount" (Willer &
Corrigan, p.656-657, 1994)*

Willer and Corrigan (1994) have said the following with regard to the consumer developing self-respect: "We would add that a critical feature of everyone's satisfaction is the extent of choice we feel we have exerted in arriving at our particular place in life" (p.657). At **BIHL**, the consumers and their families are provided with several options on the services that they can use, what goals they want to set, etc. They are given many opportunities to make choices for their therapy.

*Principle #10: "Needs of individuals last a lifetime; so should their
resources" (Willer & Corrigan, p.657-658, 1994)*

BIHL monitors their consumers for the long-term in the community. The consumers are able to come back for therapy if needed. Ongoing support is given in an individual's home and/or place of employment/volunteering.

Conclusion

BIHL fosters community participation as a community-based facility providing a continuum of services to the entire community that facilitate on-going interactions between TBI survivors and members of the community. The therapy and care of the TBI services are aimed at helping consumers overcome emotional, behavioural and social consequences of TBI, allowing them to re-integrate and participate successfully in the community. **BIHL** implements three stages of therapy in the Adult and Pediatric TBI services that focus on skills development, skills solidification, and skills implementation in the community. The therapy is supplemented with primary care, well-being and health promotion services, and ancillary programs. The most important aspect of **BIHL** is its commitment to individuals for the long-term. Progress of the consumers is tracked and supported during the "Life After Rehab" stage where individuals implement their acquired skills and knowledge. Support in work and volunteering placements is provided and necessary adjustments are made to the positions.

When evaluated according to the WIT model proposed by **Willer and Corrigan (1994)**, **BIHL** does a notable job in addressing the outlined principals and services mandated for a program that successfully integrates its consumers. The outcomes of **BIHL**, in terms of community participation, is better understood by analyzing the **ICF** measures in conjunction with the case studies of TBI survivors. The measures monitored long-term (even in stage 3) include learning, general tasks and demands, communication, mobility, interactions and relationships, self-care and domestic life. The cases, similar to the seven provided in this chapter, provide real-life examples of TBI survivors that have undergone long-term rehabilitation at **BIHL** and demonstrate how they have successfully attained community participation. Further, **BIHL**'s success is featured in various publications, including in an article by **Tisha Nickening (2004)** that looked at how to successfully integrate TBI survivors back in the community. Consumers, moreover, view **BIHL** as a place of hope, and many, including "L" from case 1; have become strong advocates for **BIHL**'s rehabilitation services and their dedication to fostering community participation.

REFERENCES

Biscayne Health and Living Institutes Inc. (2009). Adult Brain Injury Team Fact Sheet. Retrieved via personal communication on October 31, 2009.

Biscayne Health and Living Institutes Inc. (2010). BIHL IOM Report. Retrieved via personal communication on October 31, 2010.

DiCowden, M. A. (2004). Shattering Myths. *Advance for Directors in Rehabilitation*, *13* (12): 25-26.

DiCowden, M. A. (2007). Healthcare for the twenty-first century. In I.A. Serlin (Ed.) *Whole Person Healthcare*, Connecticut: Praeger Press.

DiCowden, M. A. & DeGrand, T. (2010). Using the international classification of functioning (ICF) to track interdisciplinary health outcomes for the whole person.

2010 North American Collaborating Center (NACC) Conference on The International Classification of Functioning, Disability and Health (ICF). Retrieved via personal communication on August 12, 2010.

Nickening, T. (2004). Finding the Way Back. *Advance for Directors in Rehabilitation*, *13* (2): 30-36.

Ontario Neurotrauma Foundation. (2010). Draft outcomes of ABI programs and services supportive of meaningful community participation. Development and Uses: ONF Community Practice in Community Participation Outcomes Framework.

Volpe, R. (2009). The conceptualization of injury prevention as change in complex systems. Life Span Adaptation Projects [not in submission - Draft].

Willer, B. & Corrigan, J. D. (1994). Whatever it takes: a model for community-based services. **Brain Injury**, 8: 647-659.

CHAPTER 15

THE BRAIN INTEGRATION PROGRAMME

A residential community reintegration program
for severe chronic brain injury

By Negar Ahmadi

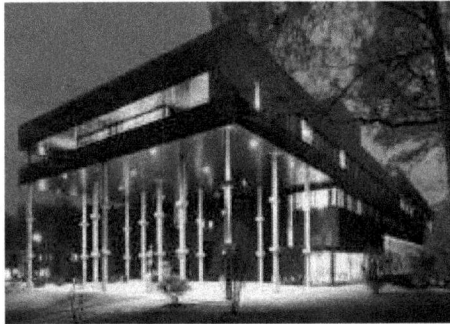

Population Served : Life Span
Contributing Author Contact Information
Mr. Gert J. Geurtsen Rehabilitation Centre Groot Klimmendaal Department for Acquired Brain Injury PO Box 9044, 6800 GG Arnhem, The Netherlands Tel: 31-26-3526145 E-mail: **g.geurtsen@grootklimmendaal.nl**

Casebook of Exemplary Evidence-Informed Programs that Foster Community Participation After Acquired Brain Injury
Copyright © 2013 by Information Age Publishing

BACKGROUND

Individuals with an Acquired Brain Injury (ABI) can suffer a range of disabilities. Physical disability has often been cited as one of the important consequences of ABI, making individuals incapable of performing many activities. In addition, many survivors of ABI experience emotional problems, behavioural disturbances and psychiatric disorders (**van Reekum, Bolago, Finlayson, Garner, & Links, 1996**; **McBrinn, et al., 2008**; **Kelly, Brown, Todd, & Kremer, 2008**; **Ownsworth, Little, Turner, Hawkes, & Shum, 2008**; **Vaishnavi, Rao, & Fann, 2009**; **Velikonja, Warriner, & Brum, 2010**). Traditionally, survivors of ABI receive therapy shortly after their ABI in order to deal with the consequences of their condition (**Teasell, et al., 2007**; **Turner-Stokes, Disler, Nair, & Wade, 2005**). However, in some instances the emotional and behavioural consequences of ABI may not respond positively to initial rehabilitation programs, and thus become chronic. In fact, many studies have shown that a large proportion of individuals with ABI experience chronic behavioural and emotional consequences and may not benefit from traditional rehabilitation programs (**Colantonio, et al., 2004**; **Evans, 2001**; **Jackson, 1994**). Therefore, programs that specifically target those with such complex behavioural or psychiatric problems long after their ABI may prove effective in enhancing community participation of these individuals.

The **Brain Integration Programme** (BIP) is such an example. Initiated in the Netherlands in response to a number of studies reporting high prevalence of emotional/behavioural disabilities following ABI (**Knottnerus, et al., 2007**; **Ribbers, 2007**), the BIP utilizes a comprehensive therapy program to target the various needs of this group of individuals. The complex nature of the chronic problems faced by these ABI survivors necessitates the use of a structured comprehensive therapy program. The BIP was developed in the **Rehabilitation Center Groot Klimmendaal** in the Netherlands on the basis of achieving optimal community integration for ABI survivors with complex behavioural or psychiatric problems (**Geurtsen, Martina, Van Heugten, & Geurts, 2008**). Groot Klimmendaal provides a wide range of programs for individuals with various conditions and disorders. **BIP** is a residential program tailored to the individual chronic needs of ABI survivors. The **BIP** goes beyond a simple rehabilitation program and takes on a more community-oriented approach towards survivors of ABI. The main objective of the program is for individuals with chronic brain injury to participate and achieve a balance in daily activities—domestic life, work, leisure, and social interaction (**Geurtsen, et al., 2008**).

The target group can be divided into the following three categories (**Geurtsen, Martina, & Voerman, 2004**):

1. People who have finished primary rehabilitation, but who need further training and supervision in order to accomplish re-integration, for which the regular Rehabilitation Centres have insufficient possibilities.

2. People who, after adolescence, are not cable of shaping their lives in the areas of public and/or social-emotional functioning, mostly at the point of transition to a new stage of life.

3. People that have or have not received primary rehabilitation, and have got stuck at a later point in life in the areas of societal or emotional functioning.

Participants in the **BIP** may be referred by regional rehabilitation centres that offer standard post-acute programs as well as neuropsychiatric departments (Geurtsen, et al., 2008). In order to better achieve the objectives of the program, the BIP imposes the following inclusion criteria (**Geurtsen, et al., 2004**):

➢ Brain injury

➢ An acceptable degree of insight in limitations and possibilities

➢ An acceptable degree of motivation

➢ Learning ability

➢ Ability to function within a group

The BIP involves the relatives of the ABI survivors as well as community members (such as employers). The program was well accepted within the community once it was developed. According to **Geursten and colleagues (2004)**, the approach taken by the BIP "introduces a new standard for delivery of rehabilitation services by shifting the rehabilitation focus from a *medical* perspective to a *psycho-pedagogic* holistic oriented approach, an approach which is believed to benefit the brain-injured individual and his family".

In addition to the community involvement, the **BIP** involves a wide range of personnel and professionals with different expertise. Both the personnel and the professionals involved perceive the program as being very effective in integrating chronic brain injury survivors with complex problems back to the community. The BIP is currently a nationally recognized program and the funding is covered by all healthcare insurance companies in the Netherlands (**Ribbers, 2007**). In fact, achieving such level of acceptance within the community speaks to the sustainability of the BIP. Another important indicator of the sustainability of the program is the strong evaluation component of the program (discussed later in the report), which has shown short-term as well as long-term benefits of the program.

RESOURCES

The **BIP** consists of a team of professionals that run the program and includes a neuropsychologist, a physiatrist, a neuropsychiatrist, occupational therapists, cognitive therapists, social workers, speech-language therapists, physical therapists and rehabilitation nurses/coaches (**Geurtsen, et al., 2008**). With such an expanded team of professional, effective teamwork becomes essential to the success of the program. The staff closely work together to monitor the progress of the participants throughout the program and provide feedback along the way. Each staff member is responsible for a specific aspect of the program and will liaise with other members to ensure that each participant is moving along the program at a reasonable and suitable pace. For instance the neuropsychologists and cognitive therapists work closely with the occupational therapists to ensure that each participants is ready to start the work module. The therapists also work closely with social workers to ensure that the families and friends of the participants are well educated about ABI and the specific needs and abilities of individuals with ABI. In addition, the complex nature of these individuals in terms of the chronic nature of their conditions requires extensive and structured therapy to allow for further community participation. Such individualization of the program contributes to its effectiveness and results in better outcomes.

The success of the **BIP** lies at least partly in the effective design of the program as well as the various resources allocated to the program. The BIP is a residential program, which allows the participants to better experience a sense of community during weekdays while taking part in the program; they learn to live with other ABI survivors and share responsibilities while in the residential program. On the weekends, participants go back to their homes, which allows them to practice their acquired skills in a different setting and which ultimately results in better community reintegration. The **BIP** is a structured program and consists of three modules: independent living, social-emotional, and work (**Geurtsen, et al., 2008**); however, the program still allows for individualization by tailoring each module to the specific needs of each participant. The structured nature of the program is unique and important as each participant has different complexities and needs.

Independent living: the main objective of this module is to train participants in performing various domestic tasks. The participants learn these tasks step-by-step and separately before executing them all together. All participants take part in the various activities, however, there is room for personal modifications if, for instance, a participant needs more time in one area as opposed to another. This module involves increased initial supervision and guidance, which is gradually reduced as participants begin to master each task. The following is a list of skills taught in this module (**Geurtsen, et al., 2008**):

➢ Home cleaning (cleaning room, doing laundry, ironing, etc.)

➢ Grocery shopping

➢ Cooking

➢ Planning and taking care of breakfast and lunch

➢ Taking care of day/night rhythm

➢ Travelling by public transport

➢ Budgeting

➢ Administrating (handling of letters, bills, archiving).

Social-emotional module: as discussed earlier, survivors of ABI are faced with great social and emotional challenges when dealing with their new condition. The social-emotional module is set to deal with such challenges by training participants to set new, adjusted, and achievable goals in life. Participants also receive education about brain injury and gain insight about their condition and their limitations. Counseling is provided to the participants and social skills are practiced to allow them to form new relationships or strengthen old ones. Furthermore, the social networks and families of the ABI survivor are also involved in this module—they receive education and counseling in order to learn about brain injury and to help set realistic goals for themselves and their family member with ABI. Therefore, this module provides ABI survivors and their families with a more realistic view about the future and helps towards a smoother re-integration into the community. The following are the specific components of this module (**Geurtsen, et al., 2008**):

➢ Education on brain injury and its individual consequences

➢ Cognitive training directed at compensation and coping strategies

➢ Social skills training with video feedback in groups

➢ Day-to-day feedback and advice on social behaviour

➢ Individual counseling to accept limitations and their consequences

➢ Group therapy directed at acceptance of long-term consequences of brain injury

➢ Individual counseling directed at substance abuse prevention

➢ Family brain injury education group

➢ Individual counseling of relatives to enhance acceptance and to develop coping strategies

Work module: many survivors of ABI may never be able to return to work after their ABI. This may result in various emotional or psychiatric disorders and further isolation from the community. Holding a job and contributing to society is an important component of community participation. The work module of the BIP provides participants with support towards this aspect of community participation, and further stresses one of the main points of the other modules: gaining insight into one's condition and becoming aware of possibilities and the limitations. It is only after such insight has been gained that participants can effectively start the work module.

Participants are provided with access to a vocational assessment unit where their abilities are individually assessed and employment in the community is arranged. Working tasks are performed and practiced in groups. For some individuals, independent paid work may not be an option, in which case other opportunities are explored, such as supported or sheltered paid work, volunteer work, or sheltered activities. The following are further details about the components of the work module (Geurtsen, et al., 2008):

➢ Neuropsychological assessment

➢ Work practice in groups

➢ Evaluation of working abilities in a vocational assessment unit

➢ Evaluation of abilities to perform supported/sheltered work, volunteer work or sheltered activities (when paid work is not possible)

➢ Free time evaluation and support to give advice about leisure time activities.

The following figure adapted from Geurtsen et al. (2008) summarizes the modules described above.

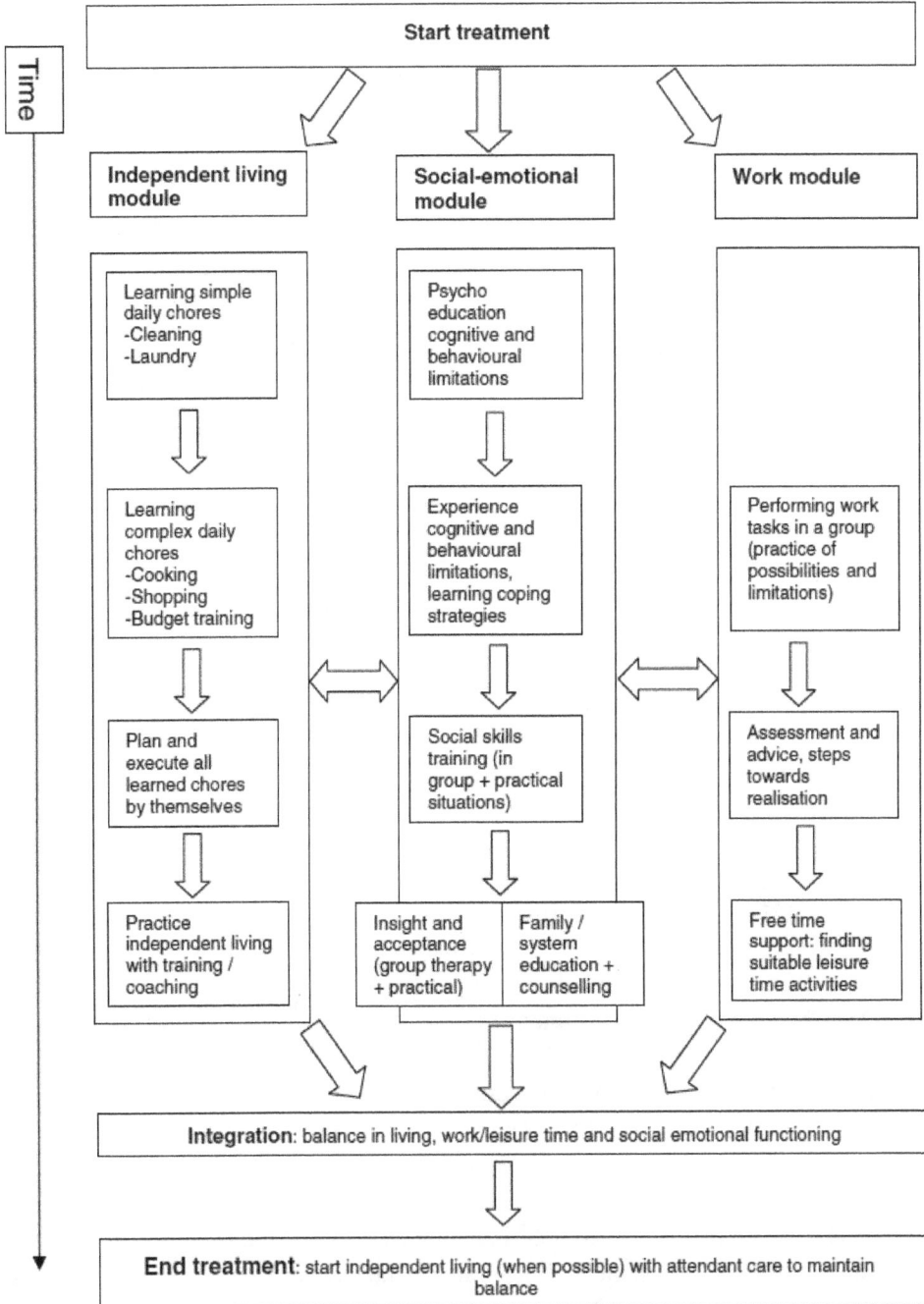

Figure 1: Three modules of BIP, dependent of participants characteristics the order can be different (**Geurtsen, et al., 2008**)

IMPLEMENTATION

The three modules of the **BIP** target different aspects of community re-integration for participants of the program. The modules are structured with set objectives; however, they allow for a certain degree of flexibility and in many instances are tailored to the particular needs of the individuals. Participants each spend a certain amount of time in each module. For the independent living module the average amount of time spent is around 100 hours per person. This module involves small group sessions where theoretical aspects of living skills are discussed, however, the majority of the training module is in individual sessions. The average amount of time spent in social-emotional module is about 110 hours per person. Similar to the previous module, the majority of the training is on an individual basis, yet there are some small group sessions for participants and some sessions for the participants' family and social contacts.

A common objective of the first two modules is for participants to gain insight about their condition and become aware of their limitations. Once they have achieved this stage, they will go through the work module. Therefore, the work module might begin later than the other two modules for some individuals. On average, participants spend about 44 hours per person in the work module, and similar to the other two modules, the time is tailored to the specific needs of the individuals. Most of the training in this module is through individual sessions, which occur after participants have been provided with vocational assessment to determines the tasks each participant can perform, as well as the number of hours per week they can contribute. This module also involves the participation of the community in the sense that community employers provide work opportunities for these individuals. Participants may have certain physical disabilities limiting them from obtaining a job despite intact intellectual capabilities. Such limitations can prevent individuals from returning to the community and obtaining a job. To help accommodate these participants, the assessment vocational unit arranges for any necessary adjustments to the workplace and any personal assistant needed while on the job. In other words, the vocational assessment ensures that the participants understand their limitations but at the same time are able to use the skills they have towards a career in the community. The vocational assessment unit also acts as an advocate on behalf of the ABI survivors to ensure that community employers realize the work potential in these individuals. However, in instances where participants are not able to obtain paid work, alternative arrangements for volunteer or sheltered activities are made. An inability to obtain a paid job does not prevent survivors of ABI from returning to their communities.

The essence of the BIP program is for participants to learn how to achieve a balance in their daily living activities (domestic life, work, leisure time and social interaction), while at the same time taking into account their capabilities and limitations. The fact that the program is individually tailored to each participant's needs is an important element in its success—progression throughout the different modules is adjusted in order to avoid frustrations and failures.

To further achieve the goal balancing life activities, participants are continually given feedback on their behaviour throughout the program. An important aspect of any community integration program is the ability of the participant to apply the learned skills in a new environment. Since BIP is a residential program, it is essential that participants practice applying their learned skills outside of the residential complex. To help with this, as part of the program participants return home on the weekends to further practice the acquired skills in their home environment. The return home not only allows the participants to practice their learned skills, but it also engages the family members in the rehabilitation process (**Geurtsen, et al., 2008**).

OUTCOME

Strengths of the **Brain Integration Programme** are its sound research and evaluation components.* Two evaluations have been conducted since the program was initiated and the results of the evaluations are used to enhance and provide feedback about the BIP. Results of the evaluations are published in an article by Geurtsen and colleagues (2008) and have been presented at a number of conferences. Two prospective cohort studies have been conducted to assess the effectiveness of the program. The first study included 24 participants who were assessed before the start of the program (T0), at the end of the program (T1) and one year after the end of the program (T2). The study investigated a number of parameters including participants' characteristics such as age, time since onset, living independently, etc. The following table summarizes the findings of the study with regard to the study population (**Geurtsen, et al., 2008**).

Table 1: Participants' characteristic on admission (Geurtsen, et al., 2008).

Variable	Mean (Standard Deviation)	Range
Age at admission (years)	28.5 (10.3)	17-51
Time since onset (years)	4.5 (7.0)	0.5-31.4
Living independently (with/without care: n)	10 (41.6%)	
Work (n)	9 (37.5%)	
Work (hours per week: mean of all 24 participants)	8.1 (14.2)	0-43

---

* Since the completion of this case, Geurtsen's May 2011 doctoral thesis on the effectiveness of BIP is available at **http://repository.ubn.ru.nl/bitstream/2066/87166/1/87166.pfd**

This study found improvements in emotional well-being, quality of life, and levels of community integration. There was also a significant drop in the number of depressed participants after completing the program compared with before commencing the program. At the time of the follow up (i.e. one year after the program), significantly higher number of participants had jobs (58% from 38% before the program), which speaks to the success of the program in community reintegration. This study also reported that eight participants (33%) who had alcohol and drug abuse problems before enrolling in the program no longer had such problems by the end of the study. Furthermore, this study found that participation in the program resulted in significant improvements in a number of different domains, including living independently, holding a job, and the number of work hours per week. Based on the results it is apparent that the improvements in community participation were seen at one-year follow up. The following table (Table 2) adopted from **Geurtsen et al. (2008)** summarizes these findings at the different timelines (T0, T1 and T2).

Table 2: *Living situation and work status before and after the BIP (Geurtsen, et al., 2008).*

Variable	T0	T1	T2
Living independently (with/without care)	10 (41.6%)	18 (75%)	17 (71%)
Living with parents	13 (54.2%)	2 (8%)	5 (21%)
Work (n of participants)	9 (37.5%)	11 (46%)	14 (58%)
Work (hours per week: mean of all 24 participants)	8.0 (SD 14.2)	7.4 (SD 11.2)	15.5 (SD 12.9)

T0= time at admission, T1= time at the end of the program, T2= time at one year after the end of the program

A second similar study has also been conducted recently with greater number of participants (n=70). The following two tables (Tables 3 and 4) summarize the findings of this study with regards to the study population as well as the outcomes. At the one year follow up, this study also found a significant increase in participants living independently, participants working, as well as an increase in the number of work hours per week (**Geurtsen, Heugten, Martina, Meijer, & Geurts, 2009**). The second study also showed that the results of the study were not simply due to passing of the time. This study assessed individuals before being placed on a waitlist (T0) for the program and just before starting the program (T1) and found no significant difference in all the outcomes measures between the two times. Therefore, the improvements in the community participation outcomes observed are primarily due to participation in the program. Similarly, this study measured the outcomes at the end of the program (T2) and one year after the program was ended (T3) and found both short-term and long-term benefits of the program.

Table 3 : *Participants' characteristics (**Geurtsen, et al., 2009**).*

Variable	Mean (SD)	Range
Age at admission (years)	25.1 (7.9)	18-49
Time since onset (years)	5.2 (5.4)	0.5-26.3
Living independently (with/without care: n)	19 (27.1%)	
Work (n)	12 (17.1%)	
Work (hours per week: only those working)	14.3 (11)	

SD= Standard Deviation

Table 4: *Living situation and work status before and after the BIP (**Geurtsen, et al., 2009**).*

Variable	T0	T1	T2	T3
Living independently (N/%)	19 (27.1%)	20 (28.6%)	50 (72.4%)	44 (65.7%)
Work (N/%)	12 (17.1%)	11 (15.7%)	23 (32.9%)	36 (53.7%)
Work hours for working participants (hr/SD)	14.3 (10.8)	12.9 (16.3)	18.1 (11.3)	18.8 (11.2)

T0= time at waitlist, T1= time at admission, T2= time at the end of the program, T3=time at one year after the end of the program

Based on the results of the two studies, it is evident that the target population of the BIP is mainly young individuals (in their 20s), however the age range is fairly wide and includes participants of various ages. A unique aspect of this program, which makes it differ from a traditional rehabilitation program, is the fact that it helps integrate individuals back into their communities even years after their brain injury. Both studies include individuals who suffered ABI two or three decades before they were enrolled in the BIP. The results of both studies showed that the program increased independent living and working both in the short term as well as in the long term. Furthermore, the program proved effective in helping participants with their psychiatric and emotional problems (such as depression or substance abuse).

Conclusion

ABI can result in a number of different impairments such as physical, emotional or psychological. Consequences of ABI in many cases will be long term and will impede on individuals returning to their communities after their ABI (**Jackson, 1994**). The Brain Integration Programme was initiated in the Netherlands to specifically target chronic brain injury survivors who have complex behavioural or emotional disturbances. The BIP is a residential program for such individuals with complex disabilities and is composed of three modules: independent living, social-emotional, and work. The participants go through the modules and receive training and consultation in both small group and individual sessions. Each module is personalized to the needs of each individual in terms of the content as well as the length of time spent in each module. A common goal among the three modules is for participants to gain insight about their condition and understand their abilities. Participants return home every weekend and practice the acquired skills in their home environment. Through these modules, the participants acquire the necessary skills to achieve a balance in their daily activities between domestic life, work, leisure, and social interaction (**Geurtsen, et al., 2008**).

The program also includes members of the community in the attempt to reintegrate chronic brain injury survivors back to their communities. For instance, family members of ABI survivors will attend workshops and educational sessions to learn about ABI and their role in the re-integration process. The program also involves the support of the businesses and employers in the community as the ABI survivors obtain suitable job opportunities matching their skills. Furthermore, the necessary adjustments are made to the work environment to better accommodate participants. Multiple evaluations have proven the program to be successful in the short run as well as long term in various domains including independent living or working. The BIP has become nationally recognized in the Netherlands and has proven successful in reintegrating individuals with chronic brain injury back to their communities. This program has the potential of replication and transfer to other countries to enhance community participation of ABI survivors.

REFERENCES

Colantonio, A., Ratcliff, G., Chase, S., Kelsey, S., Escobar, M., & Vernich, L. (2004). **Long-term outcomes after moderate to severe traumatic brain injury**. *Disabil Rehabil, 26*(5), 253-261.

Evans, R. W. (2001). What can we do about long-term sequelae of traumatic brain injury? *N C Med J, 62*(6), 373-375.

Geurtsen, G. J., Heugten, C. M., Martina, J. D., Meijer, R., & Geurts, A. C. (2009). Prospective programme evaluation of a new residential community reintegration programme for severe chronic brain injury. *Brain Impairment, 10(2),* 264.

Geurtsen, G. J., Martina, J. D., Van Heugten, C. M., & Geurts, A. C. (2008). A prospective study to evaluate a new residential community reintegration programme for severe chronic brain injury: the Brain Integration Programme. **Brain Injury**, *22*(7-8), 545-554.

Geurtsen, G. J., Martina, J. D., & Voerman, V. F. (2004). The "Brain Integration®" rehabilitation program. A new holistic treatment approach in the Netherlands. Description of the program and research. *Int J Rehabil Res, 27*(S1), 52-53.

Jackson, J. D. (1994). After rehabilitation: meeting the long-term needs of persons with traumatic brain injury. *Am J Occup Ther, 48*(3), 251-255.

Kelly, G., Brown, S., Todd, J., & Kremer, P. (2008). Challenging behaviour profiles of people with acquired brain injury living in community settings. **Brain Injury,** *22*(6), 457-470.

Knottnerus, A. M., Turner-Stokes, T., van de Weg, F. B., Heijnen, L., Lankhorst, G. J., & Turner-Stokes, L. (2007). **Diagnosis and treatment of depression following acquired brain injury: a comparison of practice in the UK and the Netherlands**. *Clin Rehabil, 21*(9), 805-811.

McBrinn, J., Colin Wilson, F., Caldwell, S., Carton, S., Delargy, M., McCann, J., et al. (2008). Emotional distress and awareness following acquired brain injury: an exploratory analysis. **Brain Injury,** *22*(10), 765-772.

Ownsworth, T., Little, T., Turner, B., Hawkes, A., & Shum, D. (2008). Assessing emotional status following acquired brain injury: the clinical potential of the depression, anxiety and stress scales. **Brain Injury,** *22*(11), 858-869.

Ribbers, G. M. (2007). **Traumatic brain injury rehabilitation in the Netherlands: dilemmas and challenges**. *J Head Trauma Rehabil, 22*(4), 234-238.

Teasell, R., Bayona, N., Marshall, S., Cullen, N., Bayley, M., Chundamala, J., et al. (2007). A systematic review of the rehabilitation of moderate to severe acquired brain injuries. **Brain Injury,** *21*(2), 107-112.

Turner-Stokes, L., Disler, P. B., Nair, A., & Wade, D. T. (2005). Multi-disciplinary rehabilitation for acquired brain injury in adults of working age. *Cochrane Database Syst Rev*(3), **CD004170**.

Vaishnavi, S., Rao, V., & Fann, J. R. (2009). **Neuropsychiatric problems after traumatic brain injury: unraveling the silent epidemic**. *Psychosomatics, 50*(3), 198-205.

van Reekum, R., Bolago, I., Finlayson, M. A., Garner, S., & Links, P. S. (1996). Psychiatric disorders after traumatic brain injury. **Brain Injury,** *10*(5), 319-327.

Velikonja, D., Warriner, E., & Brum, C. (2010). **Profiles of emotional and behavioural sequelae following acquired brain injury: cluster analysis of the Personality Assessment Inventory**. *J Clin Exp Neuropsychol, 32*(6), 610-621.

CHAPTER 16

INSIGHTS ABOUT COMMUNITY PARTICIPATION AFTER ACQUIRED BRAIN INJURY

By Richard Volpe

This concluding chapter discusses some insights derived from casing exemplary community participation programs. Although the Arnstein scheme presented in Chapter 1 may have been useful in highlighting the power dimension in community participation, Malec and Basford (2008) provide another approach to classifying the cases. Their framework alternatively allows us to look at the reviewed cases by placing them on a continuum from more or less traditional services to community-based programs. This approach to the classification of the cases takes into account their location, actual physical relationship to traditional rehabilitation settings, complexity and the extent to which they are actually in/part of the communities of survivors. They classify programs for the chronic psychosocial period after acquired brain injury in five categories:

1. Neurobehavioural programs;

2. Day treatment programs;

3. Outpatient community re-entry programs;

4. Residential community re-integration programs;

5. Community-based programs.

The first two types of programs attempt to deal with a wide range of problems in largely traditional settings. These programs are often both comprehensive and highly targeted in their treatments. Moreover, they have the most evidence supporting outcome effectiveness. The last three kinds are harder to sustain and evaluate. They tend to appear less frequently in reviews and program descriptions. The focus of this review has been on community-based programs, the last three types of services. They are apt to be for

303

individuals who have the potential for some sort independent living, but require a variety of both short and long terms supports.

1. Neurobehavioural programs:

All the programs reviewed have cognitive/behavioural elements that are described in a variety of ways. However, none of the cased programs have cognitive/behavioural treatment as their exclusive focus.

2. Day treatment programs - Comprehensive (holistic):

The *communityworks, inc.* services are tailored to meet the individual needs and goals of each consumer. Services include case management, independent living training, information about and referral to community resources, peer support, physical therapy, occupational therapy, cognitive therapy, speech therapy, personal care, drug and alcohol counseling, overnight support and employment support. At *Krempels Center* clients live outside of the program and are supported in learning skills to live independently. Field trips and community events are encouraged to broaden the client's physical environment and ties to the community. Community outings help to increase the client's knowledge of various societal and cultural norms. *Simply Self-sustaining System* services aim at providing persons with an ABI the opportunity to relearn skills, re-access social groups, and modify behaviour sufficiently to be able to be included in work; namely, a small business. Workshops centre on the performance of simple and repetitive tasks (i.e., how to make items for sale) and the development of functional and self-sustaining skills. The *Skills to Enable People and Communities* consists of 2 phases (the STEPS Skills Program and STEPS Network Groups), which aim to facilitate the development of social support networks.

3. Outpatient community re-entry programs:

The *Community Approach to Participation's* home-centred therapies eliminate geographic disadvantage to rural clients and allow for services to fully incorporate the client's family, friends, neighbours, and other community members. The *Pediatric Acquired Brain Injury Community Outreach Program's* Travelling Acquired Brain Injury Rehabilitation and Reintegration Team provides case specific consultation, telephone consultation, community liaison visits and educational programs to clients. Home visits, school visits, clinics and follow-up appointments are available to each client. *School Transition and re-Entry Program* uses a multi-faceted approach to facilitate communication and cooperation between all points of contact in the child's community: hospital, school, and parents (family). A comprehensive hospital-school transition intervention provides a systematic and coordinated approach to the development, validation and dissemination of effective measures and transition intervention practices, such that the clients may participate in their schools and communities. *TIRR Memorial Hermann's Challenge Program* is a specialized outpatient program for persons with a TBI or an ABI. Community participation becomes a key focus as compensatory strategies are learned, following a focus on restoration therapy.

4. Residential community re-integration programs:

Biscayne Institute of Health and Living offers a full continuum of services ranging from primary care to health and wellness promotion in the form of a 3-stage residential program. Clients are followed long-term in the community and are able to return to BIHL (even as volunteers), if they so choose. *Brain Integration Programme* is a structured residential program. The program allows participants to achieve a balance in their daily activities between domestic life, work, leisure and social interaction, through participation in three modules.

5. Community-based services:

Acquired Brain Injury Ireland's Side by Side Day Resource Service provides a range of flexible and tailor-made community-based services to its clients. Local businesses and facilities assist in the provision of service. The *ABI Partnership Project* provides a broad range of community-based services. Two specific services offered are Outreach and Aboriginal ABI Community Support. *Community Head Injury Resource Service's* Adult Day Services provides mentorship and offsite programming opportunities to clients. Many of the programs are run in partnership with local organizations and private businesses that provide their expertise, equipment, and facilities (e.g., Continuum of Vocational Placements Program). *Clubhouse* activities are dynamic in nature. Eliciting the support of local businesses, employers and community partners, the Clubhouse's community participation strategy is enhanced by increased awareness among the public of the lifelong effects of brain injury. Roles, tasks and relationships grow out of the need to operate the Clubhouse.

Conclusion

Brain injury can produce a wide range of challenges for survivors, who may exhibit physical, cognitive, emotional, and behavioural changes that persist long after acute treatments and primary rehabilitation. Each of the ways exemplary programs have examined these challenges emphasize how tightly individuals and their communities are intertwined. They draw attention to the seat of power in relationships, program geography, the locus of decision-making, associated values and ideas, and analytic efforts to measure community participation. Traditional treatment settings are usually not designed to provide opportunities to optimize community participation, client control, and decision making. Power is held and exercised by the bureaucracies for their greater ends, not an individual's self interest. It is in these settings—treating those in need of services as if they are sick— that the traditional medical model is supported. This may be manifest in the technical focus on the person as an object to be cared for, looked after, treated, and rehabilitated. In terms of the requirements of professional ideology, the individual, technically manipulated, is objectified and personally externalized. The patient is managed by others as an object and not as an agent with self-direction. They are not expected to cure themselves and are seen as objects to be treated. In contrast, the exemplary programs cased here define clients not as helpless and dependent, but as independent active agents. The agent, in contrast to the patient, is a role in which the client is enabled in community participation. The agent acts on his or her environment in contrast to the patient who is acted upon. A consistent practice principle of exemplary programs that foster community participation is not that they empower individuals; rather, they organize their efforts to *enable* survivors to obtain and to exercise power in their lives. People cannot be given power. They may take it if they are enabled to so choose.

The programs in this casebook appear to be successful because they directly address the need for complex system change. While many treatment models address physical needs, less attention is given to social psychological components. However, it is this dimension that usually means the most to survivors. Being part of a community is how humans make and derive meaning in life. Connecting to those around us may require extra effort after a brain injury, different approaches, new connections, and novel approaches to engagement. The sum of these factors means that programs aiming to build networks as well as maintain and facilitate friendships offer individuals with brain injury a chance to feel valued, connected, and engaged with their community. Moreover, this involves recognizing how important it is that power be understood and distributed in the practices associated with the provision of human services.

Community participation is by nature inclusive and iterative, leading to positive cycles of social interaction. Participation boosts confidence, returns meaning to activities, and lends individual's social and emotional capital. Engaging in participation also denotes acknowledging that others have as much to gain from survivors of acquired brain injury as they have to gain from anyone—that is to say, it is a process that is not hierarchical, but demands that we respect the dignity of every individual. Participation is also not individualistic, prescriptive, or dogmatic with individuals defining for themselves the level of engagement and network they desire for themselves. In short, community participation is a human rights concept—it is respecting that every single person has something to contribute. Valuing that contribution should be expected of everyone in the spirit of reciprocity and community.

REFERENCES

Malec, J. F., & Basford, J. S. (1996). **Post-acute brain injury rehabilitation**. *Archives of Physical Medicine and Rehabilitation*, (77), 198-207.

Appendix A : BRIO Summaries

communityworks

Background	Resources	Implementation	Outcome
In 1991, communityworks founder and owner, Dr. Janet Williams, established the program to address the need for a new approach to rehabilitative services—one that gives control back to the individual. The program objectives of communityworks are informed by the previous research Dr. Williams conducted on rehabilitation systems in Canada, Norway, Denmark, The Netherlands, Germany, Italy, India, and 48 states in the U.S. Communityworks provides "whatever it takes" for consumers to live in the community. Service programs are tailored to meet the individual goals of each consumer. Communityworks provides services to individuals of all ages with TBI (full range of injury severity), cerebrovascular accidents, multi-diagnosis situations, CNS disorders, and spinal cord injuries.	In 1991, Kansas implemented the first funding in the US to support people with brain injuries to live in the community through a Medicaid Home and Community Based (HCBS) waiver. This HCBS funding specifically stated that people had to live in their own home and receive services in the community. Communityworks has received reimbursements from a variety of sources (e.g. Blue Cross & Blue Shield of Kansas City, TRIWEST, United Healthcare, etc.). When funding from private sources runs out, communityworks assists the consumer in identifying and accessing funds from federal, state, and community resources. Staff remains focused on designing a system that will continue working for the consumer even when professional services are no longer need. Consumers have long-term access to services, and are able to reenter the program if new needs/ goals emerge.	Consumers are in control of their own rehabilitation programs and do all of the decision-making, i.e., consumers interview and choose their own staff, decide where they want to live and work, and decide on their own rehabilitation goals. Communityworks collaborates with consumers, their families, physicians and hospitals, and government and mental health agencies to insure that the consumer is connected to all possible community resources. Communityworks uses a multidisciplinary framework and offers a variety of services depending on the individual needs of consumers. Services include: case management, independent living training, info and referral to community resources, peer support, physical therapy, occupational therapy, cognitive therapy, speech therapy, personal care, drug and alcohol counseling, overnight support, and employment support.	The Kansas Department of Social and Rehabilitation Services reports a saving of $40, 000 per person per year for individuals using communityworks services paid for by Medicaid as compared to individuals in institutional settings. Thus, the costs of providing services in the home and community are far less than the cost of care provided in TBI institutional facilities. Consumer satisfaction surveys are completed 3 times a year. The survey consists of two questions, and is designed to provide the staff at communityworks with a sense of consumers' overall satisfaction with services, as well as the levels of satisfaction concerning assistance from case managers. The survey also includes a section for consumers to contribute feedback. The ultimate goal of this survey is to assess whether services have been successful in achieving community connections from the consumer's perspective. Services are further evaluated by measuring goal attainment. All goals are decided upon by the consumer, and many intrinsically relate to making community connections. The purpose of staff is to help the consumer get connected, and then fade out of the task.

Cornerstone Clubhouse

Background	Resources	Implementation	Outcome
Many individuals have completed intensive rehab, been discharged, and then found no community left for them in the real world. By focusing on each individual's abilities and unique contributes, the Clubhouse model provides normalized, inconspicuous support that members use to improve his or her quality of life. Cornerstone Clubhouse is the first Acquired Brain Injury Clubhouse in the world to be certified through the International Center for Clubhouse Development (ICCD) in New York. Cornerstone recently underwent the recertification process. Cornerstone Clubhouse has been in existence since the late 1990s.	Small staff of seven people plus the Executive Director. The Clubhouse model dictates the organization is not staff-heavy in order to keep members driving the organization. Physically located in an area where access to local transportation can be assured, both in terms of the program and Transitional Employment (TE) opportunities. The convenient location is helpful in terms of members' independent access to the Clubhouse and TE. Offered under the auspices of Dale Brain Injury Services. Funded by the Ministry of Health. The Clubhouse maintains its own budget.	The Clubhouse model is flexible in terms of the size of community it can serve. The activities done in a clubhouse are dynamic. Without the work and input of the members, a clubhouse could not operate. Roles, tasks, and relationships grow out of the need to operate the Clubhouse. Members have the opportunity to participate in all the work of the clubhouse, including administration, research, outreach, HR issues, advocacy, education, and orientation. Members are involved in all projects because they take responsibility for their clubhouse and its direction. The Clubhouse facilitates return to paid work through Transitional Employment, Supported Employment and Independent Employment. No employment is offered through in-house businesses or sheltered settings.	The Clubhouse conducts two member satisfaction surveys, one family satisfaction survey, one community partners' survey, and an employment placement survey annually. Evaluation results are both qualitative and quantitative. Survey results indicate members, families, and community partners are satisfied with the community participation aspects of the program. A recent Life, Work, Love, Play survey represented quality of life prior to and after becoming a Clubhouse member. In the Life, Work, Love and Play domains, the members surveyed displayed a quality of life improvement postmembership (e.g., 30% satisfied premembership to 80% satisfied postmembership).

Side by Side Brain Injury Clubhouse (SxS)

Background	Resources	Implementation	Outcome
In the early '90s the brain injury community said it would be good for people to have a place to go to be themselves. Cindi Johnson (Executive Director and Rehab Therapist) is associated with individuals who spearheaded the clubhouse movement. Lessons learned suggest that the model works best when everything that is done in the clubhouse, is for the clubhouse. As a consumer driven program, members do hiring and fundraising. Shepherd Center and Emory Healthcare, Rehab Hospitals, agreed to sponsor the start-up of the Clubhouse in July 1999. The two Rehab Hospitals maintained oversight of the clubhouse for the first 2 years.	The only Clubhouse resource for people who are not in rehab within several hours drive. Very active fundraising. Applications to rotary community service grants, foundations, the local business community and local government. SxS raises between 1/4 and 1/3 expenses from the public. They also have 3rd party payers. In recent years SxS was able to purchase and renovate a free standing facility. Members may not be able to coordinate their own transportation. Some take public transport directly or their families bring them, or some have paid transport providers thru Medicaid or Workers Comp. A lot of coordination is required by staff to help with transport.	SxS follows a best practice model that is outlined in the CARF standards for employment in community services. The members are part of a larger community in addition to participating in an individualized approach that assists them with their lives outside of the clubhouse. The Clubhouse exists to support the members and the members can use it voluntarily for the purpose that they need. The Clubhouse is not to create artificial jobs; it encourages people to work in the community. The community participation strategy is enhanced by increased awareness among the public of the lifelong effects of brain injury; thus, advocacy is underway. Culture is celebrated. SxS serves individuals of 14 different ethnicities.	Among members who attended 30 or more days, 61% who have ever attended Side by Side with a goal of paid or unpaid work met their goal. This goal includes community volunteer activities. Eighty-nine percent of ABI Clubhouse members who participated in the vocational services track of the program either became job ready or obtained a job or volunteer placement. The Social Outing Survey administered to families suggested that 86% of members represented enjoyed the outings they attended very much; and that 50% of families are willing to help organize or host an event. Advocacy and dissemination efforts are on track. Members, volunteers, staff, and Executive Director all play a role.

Skills to Enable People and Communities (STEPS) Program

Background	Resources	Implementation	Outcome
The Skills To Enable People and communities (STEPS) program aims to develop social support networks for people with brain injuries and their families in order to enhance quality of life and community participation.	There are two main directors of the program—one has a background in physiotherapy and the other in occupational therapy (however neither are working in this capacity) and both are employees of ABIOS. There is also some administrative support.	Program development was informed by relevant literature, ABIOS' community rehabilitation experience, input form key community and rehabilitation stakeholders, and was enhanced by focus groups of individuals with ABI over a 6-month period.	A total of 616 people attended the STEPS Skills Program from 2006–2010. There are now 18 Network groups that meet regularly and these groups are open to new members. A further 4 groups continue to maintain connections but decided not to be open to new members.
The Networks of Support (the original name of the project) was established in 2005, and was funded for 3 years by the Pathways Home initiative of the Australian Commonwealth Department of Health and Ageing, and administered by Queensland Health. It was a project of the Acquired Brain Injury Outreach Service (ABIOS). Today STEPS is permanently funded by the state health department, Queensland Health, and remains a service arm of ABIOS.	All of the program leaders (both peer leaders and professional leaders) are essentially volunteers; however there is a small stipend available for peer leaders for leading the 6-week program and catering costs and hire of meeting places are met by the STEPS Program.	The STEPS program consists of 2 phases (1) the STEPS Skills Program and (2) STEPS Network Groups.	71 % of clients were still meeting with their groups at 3 months post-course completion, with 67% still meeting at 6 months.
	All resources required to participate in the STEPS Program Leader Training, deliver the STEPS Skills Program and coordinate a Network Groups are provided by the program. They include brochures, leader manual, poster, activity planner, DVD, group workbook, referral forms, attendance records etc.	The STEPS Skills Program is a 6-week group program (i.e., one 2-hour session per week for six weeks) that is led by leaders/facilitators. One leader is a "peer leader" with lived experience of ABI, while the other is a "professional" leader, usually an allied health professional with an interest in community rehabilitation.	Independent evaluation of the project phase was conducted by Griffith University. Nonparametric analysis showed significant client outcomes in the areas of independence, goal formation, coping and stress. Clients reported significant differences across time in their dependence on others, their long-term outcomes reflected a stronger sense of autonomy, client perceptions of coping effectiveness were enhanced and they felt more capable of coping.
It is now a Queensland state-wide initiative serving adults 18-65 years and their families and friends. Among participants, 55% have incurred a TBI as a result of a MVA, fall or assault, and 35% from stroke. Males make up 68%, with an average age of 35 years, 43% had never married and 80% are currently in receipt of a pension.		The Program adopts a self-management approach sequentially exploring 3 themes: how I look after myself, how I live in my community and how I work with services. The sessions contain participation and discussion in groups, a workbook and reflection on a range of topics relevant to these areas. The workbook is written in such a way that caregivers and friends can also participate. The Program culminates in a community outing organized by participants during the previous 5 sessions. A plan is then made to decide if the group wants to continue	Supporters (caregivers/friends) surveyed were less likely to report stress and feelings of depression.
Service and support opportunities in Queensland are limited, further complicated by the geographical dispersion of available services (i.e., concentrated in the			

(continued)

Skills to Enable People and Communities (STEPS) Program (continued)

Background	Resources	Implementation	Outcome
densely populated south-eastern corner of the state, more limited in regional and rural areas). STEPS grew out of this paucity of community services and has now been delivered across 85 sites (at the end of 2010), by 102 leaders in metropolitan, rural and remote locations.		meeting and in what capacity, and the group becomes their own Network Group. Individuals who have completed the 6-week program form the STEPS Network Groups. This provides an ongoing source of support for group participants. Groups assume ownership of their STEPS Network Group and the group makes key decisions such as the format of group meetings, topics, frequency of meetings and whether newcomers can join the group or not. Most groups welcome newcomers.	

A Simply Self-Sustaining System, Community Based Reintegration Post ABI Program

Background	Resources	Implementation	Outcome
Focuses on survivors of ABI predominantly in the rural areas. Can host 3 residential, short-term persons. Population selected b/c of need for services for ABI survivors after they leave acute care. Started 20 months ago after 10 years of planning. A non-medical rehabilitation service. Rehab model is not connected with the hospital. However all the survivors are medically stable. Program is in its infancy and can only survive if there is work, items to be produced, a market for these items, and a readiness to sell. Program also educates mentors, the survivors themselves and the community on ABI and TBI.	Program founder is a clinical neuro-psychologist with a commitment of functional rehabilitation in the community. Aim is to transfer the responsibility to the community coordinators, who are highly skilled local people, yet underemployed. Hope is to have them take on the management of the business in conjunction with the community. Community members are also involved and provide support for free. i.e., Farmers drop off food, local community members who drop off their services and handyman skills for free. Facility is now housed in a rural town in renovated stables for workshops.	Rehab is usually done in homes or in community workshops. Service aims at providing an opportunity to ABI (both traumatic and non-traumatic) for relearning skills, re-accessing social groups and modifying behaviour sufficiently to be able to be included in 'work', namely a small business. Clinical assessment sets the seed, after that local community members as mentors take over, creating the actual business structure. Program is coordinated by sympathetic but not professional, mentors in 'workshops' who are equipped with a specific skill. They sew, design, cook, do woodwork, etc. and have to teach, guide, alter behaviour, etc at the same time. Workshops focus on simple and repetitive tasks on how to make items for sale. Functional skills are developed as well as self-sustaining skills. i.e., learning punctuality, task completion, safety, respectful behaviour and social conflict resolution. Moves away from rehab of deficits to development of capacity. Buddying system used to integrate client into applicable social settings.	Qualitative testimonials of clients show a noticeable positive shift in the behavioural restructuring of the client, development of skill training and greater satisfaction of the client in community integration and participation. Since program is still new, it is in the process of developing a formal outcomes measure to systematically evaluate the program.

CHIRS (Community Head Injury Resource Services)

Background	Resources	Implementation	Outcome
Formerly known as Ashby House; started in 1978 as the first community-based brain injury rehabilitation program in North America. From its origins as a transitional group home, CHIRS has evolved into a multi-service agency that provides a broad range of supports to an adult clientele (aged 18–60) with diverse and complex needs. Both adults with ABI and their families are included within CHIRS' target population. Services form the basis of a comprehensive model of service delivery: Residential services offer supported living opportunities that range from twenty-four hour supervision to supported independent living. Several areas of service and community support are provided within CHIRS: Ashby Community Support Services (ACSS), Employment Support Services, Adult Day Services (ADS), Family-Centered Services, Aging at Home, Residential Services. The Ashby Community Support Services (ACSS) program provides highly specialized Employment and Education Services, assisting clients to participate in a variety of work and learning opportunities, which challenge their unique abilities.	A registered not-for-profit charitable organization primarily funded by the Central Local Health Integration Network (LHIN) through the Ontario Ministry of Health and Long-Term Care. Many of the programs are run in partnership with local organizations and private businesses that provide their expertise, equipment and facilities. These relationships are mutually beneficial in allowing participants to try new programs and in helping to create a profile for brain injury within the greater community. For example, the Continuum of Vocational Placements (from an error-free workshop setting to competitive supported employment) was developed by CHIRS program managers. This program has resulted in numerous community collaborations, including charitable groups and commercial enterprises (e.g., IKEA and Sheridan nurseries). CHIRS provides leadership in the development of brain injury services across the province and participates in regional and provincial planning for government-funded ABI services.	In conjunction with the Supported Employment Program, a CHIRS' Job Developer works with clients to determine their areas of interest and to design individualized work assessments enabling the client, his/her family, and CHIRS staff to assess their vocational skills. The Job Developer also undertakes an extensive job search, partnering with interested community employers. Once a client obtains a placement, a trained Job Coach provides a variety of work site supports to assist the client in learning his/her job and maintaining employment. Work site supports can include travel training, job-site and task analyses, ongoing assessment, the development of individualized strategies, employer education, social skills training, and other such supports relevant to human development within the physical environment. Adult Day Services (ADS) provides mentorship and offsite programming opportunities: Clients are able to volunteer their time to see what strengths and interests they have. Having volunteered, they are invited to become mentors, and may assist with the lunch preparation, club coverage and operations of the Club. Programs are developed and coordinated offsite in efforts to launch clients into the community. Clients and their families	Client satisfaction surveys, constructed of five to seven questions, are disseminated (via email) once a year to clients of the Adult Day Service (ADS) program. Clients are approached by persons who are not members of their care team and asked to complete the surveys by a scheduled date. Client satisfaction is operationalized in terms of 'respect', 'community participation', and 'contentment with programming' and 'clientcentered care', among other things. Practical questions pertaining to cleanliness and fee structures are also included in the client satisfaction survey. Clinical statistics are collected on client goal attainment, use of ethical framework and client complaints. Client safety data pertaining to falls, medication errors, incident of choking, adverse events and infectious diseases are also assessed. A formalized performance management system is maintained and formal written feedback is provided to staff and managers. Regular supervision at meetings provides a forum for ongoing feedback throughout the year. Service agreements—in place for all clients— outline CHIRS' code of ethics and code of conduct, program expectations and other aspects of service. CHIRS uses an active quality assurance program that

(continued)

CHIRS (Community Head Injury Resource Services) (continued)

Background	Resources	Implementation	Outcome
		play a large role in the decisions made around the services and supports provided.	tracks service planning, documentation and service delivery. Benchmarks have included the timeliness of service planning meetings and completion of periodic reporting. CHIRS has earned its fourth three-year accreditation award from the Accreditation Canada.

The Community Approach to Participation (CAP) Model

Background	Resources	Implementation	Outcome
Worked with similar patients in hospital setting Observed that patients with severe symptoms and years after ABI acute phase still capable of achieving improvements incrementally Health care reforms paved way for private services Private practice represented a timely opportunity to pursue methods to rehabilitate ABI survivors more completely & within own communities Private Practice of Occupational Therapists & neuropsychologists established Met with M. McColl (CDN) to discuss progression of the CAP model	Clinical experience 30 years Flexible, creative approach Variety of insurance funders Entrepreneurship Family help in business start-up Links to academia: network, University teaching Use of a range of Measures for Participation & Activity Home-centred therapy eliminates geographic disadvantage to rural clients	Primacy of social roles participation (friend/ worker/student/volunteer, for example) importance to individual client forms the basis for planning therapy collaboratively Positive, individualized support that is flexible, goal-oriented and balanced delivered in client homes or environment where valued role is experienced involving friends, neighbours & other community members. Focus on individual's strengths, building self-identity. (e.g., finding one's own way by transit to a gym, living apart from family, or shopping for groceries alone) Informal SWOT-style Analysis at Intake Desired participation is subject to trials/ assessment cycle for iterative progress Team of Occupational therapist, neuropsychologist, physiotherapist, family therapist, dietician, speech pathologist, M.D., G.P., Case manager	Community participation facilitated by coping mechanisms, use of cues, or environmental modifications to barriers Over long-term, shaping of social behaviours, adaptive skills learned Participation builds from experience of achievements and sense of belonging Increase in number of life roles. Decrease in incidence of challenging behaviour (e.g., verbal aggression) Latest study (2009) shows improvements continue with longer duration of therapy such as 3 years. Decrease in hours of care was sustained in approx. 42% subjects. Improvement possible 6 years post injury Long-term intermittent support available to clients

ABI Partnership Project (highlighting Outreach & Aboriginal ABI Community Support)

Background	Resources	Implementation	Outcome
Yearly in SK, approx. 2,200 people sustain ABI. Of these, SK estimates 150 will need multiple services & lifetime support. SK Health & SK. Govt. Insurance (SGI) est. partnership (1996) to create coordinated continuum of comm-based services for people with ABI & their families, so that they "may live successfully in their communities with improved quality of life." ABI Partnership Project includes 36 comm.-based programs throughout SK: Outreach Teams, Regional Coordinators, Rehab. Programs, Residential Options, Education & Prevention Services, Life Enrichment Programs, Children's Program, Independent Living Worker Programs, Vocational Programs, Crisis Management, Day Programs. In 1999 SK Abilities Council (SAC) recognized the demand for a program for ABI survivors whose needs went beyond scope of a vocational service. In 2000, Community Support Program approved and began to be offered by the SAC. In 2006, Aboriginal ABI Comm. Support offered. Services & programs enable clients, fams, & caregivers to get ed., rehab, life enrichment, respite, residential & vocational services as close to home as possible.	Members of Outreach Team meet with clients to establish and maintain relationships, learn clients' goals, & connect clients with services that help clients meet individual goals. Aboriginal Community Support Program: – Candidates must have documented brain injury, be over 18, & be emotionally stable. – Enrollment based on available funding, as services are free of charge to participants. Participants enrolled for as long as funding permits. – Group meetings and outings in the community with a focus on cultural activities. SAC, Saskatoon pays salary & benefits of a Program Supervisor on half-time basis.	Allows clients to make own choices about program activities. Services are individualized to meet expressed needs & goals. Client goals revised yearly or new goals set when current goal has been achieved. Community Support Worker maintains goals with client and reports to supervisor monthly. Advisory Group for Partnership Project (made up of survivors, family, rehab profs., agency reps, etc.) in place since program inception. Their input has helped shape the program. (Difficulty maintaining Aboriginal representative in Advisory Group). Staff members work 'with' not 'for' clients in terms of general skill development and social integration. Promotional materials translated into Cree, & Dene for northern clients. Aboriginal ABI Group makes new connections in community w/elders, ceremonial groups from various reserves, cultural centres, urban services, Aboriginal agencies, & Aboriginal community programs. Aspires to decrease Aboriginal clients' isolation, helping them feel more part of community, along with strengthening their spirituality by participating in traditional practices.	Use website, brochures, word of mouth, education & prevention program to disseminate program info. Positive outcomes: making connection with new groups in the community. Challenges for whole partnership to work as a team because so spread out throughout province. Meet twice/year to work as a team. For each client , Goal Attainment sheets completed on regular basis & Mayo Portland Inventory Assessment (MPAI-4) done at intake & discharge. Partnership Project's 2007–10 Review (unpublished), shows significant improvements in participation & total scores of MPAI-4. In terms of Goal Attainment, of 4,426 goals submitted, 62% achieved, 28% partially achieved (withdrawn goals not included in percentages), & 10% were not achieved. Goals are divided into 5 categories: Cognitive, Functional Independence, Psychosocial/Emotional, Community Activities, & Other.

Acquired Brain Injury Ireland

Background	Resources	Implementation	Outcome
Established in 2000, Acquired Brain Injury Ireland (formerly the Peter Bradley Foundation) was set up to provide a range of pioneering, flexible and tailor-made services for adults (18–65) with Acquired Brain Injury. The Foundation develops and provides services *nationwide*. Acquired Brain Injury Ireland provides a flexible approach, focusing strongly on individual development and incorporating *person centred planning* (PCP)—an internationally recognized *best practice*. Person Centred Planning ensures that the person served is fully involved in all decisions that affect his or her life. A personal profile is drawn up for each person that identifies their current abilities and their support needs. Mission: to enable people with an acquired brain injury to live an independent life within the community, by providing and maintaining a supportive living environment.	**Human Resources** – ABI Case Manager, ABI Local Services Managers, Rehabilitation Assistants, ABI Social Work—Family Liaisons, Occupational Therapists, Clinical Psychologists, – Many board members/ stakeholders have personal experience with ABI. Board members include healthcare professionals and business people. **Financial Resources** – Core funding from the Health Service Executive (HSE) is provided to ABI Ireland.	Side by Side Day Resource Service: provides clients with a work-ordered day filled with meaningful activities. A *holistic model* is followed, which enhances self-esteem, independence, community involvement and personal growth. The Day Service provides resources, support and advocacy to assist members in achieving their personal goals for living and participating in the broader community (e.g., personal care, home management, cookery, finance, accessing local community services and support, health and safety). *It is designed to help individuals move away from an environment where treatment is administered to an environment where they can once again reciprocate and contribute to the community, empowering them with responsibility in their own lives.* Where possible, Day Service staff identify work placements in the community. A personal development plan (PDP) is created in partnership with each client and clearly identifies where that individual is independent, where support is needed and any potential risks. It is then implemented and prioritised with realistic and achievable goals identified and set jointly with the individual client.	Measurements include: Individual Rehabilitation Plans, and a written service agreement for people served; Regular consultation with families/ carers; Annual Key Performance Goals; Annual Accessibility Plan; Regular consultation with funders at national and local level; Annual independent auditing of finances; CARF Accreditation. Annually, a survey of the people in the service is elicited to determine their views on a range of issues affecting the service offered. This survey is managed through an independent third party organisation called uSPEQ. The uSPEQ questionnaire asks respondents to rate their experiences related to access to services, the service process, the way the programmes meet their needs, and their perception of the outcomes they have attained. *uSPEQ operationalizes and measures 'community participation'.* The 2009 survey indicates a very high positive response from the clients. Client testimonials include: A Different Light—But a New Light by Risteard Lloyd: Reestablishing one's identity after Brain Injury (a story of survival) (http://www. abiireland.ie/docs/ TheRisteardLloydstory 2009.pdf). ABI Ireland facilitates research projects pertaining to ABI:

(continued)

Acquired Brain Injury Ireland (continued)

Background	Resources	Implementation	Outcome
			information on current and past research projects are available to members, families and interested parties; where appropriate, *clients and their families participate in research projects.* In 2008, ABI Ireland *piloted a paediatric service* in Tullamore, Co. Offaly which could, with support from the HSE, be delivered throughout the country. ABI Ireland is currently being *replicated in Slovenia;* ongoing collaborations exist between ABI Ireland and the Ministry of Labour and Family & Social Affairs.

School Transition and reEntry Program

Background	Resources	Implementation	Outcome
This program reaches parents of school aged children with moderate to severe TBI/ABI. Program is based on "Back to School" a program which included an observational study which followed a cohort of children treated in hospital for TBI/ABI in various states. The observational study included focus groups with stakeholders regarding the services the children received, those they did not but their families wanted, challenges and concerns. Focus groups were conducted with personnel from all hospital departments in which children with TBI/ABI may have been treated and any personnel who would	A 5 year project funded by the NIDRR: National Institute on Disability and Rehabilitation Research. A website for parents is part of the program interventions: developed to help parents advocate for their children and address a range of concerns common to parents with an injured child: http://free.brain injurypartners.com/ Previous research demonstrated the importance of linking hospitals that treat clients post-injury and schools that educate them to the child's needs and consequent functioning and recovery. Program is flexible in order to accommodate different areas of the United States.	Serves children aged 5–18 who have suffered TBI/ABI. The objective of this program is to present a systematic and coordinated approach to development, validation and dissemination of effective measures and transition intervention practices for children so that they may participate in their schools and communities. The primary goal of this program is to improve identification of school aged children with TBI/ABI when they are in the hospital. The program seeks to implement a process by which hospitals communicate to local school districts when a school aged child has suffered TBI/ABI	No outcomes yet, but may be a promising practice. An RCT is underway in which 50% of participants are participating in this program and 50% are not and both are receiving traditional treatment. There are approximately 70 children in each condition, 50 have completed the program and initial data is being analyzed. Rolling enrollment for this RCT began in late 2008, recruitment ended March 2011. Measures include: Child and Adolescent Scale of Participation; Child and Adolescent Scale of Environment; Child Behavior Checklist; Behavior Rating Inventory of Executive Function; a State/Trait Anxiety Index;

(continued)

School Transition and reEntry Program (continued)

Background	Resources	Implementation	Outcome
provide information to parents including: social workers, nurses, physicians and hospital administrators.		(informing their teachers) so that teachers may work with families to improve the educational experience of the child. This goal is being met through STEP: a comprehensive hospitalschool transition intervention, which includes hospital, school and family components. Project recruiters are placed in the hospital to recruit families with children who have suffered a TBI/ABI. Within STEP, "Transition facilitators", mainly PTs, Special Eds or Social Workers (who already work for the Board of Education within schools) liaison with the hospital and then produce an individual educational plan for each child.	and program developer's own measures of service provision and satisfaction. Children do not fill in their own measures. The STEP program has been taken up in Tennessee and Ohio. A program modeled after STEP (facilitator works with families and teachers post injury, through the school year and potentially to the age of 18/graduation) is being rolled out in both states based on anecdotal outcomes of the original program (student, school and families experiences— no standardized outcome measures or RCT results available). The program in itself (5 year project) is not intended to be sustainable. However, it is designed in such a way that if taken up long term it can be sustainable: recruiters will be replaced by a standard discharge protocol within the hospital (a paper form faxed to point of contact at Board of Education); facilitators are persons who are already employed by a local Board of Education.

PABICOP

Background	Resources	Implementation	Outcome
PABICOP was founded in 1999. It was initiated as a partnership between the Thames Valley Children's Centre and London Health Sciences Centre. PABICOP represents an innovative approach to providing support and training to children and families with an ABI through an Acquired Brain Injury Rehabilitation and Reintegration Outreach Team. The Travelling Acquired Brain Injury Rehabilitation and Reintegration Team bridges the gap between rehabilitation services that are currently at Children's Hospital of Western Ontario (CHWO) and those in smaller rural communities in Southwestern Ontario. Three primary objectives: to improve integration and acceptance of children with an ABI into their home communities, to improve the quality of life of children and their families with an ABI, to minimize problems and maximize the quality of life of each individual child with an ABI as they enter adolescence and adulthood. PABICOP's philosophy and model of operations is holistic, parent and family/client centered, community-based, and inclusive of the community at large in the ongoing care and management of the child or youth with acquired brain injury. PABICOP also encompasses the concepts of	**Financial Resources** – Funded by the Ministry of Health and Long-Term care. – In 1999, funding from the Ministry was established at $348,000 per annum. – In 2009, funding for PABICOP service delivery is $369,000. **Human Resources** – The direct outreach consultation component is a feature that makes PABICOP's approach unique for pediatric brain injury services in the Southwest Region. The team providing services includes a Developmental Pediatrician, a Pediatric Neurology Nurse Practitioner, a Community Outreach Coordinator, 2 School Liaison Workers, an Occupational Therapist, a Psychometrist, and a Neuropsychologist. Community outreach consultation services are provided primarily by School Liaison, Occupational Therapy, Social Work, and Psychometry.	A child or youth can be referred to PABICOP for assistance with the effects of a remote brain injury, including medical, psychological and educational issues. Hospital-based criteria used for a referral include the following: loss of consciousness no matter how brief; confusion at the scene or shortly thereafter; amnesia for the event. If any one of these criteria exist, the child or youth will be seen. The Outreach Team provides several services: case specific consultation, telephone consultation, community liaison visits, educational programs. Case specific consultation: Site visits provide an opportunity for community service providers, families, and the client to raise questions about community services, and for the outreach team members to offer suggestions about the client's rehabilitation and integration. Telephone consultation: Additional telephone consultation is provided to the client and family, as requested. Community liaison visits: A community liaison person is available to provide followup site visits to schools and community groups to address specific or specialized needs that cannot be addressed during the larger outreach team visit. Educational programs: Inservices, seminars, and	An anonymous questionnaire (distributed to community representatives) assesses knowledge about head injury, to determine whether the outreach program is successful at increasing the general level of knowledge about pediatric ABI. Increases in knowledge(s) related to pediatric ABI are central to community awareness. Moreover, they are thought to facilitate community involvement and support for pediatric persons with an ABI. Satisfaction Rating Scales have been developed for parents, clients and community workers. Responses on these rating scales are used to modify and develop the outreach program. Internal evaluations of PABICOP have been completed by McDougall et al.—a research team affiliated with Thames Valley Children's Centre (2006) and Gillett—program developer and creator (2004). PABICOP has been successfully replicated in various sites across Europe and Australia.

PABICOP (continued)

Background	Resources	Implementation	Outcome
continuity, accessibility, knowledge, collaboration, empowerment, and advocacy within its services (which are individualized, inclusive of home/school environments, long-term, and centred on the needs identified by the client). Over 50% of client referrals are from Fowler Kennedy Sports Medicine, and involve children with complex concussions.		educational programs are offered in communities where needs are identified. Examples of educational programs include inservices at a school board on a professional development day, or a half-day seminar at a children's treatment centre.	

The Challenge Program—TIRR Memorial Hermann

Background	Resources	Implementation	Outcome
TIRR used to be a free standing rehab facility, however due to hard times, after 5 years bought out by Memorial Hermann (MH) Hospital. Now fall under rules and regulations under MH. Challenge Program is an inpatient Day rehab program organized in larger scale by Dr. Catherine Botke in 1988. TBI philosophy was to treat people holistically and to help them to return to work. Treatment model was emulated from Dr. Ben Yashay's Brain Injury program at the University of New York. Are seeing more clients with Acquired Brain Injury, also people with strokes. 80% of population have TBI. Program designed by emulating and travelling to see other programs. i.e., the Residential program called	Private insurance pays for the majority of the program. Partnership with Federal State Dept of Rehab Services, State agency w/ fed money. Medicare also pays for the services. Funding is getting harder and harder, Program manager finds that she has to almost everyday educate insurance providers about the required treatment for people with ABI. For instance cognitive rehab is what's getting cut. As a result managers constantly need to defend itself and the program may need to change its model to survive with the funding pressures.	Overarching belief is that people will get better if they have something to do in society. Objective of the program is to identify something the client can do and help them meet that goal at end of treatment. Everything else becomes complimentary to this objective. First focus on restoration therapy and then compensatory therapy due to acute level of clients. Within compensatory therapy community reintegration becomes a key focus. Spend a lot of time educating and working with the family so that client can be more independent at home. Family is invited and encouraged to be part of the daily therapy work and to collaborate with the members of the rehab team.	Outcomes measures are taken during the program, if not meeting goals, may need to change the approach Satisfaction survey of the client filled out at discharge and use it to change what their doing. Use 3 different outcome tools including Social Scale measure and Community Integration Questionnaire at admission and discharge and then at 3 months and 1 year after as followup. There has been a noticeable shift after a 3 month follow up. 85% of clients when graduate after program have some community integration 88% of client have significantly less need for supervision and report meeting their independence and personal safety goals. • 90% of adult clients who completed the program

(continued)

The Challenge Program—TIRR Memorial Hermann (continued)

Background	Resources	Implementation	Outcome
Transitional Learning Community in Galveston.		Very Group Therapy heavy program. In order to help clients become aware of their social skill challenges, peers provide them feedback and a sense of community to learn more strategies. Cognitive Therapy, Psychotherapy Therapy, and Community Integration and are integrated with each other, 2–4 days a week. Use a tracks based method for clients based on what clients think they can accomplish during the year i.e., employment track, volunteer ready, educational track and Independent living readiness.	met their volunteer or work goals • 80% adolescent clients who completed the program returned to school by discharge • Clients rated the program as 4.5/5 for overall satisfaction (1 being poor and 5 being excellent Also measure how clients are socially integrated within their community (i.e., leisure activities, shopping, volunteering) from the social component of the community integration questionnaire.

Krempels Brain Injury Foundation

Background	Resources	Implementation	Outcome
In 1995, David Krempels received a sizeable jury award in compensation for injuries caused by a car accident. David attended support groups following his accident, however he did not feel that this was enough support. He used some of the money from his award to rebuild a comfortable life for himself. But he also decided to invest in a new career—an organization to help these people. Four friends helped him start the Krempels Brain Injury Foundation for People Living with Brain Injury. The Krempels Center was founded in 1995, and originally focused on providing financial assistance to people who suffered a brain injury. In 2000, the Center began to expand its mission to provide better postrehabilitation to people with brain injuries. The Steppingstones program was developed in 2001, and was recently renamed the Community Program. David is still actively involved in the foundation, and runs a bookclub every Friday with members.	The Krempels Center Community Program is located in a community setting with other non-profits. This setting helps folks interact with others without a brain injury. There's a restaurant/café in the building, a health centre where some members go, and a "rebuilding of credit" place where members can go if they wish to buy a car etc. The foundation is broadening its base of financial support to include: SteppingStones member fees; Medicaid and private insurance revenue; grants from other foundations and charitable organizations; gifts from individual donors and corporate sponsors. Interns do "in kind" donations of a sort. Low income members are subsidized.	Target pop: 18+ People with a stroke or brain tumor can attend the program, not just folks with TBI or ABI. This program is run in a fairly small community so they're the only resource in town for people with such injuries. Open three days /wk and members choose from a variety of groups. Each day is structured. Members choose to attend the program according to their needs, whether it is three days a week or one group a week. There are also events to celebrate milestones. Members provide interns and researchers with insight into living with TBI. There are different types of groups: creative, emotional, functional (i.e., cooking), community outings, brain power (i.e., cognitive skills), physical activities and recreation, social, and vocational	Evaluations have been primarily qualitative in nature, which is congruent with the Krempels Center mission of being client centered and member driven. Pre/post evaluations had been done in the past, but it was found that members had memory issues. Therefore, there is always on-going discussion of which groups members find most beneficial, and which groups they would like to see added/removed. Published evaluation indicates that member needs were found to be met by the program. The needs that participants found to remain unmet include social support for caregivers, transportation issues and community education. Qualitative research done to uncover factors leading to successful recovery and productive lifestyles after ABI. Major themes emerged: • development of social support networks, grief and coping strategies, • acceptance of the injury and redefinition of self, • and empowerment

Biscayne Institutes of Health & Living Inc.

Background	Resources	Implementation	Outcome
BIHL (established in 1988) follows the Biscayne HealthCare community™ model which focuses on health care delivery for frontline community-based care; model lies in between individual practitioners and hospitals on a continuum of healthcare delivery. In its Brain Injury (day) programs involving patients with ABI/TBI, community integration is the ultimate goal. It specializes in reintegrating "difficult to treat" long-term ABI/TBI patients. The main focus is on treating the whole person via individualized treatment by a community team of professionals addressing physical, cognitive, social and behavioural aspects. BIHL as a best practice: When evaluated with WIT model and ONF's CoP framework, BIHL addresses and accounts for all the principals and services needed by a program that fosters community participation.	BIHL holds 6 accreditations (CARF, CORF, etc.) and is funded by Medicare, private insurance, private pay, grants, Dept. of Education and Florida State Brain & Spinal Cord Injury Program. **Professional Staff:** psychologists and neuropsychologists, physicians, physical therapists, occupational therapists, speech therapists, special-ed teachers, social workers, etc. **Program Strategies:** (summary) offers a full continuum of services ranging from primary care to health/wellness promotion to the community (throughout the day people with brain injuries interact with the community)	Program Details: a) STAGE 1: Assessment and Treatment Plan – evaluation performed in each case, development of interdisciplinary care plan with patient and family in mind, followed by team rounds each week held to assess progress and set new goals – tailored cognitive retraining program – biofeedback, physical, occupational and speech therapies provided in transdisciplinary manner – healing process helped with Chinese medicine – administration of modules to help with taking medication, performing activities of daily living and maintaining safety – individual, family and group (builds social skills) therapy provided b) STAGE 2: Consolidation of the Learned Skills—field trips, etc. c) STAGE 3: Life after Rehab – protected/supported work and volunteering environments – monitored at home as well – BIHL facility located in peaceful/attractive surroundings with rooms that look like rooms in a home – BIHL is community based: consumers and their families are able to participate in their own therapy (consumers/families can work with the team to choose services); clients are able to come back . . . they are followed long-term in the community and are allowed to return to BHL if they want to (even as volunteers)	Annually, an Information Outcomes Management report is made to show the goals met by the target groups and their costeffectiveness. In TBI and neurological care (data from 2009), 85% of cognitive goals met, 79% of emotional needs met, 50% of physical goals and 65% of behavioural goals met. The functional improvement of complex cases is followed using WHO's ICF (10-year case studies exist); one of the assessed domains is the individual's activities and participation (e.g., in the community). Positive outcomes documented in peer-reviewed journals and in book entitled *Humanizing Healthcare*. Functional assessment measures (COMBI) conducted pre- and post-treatment on all individuals with ABI/TBI. RESEARCH DESIGN: • case studies • questionnaires

The Brain Integration Programme (BIP)

Background	Resources	Implementation	Outcome
The BIP was developed in the Rehabilitation Centre Groot Klimmendaal in the Netherlands on the basis of achieving optimal community integration for ABI survivors with complex behavioural or psychiatric problems. BIP is a structured residential program and the main objective of the program is to re-integrate individuals with chronic ABI back to their communities. The program allows participants to achieve a balance in their daily activities between domestic life, work, leisure, and social interaction. Participants in the BIP may be referred by regional rehabilitation centers that offer standard post-acute programs as well as neuropsychiatric departments.	The BIP is a national well-recognized program covered by all healthcare insurance companies in The Netherlands. The BIP is a standardized rehabilitation program consisting of three modules: – Independent living module aims at training specific abilities in order to perform domestic tasks. – Social-emotional module: aims at setting new, adjusted and achievable goals in life. – Work module: aims at developing vocational aims. The participants start the program with simultaneously participating in all the three modules. However start of the work module requires certain level of insight and awareness of one's condition. Participants' family and social contacts are involved with social-emotional module to obtain a realistic view about the condition of the participants.	On average, participants spend about 100 hours per person in the independent living module, 110 hours in the social-emotional module and about 44 hours in the work module (hours are adjusted based on individuals' needs). The work module involves the participation of the community employers. Also, the assessment vocational unit working with participants arranges for any necessary adjustments to the workplace and any personal assistant needed while on the job. Participants return home every weekend to practice the acquired skills. The professional staff consists of a neuropsychologist, a physiatrist, a neuropsychiatrist, occupational therapists, cognitive therapists, social workers, speech-language therapists, physical therapists and rehabilitation nurses/ coaches who work closely to together to ensure that participants move along a reasonable pace.	Two comprehensive cohort studies have been completed to assess the effectiveness of the program. The results of both studies have shown that the program was successful in improving community integration in participants with brain injury at the end of the program as well as at one year follow up. The results showed that at one year follow up after completion of the program, employment significantly improved (from 38% to 58%), and hours of work increased from 8 to 15 hours. Also, living independently rose from 42% to 70%. It is concluded that even participants with complex problems due to severe brain injury who got stuck in life could benefit from the program and be reintegrated back to their communities.

Appendix B: Life Space Charts

communityworks

Sociocultural	Interpersonal	Physical Environment	Internal States
Norms and values, family, religion, communication	*Interactions with others, primary and secondary relationships*	*Housing, neighbourhood, natural objects*	*Health, self-esteem, sense of well-being, quality of life, biological*
• The strengths and personal goals of the individual are given primary importance in intervention plans. • Consumers and their families are provided with the education and tools to support themselves over time.	• Opportunities are offered that will foster community connections. • The "coach" encourages the consumer to explore new activities in the community. • Social support networks are built through living in generic housing options in the community. • Families are included as decision-makers in intervention plans.	• The environment is identified as a critical factor in skilltraining. Thus, interventions take place in the same environments in which the skills will be practiced. • The physical environment is modified to meet the needs of the individual.	• Consumers discover new meanings in their lives as they find their places in the community. • Consumers gain confidence in their independent living skills through real-life experience. • A sense of autonomy is achieved through the provision of selfdirected services.

SXS and Cornerstone Clubhouse

Sociocultural	Interpersonal	Physical Environment	Internal States
Norms and values, family, religion, communication	*Interactions with others, primary and secondary relationships*	*Housing, neighbourhood, natural objects*	*Health, self-esteem, sense of well-being, quality of life, biological*
• Elicits support of local businesses, employers, and community partners. • Addresses the stigmas and lack of resources for individuals with ABI through advocacy, education, and dissemination of information. • Clubhouse Standards codify the philosophy and practice of the Clubhouse Model for all interested parties.	• Fosters egalitarian relationships and mutual reliance between members and staff. • The Clubhouse community reaches out to members who are not attending, become isolated, or in hospital, not to see why they are not attending, but to ensure they are ok. • Acting out behaviours are dealt with in the social community context rather than treated as isolated clinical issues. • Clear conflict resolution policies.	• Space and location allows disability access wherever possible. • Members assist other members to live independently by helping with physical tasks such as shopping and laundry. • The Clubhouse has no staff only or member only spaces. • The Clubhouse has a distinct physical location separate from any other • rehabilitation facility, including its own name and telephone number.	• Individual long-term goals are broken down into smaller, more manageable pieces to give clear benchmarks for progress. • Individuals in the program are valued for their unique talents and • contributions to the Clubhouse effort (e.g., artistic, musical, computer skills). • Members select work units they feel would be a good fit given their innate abilities. • Support offered for members who are experiencing psychological distress at any point in life. • Personally relevant tasks and program content.

Skills to Enable People and Communities (STEPS) Program

Sociocultural	Interpersonal	Physical Environment	Internal States
Norms and values, family, religion, communication	*Interactions with others, primary and secondary relationships*	*Housing, neighbourhood, natural objects*	*Health, self-esteem, sense of well-being, quality of life, biological*
• Identifying and examining difficulties in the community regarding stigma and restrictive attitudes • Undertaking community awareness projects including attitudes and accessibility	• Opportunity for building social networks and forming new and supportive relationships through participation in weekly meetings • Interactions with other ABI survivors in a nonrehabilitation setting • Participate in weekly workshops focusing on relationships with family, friends, and the wider community • Potential to strengthen relationships with caregiver, family and friends through improved reflection around brain injury and coping	• Working with others to plan transportation to and from weekly meetings as well as independent planning of future network meetings • Using a space in the community to connect with other individuals with acquired brain injury and their families, friends and caregivers	• Reflect on the impact and meaning of acquired brain injury including limitations and goal setting through participation in weekly workshops • Working through specific problems after brain injury and regaining structure and balance • Learning self-management techniques to manage stress and transition toward independent living • Gain insight into changes after brain injury including stress management • Building confidence through the formation of support network

A Simply Self-Sustaining System, Community-Based Reintegration Post Acute Brain Injury Program

Sociocultural	Interpersonal	Physical Environment	Internal States
Norms and values, family, religion, communication	*Interactions with others, primary and secondary relationships*	*Housing, neighbourhood, natural objects*	*Health, self-esteem, sense of well-being, quality of life, biological*
• Family and friends are incorporated and encouraged to be part of the rehabilitation, workshops and daily activities • Local community members become part of the rehabilitation process and are employed by the program. • Local community members are trained to become social reintegration coaches/ therapists for the clients and partners with the program. • Clients are integrated into the local community markets and become normalized by highlighting their capacities and participating in the market • Clients are taught valuable skills and adopt to meaningful roles within the local communities as well as their own personal communities	• Clients interact with the program staff, community coordinators and other clients with the expectation of all members to be respectful, courteous and treat each other with value and human worth. • Clients are given some autonomy in the decision making of their rehabilitation. Although workshops are found to be most effective in matching tasks according to client capacity. • Rehabilitation is done with the client and family or friends not on them. • Family and friends are encouraged to visit and contribute to the program. • Local community members are brought in to deliver workshops and collaborate with clients which inadvertently normalizes clients with ABI and the focus of client capacity becomes highlighted	• Clients are supported by community coordinators and program staff that uphold the principal of communal respect • Workshops and rehabilitation program is situated in a safe communal farm that is located in a small rural town yet accessible to the local store and hospital • Clients are able to return to their families and homes. • Families and friends are encouraged to visit and participate • Functional rehabilitation is also done at the client's home or place of stay in order to generalize the skills learned to their relevant contexts. • Social reintegration skills are expected to extend to client's homes and place of stay.	• Clients are given the chance to practice, problem solve and use learned strategies in a safe social context with a functional relevance to their strategies. • Residential facilities are available for short term stay for clients who require additional support to encourage their independence and autonomy • Functional skills are developed alongside with social reintegration in a safe environment tailored to their capacities.

Community Head Injury Resource Services—CHIRS

Sociocultural	Interpersonal	Physical Environment	Internal States
Norms and values, family, religion, communication	*Interactions with others, primary and secondary relationships*	*Housing, neighbourhood, natural objects*	*Health, self-esteem, sense of well-being, quality of life, biological*
• Many of the programs offered by Adult Day Services (ADS) are run in partnership with local organizations and private businesses. These relationships are mutually beneficial in allowing participants to try new programs and in helping to create a profile for brain injury within the greater community. • Offsite programming is designed to launch clients into the community—participation within adapted programs promotes community participation through the building of community connections and autonomy. • A close partnership with the Toronto ABI Network helps CHIRS collaborators and stakeholders to respond to the needs of the community. • CHIRS collaborators and stakeholders are provided with educational and practical resources by which to address sociocultural considerations (relevant to their clients) across the lifespan. CHIRS has staff representation from many of the main cultural communities served	• CHIRS staff members receive intensive onsite training where they learn about client support, community-based participation, agency systems, and procedures. • Clients and their families play a large role in the planning of services and supports. • Clients are invited to become mentors, and may assist with the lunch preparation, club coverage (i.e., greeting new members of the Club, helping others to feel welcome, assisting with the gardening) and operations of the Club. • Work positions are individually designed to ensure a match between a client's strengths and the employer's needs. • Currently, CHIRS staff are looking at social enterprises and prospective partnerships.	• In addressing the perceived lack of community programs, a grass roots movement, led by Dr. Mira Ashby, designed individual CHIRS programs, which fostered community participation and support. • As the entire CHIRS staff evolved, CHIRS expanded its Adult Day Services (ADS) program to meet needs identified in the community. For example, clients asked for work programs and a partnership with IKEA soon developed. • Work site supports can include travel training, jobsite and task analyses, ongoing assessment, the development of individualized strategies, employer education, social skills training, and other such supports relevant to human development within the physical environment. • 'Enabling foundations', or mechanisms by which to achieve strategic goals, include inspired teamwork, optimal environments to meet client needs, a safety and wellness culture, enhanced information and management systems, financial sustainability, and sound governance.	• CHIRS provides services for persons who have sustained ABI based on the principle that services, supports and life opportunities must be provided to correspond as much as possible with the individual's community environment, in a manner which enhances the individual's well-being, dignity, self-respect, and physical and emotional security. • CHIRS staff strive to find opportunities for clients to address their current goals in the community, while providing a structured environment where individual skills and supports can be 'learned' or 'honed'. • The process of creating a "Service Plan" involves a comprehensive assessment of the client's goals and needs. • Client satisfaction surveys demonstrate that clients feel they are able to achieve their personal goals.

The Community Approach to Participation (CAP) Model
for Community Integration in People with Acquired Brain Injury

Sociocultural	Interpersonal	Physical Environment	Internal States
Norms and values, family, religion, communication	*Interactions with others, primary and secondary relationships*	*Housing, neighbourhood, natural objects*	*Health, self-esteem, sense of well-being, quality of life, biological*
• Client norms and values are central to customizing a mutually agreed to plan of therapy • Communications with clients are structured to be encouraging, open, and collaborative • Family belonging, if important to a client is leveraged to assist with community integration • Opportunities for participation are explored, perhaps adding new focus for clients	• By reducing incidents of challenging behaviour, therapy following the CAP model evens a client's temperament, reducing stress in primary relationships • Friends and family forming primary relationships in a client's life are included in plans for therapeutic interventions and trials of activities • The therapeutic relationship formed between client and therapist provides a bond for trust, feedback, and support over the long term as client needs may change over the life span.	• Functional abilities to manage everyday tasks are within the scope of the CAP model if this is part of a client's desired goals and may lead to the ability to live independently • The physical environment is modified where possible and appropriate to facilitate skill development to meet client goals • Support systems are strengthened or created to enable a client to enjoy living within a chosen community.	• Social role development according to client-set goals builds self esteem • Holistic therapy to improve overall quality of life for client, but also for care givers & family members • Interventions seek to address both physical and psychological states of health to optimize participation within communities • Opportunity to discover personal insights building realistic selfawareness

ABI Community Partnership Project—Aboriginal Community Support Program

Sociocultural	Interpersonal	Physical Environment	Internal States
Norms and values, family, religion, communication	*Interactions with others, primary and secondary relationships*	*Housing, neighbourhood, natural objects*	*Health, self-esteem, sense of well-being, quality of life, biological*
• Clients connected to services and programs within community but outside ABI Partnership Project, who work with already existing programs.	• Meaningful relationships between client and outreach worker formed and maintained. • Activities and outings assist clients in making social connections	• Space for traditional teachings, sacred ceremonies, and gatherings. • Outings provide for varied physical environment.	• Goals set by clients as they work toward independence and skill attainment

ABI Community Partnership Project—Outreach Teams

Sociocultural	Interpersonal	Physical Environment	Internal States
• Clients connected to services and programs within community but outside ABI Partnership Project, who work with already existing programs.	• Meaningful and longlasting relationships between client and outreach worker formed and maintained. • Clients include family members and help them better understand the nature of brain injuries and ways to cope with changes in their family member with an ABI	• Flexible to meet needs and desires of client. Meetings take place in locations convenient to clients	• Goals set by clients as they work toward independence and skill attainment. • Opportunities for clients to share their personal stories provides a form of emotional therapy as well as a sense of giving back to his or her community.

Acquired Brain Injury Ireland

Sociocultural	Interpersonal	Physical Environment	Internal States
Norms and values, family, religion, communication	*Interactions with others, primary and secondary relationships*	*Housing, neighbourhood, natural objects*	*Health, self-esteem, sense of well-being, quality of life, biological*
• Side by Side Day Resource Service is designed to help individuals move away from an environment where treatment is administered to an environment where they can once again reciprocate and contribute to the community, empowering them with responsibility in their own lives. • ABI Ireland is currently being replicated in Slovenia; ongoing collaborations exist between ABI Ireland and the Ministry of Labour and Family & Social Affairs	• The Rehabilitation Team is responsible for assessing the individual needs of a client and for developing a person centred programme of rehabilitation and support. The Rehabilitation Team consists of clinical staff, Local Services Managers, ABI Case Managers, and Rehabilitation Assistants together with the person with an ABI and family members/carers affected by acquired brain injury. • Program coordinators have further developed the aspect of a workordered day, whereby the members take a more active part in practically running the Centre and participating within the larger community.	• ABI Ireland Assisted Living residences are conveniently located with access to local shops, transport and amenities. • The Side by Side Day Resource Service is 'inserted in the community', with many facilities located nearby	• As the needs of the individual client change over time, ABI Ireland provides a flexible approach, focusing strongly on individual development and incorporating person centred planning (PCP). • The role of the Rehabilitation Assistant is to facilitate and assist optimal independence and participation in activities within an individual's own home or work environment, and in the community. • The Side by Side program model is flexible, variable, person- and client-driven

School Transition and re-Entry Program (STEP)

Sociocultural	Interpersonal	Physical Environment	Internal States
Norms and values, family, religion, communication	*Interactions with others, primary and secondary relationships*	*Housing, neighbourhood, natural objects*	*Health, self-esteem, sense of well-being, quality of life, biological*
• STEP uses a multifaceted approach to facilitate communication and cooperation between all points of contact in the child's community: hospital, school, and parents (family) • STEP promotes awareness raising through information provision (in the form of brochures and the Brain Injury Partners website). • Adoption of this promising practice by both Boards of Education that have participated in STEP and those that have not, encourages policy development around the provision of educational assistance for school aged children with TBI. • Policy development is also promoted by the increased application of legal frameworks (IDEA) that promote the provision of educational assistance for schoolaged children with TBI.	• STEP encourages communication and cooperation between all points of contact in the child's community: hospital, school and parents (family). • STEP facilitates the full participation of school aged children with TBI in their communities, thereby enriching the child's peer relationships.	• By providing information on TBI, parents and teachers are made aware of risk factors associated with TBI and common causes of TBI, thereby facilitating injury prevention at home, at school, and at play. • By promoting the application of educational assistance for school aged children with TBI, STEP promotes safety in engaging with physical environments.	• Through information provision, STEP outlines constructive means of coping for parents and teachers. • Information provided by STEP promotes empowerment of parents and teachers to understand, encourage and advocate for the child over the life course, within grade school and beyond. • Constructive realtionships with parents and teachers promote a child's participation in their community and fosters greater quality of life for the child in and outside of school.

Pediatric Acquired Brain Injury Community Outreach Program (PABICOP)

Sociocultural	Interpersonal	Physical Environment	Internal States
Norms and values, family, religion, communication	*Interactions with others, primary and secondary relationships*	*Housing, neighbourhood, natural objects*	*Health, self-esteem, sense of well-being, quality of life, biological*
• Long-term care of the client with an ABI must occur within his or her own community. The family and extended community are the most important 'agencies' in assisting the client throughout his/her life. • Targeted partners include the family, hospitals, physicians, nursing, allied health professionals, the courts, lawyers, and insurance agents, CCAC's, schools, teachers, principals, educational assistants, children mental health centres, and community, recreational and religious centres. • Community participation is key to program functioning. PABICOP regards the child/family and their community as the real 'experts', encouraging and supporting as much community partnership as possible. • PABICOP has its clinic in the community to facilitate community participation.	• The PABICOP team consists of the following personnel—a pediatric neurologist, a community outreach coordinator, school liaison personnel, psychometry, neuropsychology, occupational therapy, speech language pathology, and a pediatric neurologist. • Home visits, school visits, clinics, and follow-up appointments are available to each client. • The school is considered a key component to the child's everyday functioning, as many children with an ABI demonstrate difficulty creating and maintaining peer relationships	• PABICOP is committed to influencing individuals, as well as the community at large, to play and live in as safe a manner as possible. PABICOP has made linkages with individual safety community programs, as well as provincial and national safety programs, such as THINK FIRST and SMART RISK. • It is the community or local providers of service that help shape the program, as they are the ones who are aware of what is available and what could be accomplished with local resources.	• PABICOP's practice is culturally sensitive and the client and their family help to guide its team of experts in understanding what is meaningful to them, in order to best plan, support and educate. • The Outreach Program strives to ensure that children with an ABI and their families receive all of the services they require with respect to their health, education, social and emotional development and well-being. • Psychosocial, mental, cultural, and emotional factors interact with physical factors, varying from individual to individual. • PABICOP educates families of children with acquired brain injuries, placing an emphasis on understanding a child's needs, learning to advocate for a child and learning to serve as a case manager for a child.

The Challenge Program, TIRR Memorial Hermann

Sociocultural	Interpersonal	Physical Environment	Internal States
Norms and values, family, religion, communication	*Interactions with others, primary and secondary relationships*	*Housing, neighbourhood, natural objects*	*Health, self-esteem, sense of well-being, quality of life, biological*
• Family and loved ones are incorporated and encouraged to be part of the rehabilitation process and strategies • Clients are connected with supportive community based partnered organizations in order to safely practice their skills to work towards their community reintegration goals. • Accommodations and adaptations are placed within the clients' community of involvement • Group therapy with specialized groups of clients are not only used a therapeutic strategy but also for socio-cultural support and mutual understanding and bonding	• Clients are encouraged to participate in social interactions and develop meaningful relationships with members in their specialized group settings (i.e., Group Therapy). • Clients are continuously involved in the decision making, assessment and goals of the rehabilitation program • Clients develop a deeper relationship with their therapist, who oversees most of the work other rehabilitation staff perform • Rehabilitation is done with the client and family or friends not on them.	• Clients are supported by empathetic rehabilitation staff who uphold clients in a respectful manner • Clients are encouraged to meet with other clients and made friendships and relationships using their Group Therapy • Clients are able to return to their personal communities in the evening to see their loved ones and practice their skills in their real communities in a residential facility designed for ABI survivors • Adaptations and information about Brain Injury is delivered by therapist to the clients' community for better support and successful reintegration	• Interpersonal skill awareness and social skills feedback is received through group therapy strategies • Clients are given the chance to practice their social strategies in their personal communities and real life setting in a safe manner with the feedback of their therapist. • Psychotherapy is provided for clients who require additional emotional and psychological support • Challenges in adapting the learned strategies to the client's communities are taken seriously by program staff, feedback is given to enable greater insight to social requirements

The Krempels Center

Sociocultural	Interpersonal	Physical Environment	Internal States
Norms and values, family, religion, communication	*Interactions with others, primary and secondary relationships*	*Housing, neighbourhood, natural objects*	*Health, self-esteem, sense of well-being, quality of life, biological*
• Clients' family members are encouraged to be involved in their own programming and be part of the Center. • Client values are central to the program. • Clients are directly linked with the community through education and workshop events. • Community outings occur to increase knowledge of various societal and cultural norms.	• Clients form primary relationships with other clients, program staff, volunteers, student interns, and members of the community throughout their involvement with the program. • The client's family is encouraged to be actively involved in the program and create their own relationships with clients, program staff, volunteers, and student interns, and members of the community. • Clients play an important, autonomous role in directing their recovery and goals. • Clients form relationships with the community as they participate in community education and fundraising events (e.g., marathon).	• Clients live outside of the program, and are supported in learning skills to live independently. • The physical environment of the actual Center space is modified to accommodate client's physical needs. • Field trips and community events are encouraged to broaden client's physical environment and links with the community.	• Clients increase their self-esteem as they participate in programs, direct their goals, and link with the community. • The programs offered through this center facilitate growth and improvement in various aspects of the clients' life, such as functional goals and social skills. • Holistic approach to improve the overall quality of life for clients.

Biscayne Institute for Health and Living

Sociocultural	Interpersonal	Physical Environment	Internal States
Norms and values, family, religion, communication	*Interactions with others, primary and secondary relationships*	*Housing, neighbourhood, natural objects*	*Health, self-esteem, sense of well-being, quality of life, biological*
• Ability to set attainable short- and long-term goals • Participation of family members in family therapy designed to educate and support them in understanding ABI • BIHL offers a continuum of core services and ancillary programs to the community • Work and volunteering placements within BIHL and the community • BIHL offers special financial accommodations provided for lowincome families • Training of professionals (e.g., from medical schools) in TBI services	• Opportunities for social interaction with other program participants (i.e., individuals with ABI), members of the community, staff and family members • Ability to develop social skills in individualized treatment plan • Social ability/behaviour monitored throughout stages of treatment (including the last stage: "Life After Rehab") • Family and group therapies strengthens/develops relationships that support individuals with ABI	• Facility designed to advocate power of healing (does not look like a traditional treatment facility and more like a home) • Most individuals are admitted to the Day program, thus able to live at home, apply the learned modules and make the necessary adjustments on a daily basis • Supported work and volunteer placements with the necessary adjustments and progress monitored by BIHL • Biscayne Academy, a school part of BIHL, provides education and treatment for the pediatric individuals with TBI	• Being aware of health status, abilities and limitations throughout the treatment stages • Understanding the importance of health and well-being through workshops and classes • Achieving cognitive, emotional and behavioural goals, and overcoming the consequences of ABI • Applying skills and knowledge developed in the program in work/volunteering placements and in the home

The Brain Integration Programme

Sociocultural	Interpersonal	Physical Environment	Internal States
Norms and values, family, religion, communication	*Interactions with others, primary and secondary relationships*	*Housing, neighbourhood, natural objects*	*Health, self-esteem, sense of well-being, quality of life, biological*
• Participation of ABI survivors and their family/social network in educational sessions on ABI and its consequences • Learning to set realistic goals • Working closely with community and employers for job placements • Achieving balance in daily activities between domestic life, work, leisure, and social interaction to allow for successful community reintegration	• Opportunity for social interactions at the residential facility with the staff as well as other ABI survivors • Participate in workshops and sessions involving social skills training • Receive continuous feedback on social behaviour • Strengthen relationship with loved ones and forming new relationships	• Living in a residential facility designed for ABI survivors • Ability to adjust to the home environment during the home visits on the weekends • Adjustments to the workplace done by the program staff in cooperation with the employers to accommodate individual with ABI	• Gaining insight into one's condition and limitations by participating in individual and group workshops as well as tasks learning and performance • Overcoming emotional, psychiatric and behavioural consequences of ABI • Becoming aware of one's skills and abilities post ABI • Learning to use one's skills towards obtaining a career and living independently

Index

9 781623 962890